ary
Medical

UROLOGY
SECRETS

Third Edition

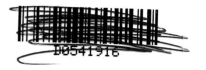

D0541916

UROLOGY SECRETS

Third Edition

MARTIN I. RESNICK, M.D.
Lester Persky Professor and Chairman
Department of Urology
Case Western Reserve University
  School of Medicine
and Director, Department of Urology
University Hospitals of Cleveland
Cleveland, Ohio

ANDREW C. NOVICK, M.D.
Chairman, Urological Institute
Cleveland Clinic Foundation
Cleveland, Ohio

HANLEY & BELFUS, INC./Philadelphia

Publisher: HANLEY & BELFUS, INC.
              Medical Publishers
              210 South 13th Street
              Philadelphia, PA 19107
              (215) 546-7293; 800-962-1892
              FAX (215) 790-9330
              Web site: http://www.hanleyandbelfus.com

Note to the reader: Although the information in this book has been carefully reviewed for correctness of dosage and indications, neither the authors nor the editors nor the publisher can accept any legal responsibility for any errors or omissions that may be made. Neither the publisher nor the editors make any warranty, expressed or implied, with respect to the material contained herein. Before prescribing any drug, the reader must review the manufacturer's current product information (package inserts) for accepted indications, absolute dosage recommendations, and other information pertinent to the safe and effective use of the product described.

Library of Congress Control Number: 2002114439

UROLOGY SECRETS, 3rd edition   ISBN 1-56053-510-5

Last digit is the print number: 9 8 7 6 5 4 3 2 1

CONTENTS

IV. INFLAMMATION AND INFECTION

V. TRAUMA

CONTRIBUTORS

Kenneth W. Angermeier, M.D.
Section of Prosthetic Surgery and Genitourethral Reconstruction, Urological Institute, Cleveland Clinic Foundation, Cleveland, Ohio

Donald R. Bodner, M.D.
Professor of Urology, Department of Urology, Case Western Reserve University School of Medicine, University Hospitals of Cleveland, and Cleveland Veterans Affairs Medical Center, Cleveland, Ohio

James A. Daitch, M.D.
Private Practice, Urology Associates, Ltd., Phoenix, Arizona

Kurt H. Dinchman, M.D.
Assistant Professor, Department of Urology, Case Western Reserve University School of Medicine, MetroHealth Medical Center, Cleveland, Ohio

Jack S. Elder, M.D.
Carter Kissell Professor of Urology, Professor of Pediatrics, School of Medicine, Case Western Reserve University, Cleveland, Ohio; Director of Pediatric Urology, Rainbow Babies' and Children's Hospital, Cleveland, Ohio

Stuart M. Flechner, M.D.
Director of Clinical Research, Section of Renal Transplantation, Urological Institute, Cleveland Clinic Foundation, Cleveland, Ohio; Cleveland Clinic Hospital, Cleveland, Ohio

Inderbir S. Gill, M.D., M.Ch.
Head, Section of Laparoscopic and Minimally Invasive Surgery, Department of Urology, Cleveland Clinic Foundation, Cleveland, Ohio

David A. Goldfarb, M.D.
Department of Urology, Cleveland Clinic Foundation, Cleveland, Ohio

Howard B. Goldman, M.D.
Assistant Professor, Department of Urology, School of Medicine, Case Western Reserve University, Cleveland, Ohio; University Hospitals of Cleveland, Cleveland, Ohio

Nehemia Hampel, M.D., F.A.C.S.
Professor of Urology, Department of Urology, School of Medicine, Case Western Reserve University, Cleveland, Ohio; Chief of Urology, VA Medical Center, Cleveland, Ohio

J. Stephen Jones, M.D., F.A.C.S.
Urological Institute, Cleveland Clinic Foundation, Cleveland, Ohio

Robert Kay, M.D.
Chief of Staff, Cleveland Clinic Foundation, Cleveland, Ohio

Eric A. Klein, M.D.
Head, Section of Urological Oncology, Urological Institute, Cleveland Clinic Foundation, Cleveland, Ohio

Elroy D. Kursh, M.D.
Urology Staff, Department of Urology, Cleveland Clinic Foundation, Cleveland, Ohio

Milton M. Lakin, M.D.
Head, Section of Medical Urology, Urological Institute, Cleveland Clinic Foundation, Cleveland, Ohio

William A. Larchian, M.D.
Associate Staff, Department of Urology, Cleveland Clinic Foundation, Cleveland, Ohio

David A. Levy, M.D.
Private Practice, St. Anthony's Hospital, St. Petersburg, Florida

Charles S. Modlin, Jr., M.D.
Staff Surgeon, Urological Institute, Transplantation Center, Cleveland Clinic Foundation, Cleveland, Ohio

Drogo K. Montague, M.D.
Head, Section of Prosthetic Surgery and Genitourethral Reconstruction, Urological Institute, Cleveland Clinic Foundation, Cleveland, Ohio

Mark J. Noble, M.D.
Staff, Department of Urology, Cleveland Clinic Foundation, Cleveland, Ohio

Andrew C. Novick, M.D.
Chairman, Urological Institute, Cleveland Clinic Foundation, Cleveland, Ohio

Jeffrey S. Palmer, M.D.
Assistant Professor of Urology and Pediatrics, School of Medicine, Case Western Reserve University, Cleveland, Ohio; Rainbow Babies' and Children's Hospital, Cleveland, Ohio

Raymond R. Rackley, M.D.
Staff, Department of Urology, Cleveland Clinic Foundation, Cleveland, Ohio

Martin I. Resnick, M.D.
Lester Persky Professor and Chairman, Department of Urology, Case Western Reserve University School of Medicine, and Director, Department of Urology, University Hospitals of Cleveland, Cleveland, Ohio

Jonathan H. Ross, M.D.
Head, Section of Pediatric Urology, Urological Institute, Cleveland Clinic Foundation, Cleveland, Ohio

Bashir R. Sankari, M.D.
Urological Institute, Cleveland Clinic Foundation, Cleveland, Ohio; Director of Renal Transplantation, Charleston Area Medical Center, Charleston, West Virginia

Allen D. Seftel, M.D.
Associate Professor of Urology and Reproductive Biology, Case Western Reserve University, University Hospitals of Cleveland; Cleveland Veterans Affairs Medical Center, Cleveland, Ohio

J. Patrick Spirnak, M.D.
Professor, Department of Urology and Reproductive Biology, School of Medicine, Case Western Reserve University, Cleveland, Ohio; Director of Urology, Metrohealth Medical Center, Cleveland, Ohio

Stevan B. Streem, M.D.
Head, Section of Stone Disease and Endourology, Urological Institute, Cleveland Clinic Foundation, Cleveland, Ohio

Anthony J. Thomas, Jr., M.D.
Head, Section of Male Infertility, Urological Institute, Cleveland Clinic Foundation, Cleveland, Ohio

James C. Ulchaker, M.D.
Staff, Department of Urology, Cleveland Clinic Foundation, Cleveland, Ohio

Sandip P. Vasavada, M.D.
Formerly Fellow, Department of Urology, UCLA Medical Center, Los Angeles, California; presently Assistant Professor of Urology, Department of Urology, Thomas Jefferson University School of Medicine, Philadelphia, Pennsylvania

Lawrence M. Wyner, M.D.
Associate Staff, Urological Institute, Cleveland Clinic Foundation, Cleveland, Ohio; Attending Staff, Charleston Area Medical Center, Charleston, West Virginia

Craig D. Zippe, M.D.
Co-director, Prostate Center, Department of Urology, Cleveland Clinic Foundation, Cleveland, Ohio

Preface to the 3rd Edition

Now in its third edition, *Urology Secrets* has been very well received by the field and has established itself as an excellent reference for medical students, residents, and clinicians. A wide range of topics is reviewed, with each chapter posing a series of key questions about the assessment and management of patients with various disorders of the genitourinary system. The clear, concise answers and the informal tone we hope make the text enjoyable as well as useful. All of the chapters have been revised and updated, and many have been expanded. Recent developments in such areas as laparoscopic surgery, chemo and immunotherapy, and erectile dysfunction have been included.

We hope that the third edition will continue to provide valuable information to early trainees and to clinicians in both the operating room and office. *Urology Secrets* is not intended to be a comprehensive text; it is, however, a user-friendly, highly readable, and valuable clinical source. The editors hope that all will find that the third edition provides a strong foundation for providing the highest quality of care to patients with urologic problems.

Martin I. Resnick, M.D.
Case Western Reserve University
Cleveland, OH

Andrew C. Novick, M.D.
Cleveland Clinic Foundation
Cleveland, OH

I. Patient Evaluation

1. PHYSICAL EXAMINATION

Kenneth W. Angermeier, M.D.

1. Are the kidneys palpable in a normal patient?

The right kidney may be palpable in children and thin adults. The left kidney is difficult to palpate, as it lies higher within the retroperitoneum than the right kidney. Examination is best performed bimanually, with one hand behind the patient in the costovertebral angle and the other anteriorly just below the costal margin. With inspiration, the kidney may be felt as it moves downward. In neonates, examination is performed by palpating the flank between the thumb anteriorly and the remaining fingers posteriorly in the costovertebral angle. Both kidneys can be outlined reliably in this fashion.

2. What is the significance of an abdominal bruit?

Although not a specific finding, auscultation of a bruit in the epigastrium or upper abdomen may suggest the presence of renal artery stenosis in the appropriate clinical setting. This finding is particularly indicative when the bruit is continuous (systolic-diastolic). A bruit may vary in intensity with fluctuation of the systemic blood pressure, or disappear if renal artery stenosis progresses to near or total occlusion. An abdominal bruit may also occur in association with a renal artery aneurysm or arteriovenous malformation.

3. Where is renal pain usually localized on examination?

Renal pain due to inflammation or obstruction may result in vague, diffuse back discomfort. A renal source often can be identified by the finding of localized tenderness in the costovertebral angle, just lateral to the sacrospinalis muscle and inferior to the twelfth rib. This is usually best elicited by percussion of the area with the fist.

4. At what filling volume can the adult bladder be detected on physical examination?

In the adult, a normal bladder cannot be palpated or percussed until there is a urine volume of at least 150 ml. For the most part, percussion is superior to palpation when a patient is evaluated for bladder distention. Patients with frank urinary retention may have visible bladder distention that may extend to the level of the umbilicus.

5. When is examination of the bladder under anesthesia important?

Bimanual examination under anesthesia is useful in assessing the local extent of carcinoma of the bladder and its mobility. In the female, this is done by compressing the bladder between one hand on the abdomen and the other in the vagina. Male patients are examined with a hand on the abdomen and a finger in the rectum.

6. What is paraphimosis?

Paraphimosis is a condition that may arise when the foreskin of the penis has been retracted beyond the corona of the glans and is not subsequently reduced. This can lead to constriction of the glans penis, resulting in pain, edema, and possible vascular compromise. Failure to reduce the foreskin after insertion of a urethral catheter is one situation in which paraphimosis may occur.

Paraphimosis is a urologic emergency that requires immediate dorsal slit or circumcision if the foreskin cannot be manually reduced.

7. What disease process is characterized by a palpable scar or "plaque" along the shaft of the penis?

Peyronie's disease is a condition in which a fibrotic scar develops within the tunica albuginea of the corpora cavernosa, and may result in curvature of the erect penis. The scar most commonly involves the dorsal aspect of the penis, although it can extend laterally or occur on the ventrum in some cases. Calcification is present in approximately 30% of patients and indicates that the scar is mature.

8. Describe the physical findings in hypospadias.

Hypospadias occurs as a result of incomplete fusion of the urethral plate during embryogenesis. The urethral meatus is abnormally located and may be present along the ventral shaft of the penis, scrotum, or perineum. The foreskin is usually incomplete ventrally, being described as "hooded." Dysgenetic tissue along the urethral plate may result in ventral penile curvature (chordee).

9. What is the appearance of genital herpes?

Genital herpes is characterized by superficial vesicles grouped on an erythematous base. The lesions are often painful and may coalesce. The incubation period is 2–7 days. The majority of patients with genital herpes have herpes simplex virus type II.

10. What is priapism?

Priapism is a prolonged, painful erection, often of several hours' duration. Physical examination reveals rigid corpora cavernosa that may be somewhat tender. The glans penis is usually flaccid. This condition is often seen in patients with sickle cell anemia, but may also be idiopathic. Priapism may occur in patients on a pharmacologic erection program. Emergent treatment is indicated, as prolonged priapism may result in intracorporal fibrosis and impotence.

11. When should a rectal examination be performed in the male?

Digital rectal examination should be performed annually beginning at age 40, or in any male presenting for urologic evaluation. It should include an estimation of anal sphincter tone, palpation of the prostate and rectum, and testing of the stool for occult blood.

12. Compare the findings on rectal examination in benign prostatic hyperplasia (BPH) and prostatic carcinoma.

In BPH, the prostate is variably enlarged and has a rubbery consistency. The enlargement is usually symmetric and may be associated with deepening of the lateral sulci and obliteration of the median furrow. Prostatic carcinoma may be palpable as a discrete, firm, or hard nodule within one prostatic lobe. This can progress to firm induration of an entire lobe or diffuse involvement of the prostate. The presence of extracapsular extension or seminal vesicle involvement should be noted. Prostatic carcinoma can also be present in a patient with a benign rectal examination, with the diagnosis usually being made because of an elevated prostate-specific antigen level or following transurethral resection of the prostate.

13. What condition is suggested by the presence of a soft, cystic mass palpable in the midline near the base of the prostate?

This finding may indicate the presence of a müllerian duct cyst or an enlarged utricle. These entities arise from remnants of the fetal müllerian system, which regresses in the male during normal development. An enlarged utricle is occasionally seen in patients with proximal hypospadias.

14. What is the significance of a palpable testicular mass?

The majority of solid testicular masses represent malignant germ cell tumors. It is important to ascertain on physical examination whether the mass is located within the testicle or is arising from the spermatic cord or epididymis. Extratesticular masses are more often benign, although malignancies may occur in these locations as well.

15. Describe the characteristics of a hydrocele and a spermatocele.

A **hydrocele** is a collection of fluid within the scrotum that is contained by the parietal and visceral components of the tunica vaginalis. It is palpable as a relatively smooth fluid collection filling the hemiscrotum and surrounding the testicle. The hydrocele may be tense or somewhat fluctuant. The testicle may be difficult to palpate in the presence of a hydrocele. A **spermatocele** is a cystic fluid collection primarily involving the epididymis, and it may be tense or firm on palpation. The diagnosis of both of these entities is confirmed by transillumination using a bright light in a dark room. A hydrocele or spermatocele should completely transilluminate, whereas a solid mass will not.

16. What is a varicocele?

A varicocele occurs as a result of enlargement of the spermatic vein (pampiniform plexus) above the testicle, more commonly on the left side. The enlarged, tortuous veins are palpable as a "bag of worms" within the superior aspect of the involved hemiscrotum. Typically, the veins fill and enlarge with the patient in the upright position or with the Valsalva maneuver, and decompress with recumbency. The ipsilateral testicle may be smaller in size than the opposite one, and in some patients, a varicocele is associated with infertility.

17. What is the significance of a varicocele that does not decompress with the patient in the supine position?

Patients with a varicocele that does not decompress with recumbency should be suspected of having obstruction of the spermatic vein where it enters the renal vein on the left, or the inferior vena cava on the right. This may be caused by a retroperitoneal neoplasm, such as renal cell carcinoma with tumor thrombus in the renal vein or inferior vena cava. Acute onset of a varicocele or a right-sided varicocele should raise similar suspicions.

BIBLIOGRAPHY

1. Brendler CB: Evaluation of the urologic patient: History, physical examination, and urinalysis. In Walsh PC, Retik AB, Vaughan ED Jr., Wein AJ (eds) : Campbell's Urology, 7th ed. Philadelphia, W.B. Saunders, 1998, pp 138–144.
2. Tanagho EA: Physical examination of the genitourinary tract. In Tanagho EA, McAninch JW (eds): Smith's General Urology, 14th ed. Norwalk, CT, Appleton & Lange, 1995, pp 41–49.

2. INSTRUMENTATION AND ENDOSCOPY

Stevan B. Streem, M.D.

1. What are the usual indications for urethral catheterization?

The most frequently performed bladder instrumentation is urethral catheterization. The indications for this can be diagnostic or therapeutic. In women, "straight catheterization" may be indicated for accurate diagnosis of possible urinary infection, especially when a voided urine shows significant vaginal contamination. In contrast, catheterization is rarely indicated for this purpose alone in men; a clean voided, midstream sample should be adequate.

Urethral catheterization also may be indicated to assess the amount of residual urine after voiding or as part of a urodynamic evaluation of bladder and urethral function. Urethral catheterization also is required for retrograde instillation of radiographic contrast medium to obtain a cystogram or voiding cystourethrogram for radiographic evaluation of the bladder and urethra.

Therapeutically, urethral catheterization is required most acutely for patients in urinary retention. In hospitalized patients, especially those who are acutely ill, catheterization is generally indicated to assess urine output on a continuing basis.

2. What catheters are best to use for such procedures?

To obtain urine for microbiologic study or to check for residual urine, straight catheters of 14–16 French size are generally sufficient. When the catheter is to be left in place (e.g., for patients with urinary retention), a self-retaining balloon catheter (Foley catheter) is used.

3. What are French sizes?

The French scale is a measure of circumference. One French is equivalent to approximately .33 mm in diameter: An 18-French catheter is approximately 6 mm wide.

4. What should be done if a catheter cannot be passed easily in a man?

Call a urology resident or a urologist. He or she will then show you how to properly use specialized catheters, such as coudé catheters with curved tips used for patients who have had prostate surgery, or filiform and follower catheters for men with urethral strictures.

5. What are "sounds"?

Sounds are specialized metal catheters most commonly used to treat urethral strictures. Only urologists or urology residents should use sounds in the urethra.

6. What if a man is in pain from a distended bladder and a catheter cannot be passed?

Sometimes the best approach in such cases is placement of a small-caliber suprapubic tube via a percutaneous approach. This requires only a local anesthetic and provides immediate relief of urinary retention.

7. What are some frequent indications for cystoscopy (endoscopic evaluation of the bladder)?

The most frequent diagnostic indications for cystoscopy include evaluation of hematuria, infection, and voiding dysfunction.

8. What are the advantages and disadvantages of flexible versus rigid cystoscopes?

In general, flexible instrumentation is more comfortable for the patient, although this is not an issue if the procedure is done under anesthesia. On the other hand, rigid instrumentation offers a greater field of vision and allows more therapeutic options.

9. What instruments are used for cystoscopy?

Usually, rigid instruments ranging from 16–22 French are used for diagnostic purposes. Two lenses with different angles of vision are used to visualize the entire urethra and bladder. Flexible cystoscopes, generally 16–18 French, are also used frequently, especially when the procedure is performed in an office setting, without anesthesia.

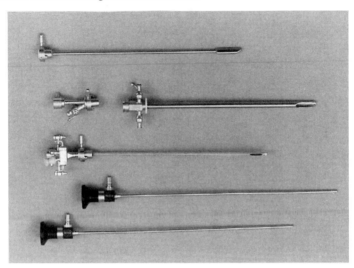

Standard rigid instrumentation for cystourethroscopy.

10. What are the main indications to perform diagnostic retrograde pyelography at the time of cystoscopy?

Retrograde x-rays of the upper tracts are performed whenever intravenous urography does not allow adequate visualization of the pyelocalyceal system and ureters, or when intravenous urography is contraindicated, such as in patients with significant renal insufficiency or a history of a significant adverse reaction to intravenous contrast.

11. What instruments are available for evaluation of the upper tracts?

Like the bladder, the ureter and pyelocalyceal system can be intubated with catheters or with rigid or flexible endoscopes.

12. What are some frequent indications for ureteral catheterization?

Ureteral catheterization is frequently indicated to obtain retrograde x-rays, to temporarily bypass obstruction (such as from ureteral calculi or strictures), and to obtain differential urine from each collecting system to further assess problems such as abnormal cytology or to localize bacteriuria.

13. Can the upper tracts (e.g., the bladder) be visualized directly with telescopes?

Yes. Upper tract endoscopy can be done for diagnostic or therapeutic purposes with both rigid and flexible ureteropyeloscopes.

14. Explain the difference between a ureteral catheter and a ureteral stent.

Ureteral catheters are placed cystoscopically to the renal pelvis and exit via the urethra. They frequently migrate distally and are a source of infection. Therefore, they are used only for temporary upper tract access. In contrast, **ureteral stents,** which are also usually placed cystoscopically, are self-retaining and completely indwelling. They are often left for several days, weeks, or even months with little risk of infection or migration.

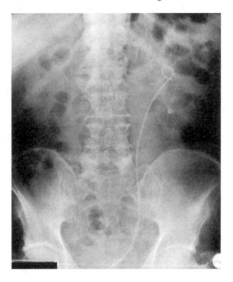

Plain x-ray demonstrating indwelling, self-retaining ureteral stent.

15. What are the indications for upper tract endoscopy?

The most frequent indications include evaluation of "filling defects" seen on intravenous or retrograde pyelography and intrinsic obstructing lesions, and management of calculi.

16. What are the indications for direct percutaneous instrumentation of the upper collecting system?

Usually, a percutaneous nephrostomy is placed for relief of ureteral obstruction in the face of infection or obstructive uropathy when retrograde catheterization is unsuccessful or otherwise contraindicated.

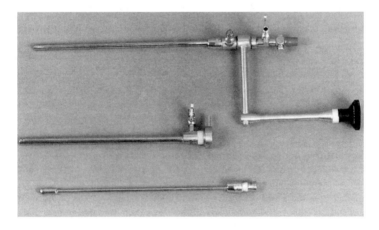

Rigid nephroscope. This instrument is similar to a cystoscope, except that it is shorter and of wider caliber. The optical system is offset to allow passage of rigid working instumentation.

17. Can endoscopy be performed via this percutaneous approach?

Yes. Percutaneous nephroscopy (*pyeloscopy* is a better term) can be performed with rigid or flexible instrumentation analogous to that used for cystoscopy and ureteroscopy. Percutaneous nephroscopy can be diagnostic or therapeutic. It is particularly valuable for management of large renal calculi, although occasionally it can be used to manage upper tract transitional cell carcinoma in select patients.

BIBLIOGRAPHY

1. Bagley DH, Huffman JL, Lyons ES: Flexible ureteropyeloscopy: Diagnosis and treatment in the upper urinary tract. J Urol 138:280–285, 1987.
2. Blute ML, Segura JW, Patterson DE, et al: Impact of endourology on diagnosis and management of upper urinary tract urothelial cancer. J Urol 141:1298–1301, 1989.
3. Carter HB: Instrumentation and endoscopy. In Walsh PC, Retik AB, Vaughan ED Jr., Wein AJ (eds): Campbell's Urology, 7th ed. Philadelphia, W.B. Saunders, 1998, pp 159–168.
4. Guz B, Streem SB, Novick AC, et al: Role of percutaneous nephrostomy in patients with upper tract transition cell carcinoma. Urology 37:331–336, 1991.
5. Huffman JL, Bagley DH, Lyon ES: Extending cystoscopic techniques into the ureter and renal pelvis. JAMA 250:2002–2005, 1983.
6. Smith AD, Reinke DB, Miller RP, Lange PH: Percutaneous nephrostomy in the management of ureteral and renal calculi. Radiology 133:49–54, 1979.
7. Streem SB, Pontes JE, Novick AC, et al: Ureteropyeloscopy in the evaluation of upper tract filling defects. J Urol 136:383–385, 1986.

3. URINALYSIS AND URINE FUNCTION STUDIES

Kurt H. Dinchman, M.D.

1. What types of information can be obtained from a urinalysis? What is their importance?

Urinalysis is the most commonly performed laboratory test in a general medical practice. It is routinely performed in two parts: (1) use of a dipstick and (2) microscopic examination of spun urine. The most common dipsticks give results such as pH, specific gravity, presence or absence of blood, protein, and leukocytes, and various other tests, including assessment of glucose, ketones, bilirubin, and urobilinogen.

2. What is the normal pH of urine?

The normal pH of urine is between 5 and 8, depending on diet and other factors. Urine pH is important in determination of renal tubular acidosis, which may cause a pH below 5.5. Uric acid stones may be suspected with acidic urine. Alkaline urine may be observed in the presence of urea-splitting organisms, such as *Proteus* sp.

3. What is the significance of abnormal findings on a urine dipstick examination?

The presence of glucose in urine may indicate glycosuria secondary to undiagnosed diabetes mellitus. Leukocytes may indicate an inflammatory or infectious process within the urinary tract; interpretation, however, must be verified by microscopic examination. Protein in the urine may indicate a reabsorption problem in the kidneys, whereas ketones may indicate ketoacidosis, as seen with diabetes or a state of starvation or malnutrition. Bilirubin may be seen in the urine of patients with early stages of liver abnormalities. Erythrocytes or free hemoglobin from lysed erythrocytes should alert the investigator to examine the urine microscopically for red blood cells.

4. How is a clean specimen obtained for microscopic examination of urine?

It is important for the investigator to obtain a "clean-catch urine." Women should clean themselves with a sanitary wipe and spread the labia to get a clean, clear stream into the specimen bottle. Uncircumcised men should retract the foreskin before giving the specimen.

5. How is a proper microscopic examination of urine performed?

The clean-catch specimen is centrifuged for approximately 3–5 minutes at 2–3,000 rpm. The sediment (button) at the bottom of the centrifuge tube is suspended in approximately 0.2 ml of urine. The resuspended button then is poured onto a glass slide and covered with a coverslip. First a low-power scanning of the specimen is performed to detect red blood cell casts, crystals, and pathogens such as trichomonads. High-power analysis identifies bacteria, yeast, red blood cells, and white blood cells.

6. What is the significance of findings in a microscopic urine examination?

High-power examination may reveal urine casts that contain erythrocytes encased in a noncellular matrix. This finding may indicate glomerular hemorrhage, as seen in glomerulonephritis. Other casts with renal tubular cells may indicate renal tubular damage. The examiner also may observe urinary crystals of phosphate, oxalate, and cystine in stone-forming patients; however, crystals also may be seen in non–stone-forming patients. Leukocytes in the urine sediment may indicate an inflammatory process secondary to infection, calculi, or interstitial renal disease. Microscopic examination also may reveal erythrocytes. The differential diagnosis for erythrocytes in urine is quite extensive. Patients with microhematuria should be evaluated for infection, calculus disease, carcinoma, inflammatory process, trauma, sickle-cell anemia, bleeding disorder, and glomerulonephritis. Epithelial cells are seen frequently in urinalysis, especially squamous epithelial cells in postpubertal and nonmenopausal women. Abnormal transitional cells in the urine indicate malignant transitional cell carcinoma.

7. What are the most commonly used renal function tests?

The most commonly used renal function tests are urine specific gravity, serum creatinine, blood urea nitrogen, serum electrolytes, and complete blood count.

8. How is urine specific gravity used to test renal function?

Urine specific gravity is a simple test of the ability of the kidneys to concentrate urine. Decreasing ability to concentrate urine parallels a decrease in overall renal function. Urine specific gravity remains the simplest method of determining the ability to concentrate and dilute urine.

9. How is serum creatinine helpful in determining renal function?

Creatinine, an end product of metabolism in skeletal muscle, is excreted by the kidneys and is not influenced by hydration status. Because of the constancy of daily creatinine production in a normal, active patient, levels of serum creatinine remain within a fairly reliable range and therefore can be used to determine renal function.

10. How is creatinine clearance calculated? What does it mean?

Calculation of creatinine clearance requires determination of the concentration of creatinine in urine and in plasma and the volume of urine excreted per minute. Creatinine clearance is calculated by the formula: clearance = UV/P, where U is urine creatinine concentration, V is urine volume, and P is plasma creatinine concentration. Creatinine clearance of 90–110 ml/min is normal. Because creatinine production is stable and filtered through the glomeruli, creatinine clearance is close to the glomerular filtration rate. Therefore, decreased creatinine clearance indicates a decrease in the glomerular filtration rate.

11. How is blood urea nitrogen (BUN) related to glomerular filtration rate?

Urea, an end product of protein catabolism, also is excreted by the kidneys, but is not as accurate as creatinine clearance in determining glomerular filtration rate. The BUN-to-creatinine ratio, however, may be used to obtain certain clinical information. A classic example is seen in dehydrated patients with prerenal azotemia, in which the BUN:creatinine ratio may be 10:1. Patients with obstruction or postrenal azotemia may have a ratio of 20–30:1.

12. How are blood count and electrolyte studies helpful in assessing renal function?

Anemia may be seen in patients with renal insufficiency due to decreased production of erythropoietin. Serum sodium and potassium abnormalities are often seen in patients with renal insufficiency. The degree of hyperkalemia is paramount in determining the initiation of renal dialysis.

BIBLIOGRAPHY

1. Schrier RW, Gottschalk CW (eds): Diseases of the Kidney, vol. 1, 5th ed. Boston, Little, Brown, 1993.
2. Tanagho EA, McAninch JW (eds): Smith's General Urology, 8th ed. Norwalk, CT, Appleton & Lange, 1992.
3. Walsh PC, Retik AB, Vaughan ED Jr., Wein AJ (eds): Campbell's Urology, 8th ed. Philadelphia, W. B. Saunders, 2002.

4. INTRAVENOUS UROGRAPHY AND ANGIOGRAPHY

Mark J. Noble, M.D.

1. In what urologic conditions is intravenous urography useful?

Hematuria
Pain thought to arise from the urinary tract
Recurrent urinary tract infection
Suspected renal/ureteral calculi
Suspected renal obstruction
Prior transitional cell carcinoma of the bladder
Evaluation of postoperative complication(s)
Diagnosis and evaluation of congenital anomalies
Trauma
Renovascular disease
Baseline study before surgery on or near the urinary tract

2. What types of contrast material are available?

High osmolality (i.e., Renografin, Conray and low osmolality. The low-osmolality agents are further divided into ionic (Hexabrix) and nonionic (Omnipaque, Isovue, Optiray). The low-osmolality agents are associated with lower risk of adverse reactions.

3. What are the risks of intravenous contrast material?

Allergic reaction, renal toxicity, and local tissue reaction (if the intravenous needle infiltrates during injection).

4. Who is most at risk for an allergic contrast reaction?

Those with a prior history of contrast reaction, asthma, or other severe allergies.

5. Which diseases place patients at high risk for renal toxicity from intravenous contrast material?

- Diabetic nephropathy
- Multiple myeloma
- Hyperuricosuria
- Amyloidosis
- Preexisting chronic renal failure
- Other conditions producing severe proteinuria

6. What is the best way to prepare the patient for urography?

Administer clear liquids beginning the evening before the study and give nothing by mouth for 6 hours before the study. Laxatives are rarely needed.

7. What drug should be avoided, and for how long, when a diabetic is to receive intravenous contrast?

Glucophage should not be taken when intravenous contrast will be used for any x-ray study. It should be stopped at least 24 hours before, and the patient should wait at least 24 hours after the intravenous contrast to resume it.

8. What is the usual film sequence for urography?

1. **Plain film**—the kidneys, ureters, and bladder (KUB) must be visualized to evaluate calcifications and bony structures.
2. **1 minute**—the nephrogram visualizes the renal parenchyma.

3. **5 minutes** — early visualization of the upper collecting system (calyces, pelvis, upper ureter).
4. **Tomograms** — performed to assess renal outlines and fine calcifications. Routine on patients > 40 years old and used selectively below age 40.
5. **15/20 minutes** — late visualization should include the lower ureters and bladder.

9. **What tricks are useful to improve the diagnostic yield?**
   1. **Delayed films** — to assess the level of obstruction in hydronephrotic kidneys.
   2. **Plain tomograms** — before contrast, these are used to assess renal calcifications.
   3. **Ureteral compression** — a compression band surrounding the lower abdomen helps to better fill the upper ureters.
   4. **Prone films** — demonstrate better visualization of the pelvic portion of the ureters.
   5. **Oblique films** — help to visualize abnormalities in three dimensions.
   6. **Postvoid film** — provides a better assessment of bladder pathology and residual urine.

10. **What features of the IV urogram are useful diagnostically?**
    1. **Plain film** — to assess bony structures and any calcifications.
    2. **Nephrogram** — to assess function (normal, delayed, or not visualized).
    3. **Tomograms** — to assess renal outlines for the presence of a mass and to assess smaller calcifications within the kidney.
    4. **Early films** — to assess the kidney for hydronephrosis, filling defect, distorted calyces, malposition, mass, and renovascular disease.
    5. **Late films** — to assess the ureter for filling defects, dilation, constriction. The bladder should be assessed for size, filling defects, mucosal pattern (thickened, trabeculated), and shape (teardrop: pelvic lipomatosis; Christmas tree: neurogenic bladder).

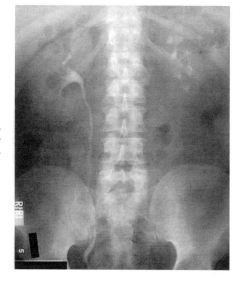

This intravenous urogram demonstrates delay in excretion of contrast on the left with a significantly smaller left kidney. This finding should raise a suspicion of renal artery disease.

11. **How can calcifications observed on plain films be localized?**
    Oblique views and plain tomography.

12. **What is the differential diagnosis of renal calcification(s)?**
    - Collecting system stone(s)
    - Tumor
    - Cyst (rim)
    - Renal artery aneurysm
    - Calyceal diverticulum
    - Parasite(s)

13. Name the causes of extrarenal calcifications seen on plain films.
Vascular, mesenteric nodes, gallstones, adrenal, and splenic calcifications are most common. Lost stone fragment(s) in a nephrostomy tract (previous renal surgery).

14. What important diagnoses can be made by plain films?
- Cancer metastases (sclerotic/lytic)
- Paget's disease (thickened cortex with coarse trabeculation)
- Myelodysplasia (increased interpedicular distance)
- Sacral agenesis (absence of sacrum)
- Exstrophy of the bladder (widening of the pubis)

15. What is the differential diagnosis of a filling defect in the kidney?
Stone, tumor, thrombus, sloughed papilla, fungus ball, vascular impression.

16. What is the differential diagnosis of a filling defect in the ureter?
Stone, tumor, thrombus, inflammation, fibroepithelial polyp.

17. What is the differential diagnosis of a filling defect in the bladder?
Stone, tumor, thrombus, middle lobe of the prostate, foreign body, ureterocele, fungus ball.

18. What is the differential diagnosis of nonvisualization of a kidney? What further studies are required?

Condition	Next step in diagnosis
Renal agenesis	Ultrasound or CT
High-grade obstruction	Ultrasound/retrograde pyelography/CT
Mass	CT or ultrasound
Vascular compromise	Renal scan
Prior nephrectomy	Confirm by history

19. List the indications for renal angiography.
- Hematuria—when noninvasive studies suggest a vascular abnormality
- Surgical planning for:
  Large renal, adrenal, retroperitoneal, or pelvic masses
  Nephron-sparing renal surgery
- To evaluate renal vascular disease
- Trauma—to evaluate vascular integrity of the kidney when this is questioned by studies such as IVP or CT
- To evaluate postsurgical vascular complications (thrombosis)
- Renal mass—to evaluate vascular pattern
- **Massive** hematuria—to locate and embolize bleeding artery branch

20. List the indications for renal venography and/or venacavography.
1. Evaluation of a tumor thrombus (renal cell carcinoma).
2. Definitive evaluation for renal vein thrombosis.
3. Renal vein renin determination in renovascular hypertension.

21. List three angiographic techniques.
1. Cut-film arteriography (standard arteriogram).
2. Intra-arterial digital subtraction angiography (IADSA).
3. Intravenous digital subtraction angiography (IVDSA).

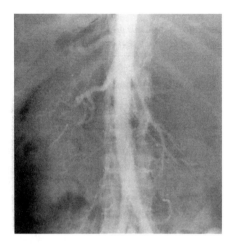

This arteriogram depicts displacement of the left kidney by a sizable, hypovascular, suprarenal mass that turned out to be a large left adrenal carcinoma. Arteriography was helpful in both its diagnosis and its surgical management.

22. Describe the advantages and disadvantages of each angiographic technique.

	CONTRAST DOSE	INVASIVENESS	IMAGE QUALITY
Standard arteriogram	↓ ↓ ↓	+++	+++
IADSA	+	++	+++
IVDSA	+++	+	+

23. What are the complications of angiography?

Hematoma	Allergic reaction to contrast	Tissue injury (if extravasation occurs)
Pseudoaneurysm	Nephrotoxicity from contrast material	Hypertension (if renal artery injury)
Atheroembolism	Vessel dissection	

24. Describe the indications for angiographic renal embolization.
- Renal cell carcinoma—to facilitate operative management of large tumors with vena caval thrombi
- Control hemorrhage from: Percutaneous biopsy, arteriovenous malformation, or primary or metastatic tumor

BIBLIOGRAPHY

1. Bradley AJ, Taylor PM: Does bowel preparation improve the quality of intravenous urography? Br J Radiol 69:906–909, 1996.
2. Papanicolaou N: Urinary tract imaging and intervention: Basic principles. In Walsh PC, Retik AB, Vaughan ED Jr., Wein AJ (eds): Campbell's Urology, 7th ed. Philadelphia, W.B. Saunders, 1998, pp 170–177, 221–224, 256–257.
3. Hartman GW, Hattery RR, Witten DW, Williamson B: Mortality during excretory urography: Mayo Clinic experience. AJR 139:919–922, 1982.
4. Kinnison ML, Powe NR, Steinberg ED: Results of randomized controlled trials of low vs. high-osmolality contrast media. Radiology 170:381–389, 1989.
5. Little MA, Stafford Johnson DB, O'Callaghan JP, Walshe JJ: The diagnostic yield of intravenous urography. Nephrol Dial Transplant 15:200–204, 2000.
6. Yalcinbas YK, Sasmaz H, Canbaz S: Thoracic left kidney: A differential diagnostic dilemma for thoracic surgeons. Ann Thorac Surg 72:281–283, 2001.
7. Pollack HM: Clinical Urography: An Atlas and Textbook of Urologic Imaging. Philadelphia, W.B. Saunders, 1990.

5. ULTRASONOGRAPHY

Martin I. Resnick, M.D.

1. What is the sound frequency of diagnostic ultrasound?
3–15 MHz.

2. How is the frequency related to depth of tissue penetration and resolution?
The higher the frequency of the ultrasound wave, the less tissue penetration but greater resolution of near objects. Similarly, the lower frequencies result in greater penetration but at the expense of resolution. Typically, abdominal ultrasound imaging for viewing the kidneys uses 3.5-MHz transducers, whereas transrectal techniques use 7.0- to 7.5-MHz transducers for imaging the prostate.

3. How do tissue interfaces affect ultrasound waves?
Ultrasound waves pass through tissue but are reflected or scattered at interfaces between tissues. This reflection of the ultrasound waves allows for the delineation of different structures. If no interfaces exist, ultrasound waves tend to pass unimpeded through the structure, which typically occurs with fluid-filled masses (e.g., simple renal cyst).

4. How are ultrasound waves generated?
An electrical current applied to a piezoelectric ceramic crystal results in vibration of the crystal with the development of ultrasound waves. Reflected ultrasound waves impinge on the crystal and generate an electrical potential that can be processed to provide an image on a cathode tube.

5. What is A-mode? B-mode?
In **A-mode** imaging (amplitude mode), the magnitude or intensity of the signal is displayed as a spike of varying height along a time or distance axis. This one-dimensional display is rarely used clinically. In **B-mode** (brightness mode), the presence of an echo is indicated by the appearance of a bright spot, while the intensity of the echo is indicated by the brightness of the spot.

6. What is gray scale?
Current ultrasound instruments usually display brightness of echoes in 64 or 128 shades of gray (gray scale). A two-dimensional, clinically useful image is obtained.

7. What is real-time imaging?
In real-time scanning, the transducer constantly changes location, providing in essence a rapid B-mode scan that gives the examiner the sense of "live" imaging analogous to x-ray fluoroscopy.

8. Explain the purpose of Doppler studies. What is color-flow Doppler?
Doppler imaging allows for simultaneous viewing in real time and evaluating blood flow. The Doppler effect or Doppler shift refers to the alteration in frequency that occurs after a sound wave is reflected off a moving target. The red blood cell is an individual moving target and each scatters a single sound wave. The combined effect of multiple sound waves is received by the transducer, and different colors (typically blue and red) are superimposed on the gray scale image, depending on whether the reflected waves are of higher or lower frequency (i.e., the red blood cells are moving away from or toward the transducer). Sophisticated instruments are able to combine both real time and color-flow Doppler studies on one image, often referred to as duplex imaging.

9. Describe the ultrasound characteristics of a renal cyst.
Typically, a renal cyst is a benign mass associated with the kidney. No internal echoes are present, the walls of the cyst are thin and can be noted circumferentially, and the transmitted waves on the back of the cyst are enhanced.

10. Describe the ultrasound characteristics of renal malignancies.

Renal malignancies are masses associated with the kidney that often distort the collecting system. They usually have a heterogeneous internal architecture with poorly defined margins that are, at times, difficult to separate from the renal parenchyma. Often calcifications with associated ultrasound "shadowing" are dispersed throughout the mass. Color-flow studies typically demonstrate increased blood flow to renal malignancies.

11. Is ultrasound helpful in detecting hydronephrosis?

The normal central echo pattern within the midportion or hilum of the kidney is hyperechoic due to the presence of fat and vascular structures. In the hydronephrotic kidney, the collecting system becomes distended with urine (fluid), which can easily be detected by ultrasound. Ultrasound imaging is very useful in detecting the presence of distention of the intrarenal collecting system to help establish a diagnosis of hydronephrosis. Such studies may not reveal hydronephrosis if the patient is dehydrated. False-positive studies can occur during periods of diuresis.

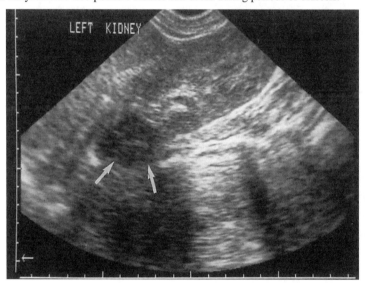

12. What are the ultrasound characteristics of a stone or calcification?

Typically, a calcification in the urinary tract appears as a hyperechoic interface with shadowing behind it due to the nontransmittal of ultrasound waves. These typical characteristics are present in calcifications throughout the urinary tract, including the kidney, bladder, and prostate. Stones of varying composition (e.g., calcium oxalate, cystine, uric acid) all will result in shadowing.

13. How is ultrasound useful in evaluating bladder outlet obstruction?

Ultrasound of the urinary bladder can detect and measure the volume of residual urine. Volume measurement can be calculated by obtaining anterior-posterior, transverse, and longitudinal (cephalad-caudad) diameters of the bladder and applying these measurements to standard formulas.

14. Describe the ultrasound characteristics of a ureterocele.

Ureteroceles are often associated with duplicated collecting systems and typically are detected in children, particularly girls presenting with urinary tract infections. Ureteroceles appear as a fluid mass within the bladder with a thin but clearly defined membrane. Many patients with ureteroceles will have associated hydroureteronephrosis of that renal segment draining into the ureterocele. Ultrasound is useful in making this determination.

15. Can ultrasound detect a testicular tumor?

Typically, the testicle is echogenic and uniform on ultrasound, and tumors within the testicle, although small, are well delineated. The tumors usually are uniform and of lower echogenicity than the surrounding testicle, but can be heterogeneous. If the tumor is large, it can replace the entire testicle so that no normal testicular tissue is evident.

16. How is the Doppler useful in evaluating varicoceles?

Doppler studies are able to detect blood flow. By checking for flow within the spermatic cord during a Valsalva maneuver, one is able to detect retrograde flow to the testicle and confirm the presence of a varicocele. Also, the dilated veins associated with a variocele will be apparent when the patient is erect but will decompress in the supine position. The clinical significance of subclinical varicoceles (i.e., those that are detected by ultrasound but are not palpable) remains controversial.

17. How is ultrasound used to assess testicular torsion?

Testicular torsion is associated with the interruption of blood flow to the testicle and, if untreated, results in infarction. Doppler studies are useful in detecting the presence or absence of blood flow when torsion is suspected. Flow studies are very useful in making this determination. Radionuclide studies have also been used to establish this diagnosis and appear comparable to the Doppler studies.

18. Are there typical ultrasound characteristics of carcinoma of the prostate?

On transrectal ultrasonography, carcinoma of the prostate typically appears as a hypoechoic area within the peripheral zone of the prostate. However, not all prostatic malignancies are associated with changes on ultrasonography. Many are isoechoic and cannot be distinguished from normal surrounding prostatic tissue, and some are actually hyperechoic. Additionally, not all peripherally located hypoechoic lesions are malignant.

19. Describe the typical appearance of benign prostatic hyperplasia (BPH) on ultrasound.

Benign prostatic hyperplasia has its origin in the transition zone of the prostate. With BPH, the anterior-posterior diameter of the prostate is increased and the gland has a more rounded appearance. The large increase in size of the transition zone results in compression of the peripheral zone, and the distinction between these zones is usually most evident.

20. How is ultrasound used to measure prostate size?

Ultrasound measurements of prostate size use the formula for calculating the volume of a prolate ellipse. The three largest diameters of the prostate (anterior-posterior, transverse, and longitudinal) are multiplied by each other and divided by 2. These measurements are usually obtained with transrectal ultrasound.

21. What is prostate-specific antigen density (PSAD)?

PSAD has been used to test for the presence of carcinoma of the prostate. The PSAD is derived by dividing the serum PSA level by the volume of the prostate (measured by ultrasound). A value ≥ 0.15 suggests carcinoma of the prostate, and these patients require evaluation.

22. Is ultrasound used in the evaluation of impotence?

Yes. Doppler flow studies are useful in measuring penile blood flow changes following injection of vasoactive substances. Patients with vasculogenic impotence will not demonstrate changes in arterial diameter or an increase in blood flow. These studies have also been used to assess for impotence secondary to venous insufficiency.

BIBLIOGRAPHY

1. Gillenwater JY, Grayhack WT, Howards SS, Mitchell ME (eds): Adult and Pediatric Urology, 4th ed. Philadelphia, Lippincott Williams & Wilkins, 2002.
2. Rifkin MD (ed): Ultrasound of the Prostate, 2nd ed. Philadelphia, Lippincott-Raven, 1997.
3. Cochlin DL, Dubbins PA, Goldberg AA (eds): Urogenital Ultrasound: A Text Atlas. Philadelphia, J.B. Lippincott, 1994.
4. Fornage BD (ed): Ultrasound of the Prostate. New York, John Wiley & Sons, 1988.
5. Pollack HM, McClennan BL (eds): Clinical Urography, 2nd ed. Philadelphia, W.B. Saunders, 2000.

6. COMPUTED TOMOGRAPHY

Nehemia Hampel, M.D.

1. What is computed tomography (CT)?

In regular radiography, a broad beam passes through the subject to produce an image on the x-ray film (detector). In CT scanning, a thin, collimated beam of x-ray is directed through the subject and is sensed on a series of x-ray detectors. During scanning, thin slices through the body are recorded. The process is repeated in consecutive slices and is later reconstructed by digital computers that assemble and integrate the data and reconstruct a cross-sectional image. The image can be displayed on screen or photographed. The reconstructed image uses measurements of linear attenuation coefficients collected from the multiple projections around the body. Usually, the images are two-dimensional; however, three-dimensional images are available.

2. When was CT scan developed?

Sir Godfrey N. Hounsfield at EMI Limited in England developed the first CT scanner in 1973.

3. What are Hounsfield units (HUs)?

HUs is a relative density scale of numbers that assigns a value of -1000 to air, 0 to water, and $+1000$ to dense bone. The density of a structure is proportionate to the amount of x-ray attenuation. The higher the density, the higher the CT number. Approximate typical values: Fat— -90 HU; soft tissue— $+40$ HU; clotted blood— $+70$ HU.

4. How wide is a CT scan slice?

CT scanning commonly uses contiguous 1-cm slices. Thinner slices of 0.5 cm can be used to obtain a more accurate delineation of small or unclear lesions. When scanning is done for urinary calculi, thin slices are used.

5. What patient positions and techniques are used in abdominal or pelvic CT scanning?

Patients are usually placed in the supine position, are kept NPO (nothing by mouth) for 12 hours, and are given a limited bowel preparation. Oral contrast media are used to avoid mistaking nonopacified loops of bowel for peritoneal or retroperitoneal masses. For most urological indications for CT scanning, a preliminary noncontrast scan before intravenous contrast media is recommended. In the evaluation of renal masses, renal or retroperitoneal calcification, suspected urine extravasation, or trauma, CT scans should always be performed both before and after intravenous contrast enhancement.

6. When is CT scan used in urology?

CT is used for the evaluation of renal, perirenal, ureteral, or retroperitoneal processes. It is effective in defining complications associated with renal transplants, assessing adrenal lesions, and detecting retroperitoneal lymph nodes and lung lesions. It has a role in staging testicular, bladder, and prostate cancer, in addition to evaluating pelvic masses. CT is used to evaluate trauma of the urinary tract, mainly the kidneys. Thin-slice spiral CT scan is commonly used for the evaluation of stone disease in acute renal colic.

7. When is CT scan used in renal and perirenal evaluation?

CT is most commonly used in detection or delineation of a renal mass. It is one of the best modalities for detecting masses and separating solid from cystic masses. It also is used in the detection and staging, as well as in the follow-up, of malignant renal tumors. In inflammatory renal, perirenal, and retroperitoneal masses, CT detects the process and defines its extent. It is the imaging modality of choice for staging renal trauma. CT scan is extremely sensitive in detecting renal calculus disease. Usually, uric acid stones are undetected on regular x-rays; however, they are intensely radiopaque on CT scans. Three-dimensional spiral CT scanning allows reconstruction of *renal, retroperitoneal* masses and renal vessels, which can be of significant assistance in the planning of nephron-sparing nephrectomy, as well as complicated renal and extrarenal surgeries.

8. Can CT scan be used as a guide for interventional procedures?

CT scan may be used as a guide for biopsy, aspiration, and drainage techniques, particularly for renal lesions. Usually, ultrasonography is faster, less expensive, and readily available, but in some cases, lesions are better demonstrated with CT. Although undetected on plain x-rays, hydronephrosis can be detected by CT scan; ultrasonography, however, is an accurate and less expensive method of detecting hydronephrosis. CT scan is somewhat less sensitive than ultrasonography in distinguishing solid from cystic masses.

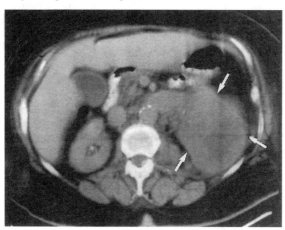

9. Is CT scan effective in the staging of carcinoma of the prostate?

CT has only a limited value for staging carcinoma of the prostate. Small lymphatic metastases in the pelvis are difficult to visualize. Differentiation of cancer from the normal gland is seldom possible in localized disease. Cancer can be detected only in advanced extraprostatic extension into the bladder base or seminal vesicles. CT scan should not be used for routine staging of prostate carcinoma.

10. What are the most important contributions of CT scan to urology?

CT is most important in the assessment of renal masses. It is the modality of choice for detecting and staging solid renal lesions and has become a standard modality in the evaluation of renal trauma and nephrolithiasis.

BIBLIOGRAPHY

1. Anderson KR, Smith RC: CT for the evaluation of flank pain. J Endourol 15:25–29, 2001.
2. Bosniak MA: Problems in the radiologic diagnosis of renal parenchymal tumors. Urol Clin North Am 20:217–230, 1993.
3. Gillenwater JY, Grayhack JT, Howards SS, Duckett JW (eds): Adult and Pediatric Urology, 3rd ed. St. Louis, Mosby, 1996.
4. Hounsfield GN: Computed medical imaging. Med Phys 7:283–290, 1980.
5. Papanicolaou N: Urinary tract imaging and intervention: Basic principles. In Walsh PC, Retik AB, Vaughan ED Jr., Wein AJ (eds): Campbell's Urology, 7th ed. Philadelphia, W.B. Saunders, 1998, pp 170–260.
6. Rubin GD, Silverman SG: Spiral CT of the retroperitoneum. Radiol Clin North Am 33:903–932, 1995.
7. Teigen EL, Newhouse JH: Imaging renal masses. Curr Opin Urol 10:421–427, 2000.
8. Urban BA, Fishman EK: Helical CT of the abdomen and pelvis: Potential diagnostic pitfalls of arterial-phase imaging in the genitourinary tract. J Comput Assist Tomogr 25:358–364, 2001.

7. MAGNETIC RESONANCE IMAGING

David A. Goldfarb, M.D.

1. What element forms the basis for MRI?
Hydrogen.

2. How does MRI work?
A large magnet aligns the hydrogen nuclei within the tissue under examination. A radio frequency pulse is applied and deflects the net magnetization of the hydrogen nuclei in the tissue. The excited nuclei precess about the axis of the magnetic field and produce an electrical signal detected in a receiver coil. The decay of the signal as the nuclei return to equilibrium is monitored. The return to equilibrium is called magnetic relaxation and is a unique property of each tissue, described by T1 and T2 relaxation times. These are important determinants of image contrast and signal intensity in MRI.

3. What pulse sequence is used for MRI?
Spin-echo.

4. What pulse sequence highlights flow in large blood vessels?
Gradient-echo.

5. Compare the advantages and disadvantages of MRI and CT.

MRI Versus CT

MRI	CT
No ionizing radiation	Ionizing radiation
No iodinated contrast	Iodinated contrast
High cost	Low cost
Less widely available	Widely available
Improved imaging of vascular structures	—
Better soft-tissue characterization	—

6. What are contraindications to MRI?
Claustrophobia, ferromagnetic prosthetic device, pacemaker, and certain intracerebral clips.

7. Outline the T1- and T2-weighted appearances of urologic tissues on MRI.

MRI Appearance of Urologic Tissues

TISSUE	T1-WEIGHTED	T2-WEIGHTED
Calcium	Dark	Dark
Fat	Very bright*	Bright
Urine (water)	Very bright	Very bright
Renal cortex	Intermediate	Bright
Renal medulla	Dark	Intermediate
Adrenal	Intermediate	Intermediate
Bladder wall	Intermediate	Intermediate*
Prostate	Intermediate	Intermediate*
Seminal vesicles	Intermediate	Bright
Blood vessels	Dark	Dark

*Asterisks indicate the best sequence for visualizing structures. No signal is obtained from flowing blood.

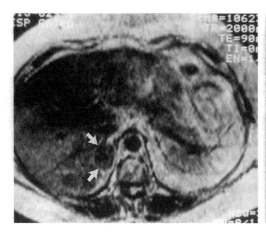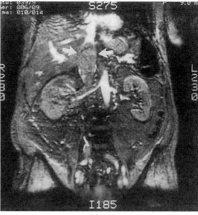

Left, T2-weighted MRI with a right adrenal mass that is iso-intense to the liver, which is an adenoma. *Right,* Gradient echo image of the abdomen. This demonstrates the full extent of a vena caval thrombus from a right renal cell carcinoma.

8. How is MRI useful in the evaluation of renal disorders?

1. **Staging of renal cell carcinoma.** MRI is comparable to CT for evaluating local tumor extension and adenopathy. Because of its ability to evaluate blood vessels, MRI can be used noninvasively to assess the precise limits of vena caval involvement.

2. **Renal masses.** Ultrasound and CT are generally better and less expensive than MRI. MRI has been used to assess renal masses in azotemic patients who cannot receive iodinated contrast. It may be used in patients with sensitivity to iodinated contrast.

3. **Obstruction.** Other methods, such as ultrasound and urography, are better and less expensive than MRI, although magnetic resonance urography may see increased use in selected patient populations (e.g., pediatrics).

9. How are adrenal masses differentiated by MRI?

Signal Intensity Compared with Liver

CONDITION	T1-WEIGHTED	T2-WEIGHTED
Adenoma	Isointense	Isointense
Carcinoma/metastasis	Isointense	Heterogeneous, intermediate increase
Pheochromocytoma	Isointense	Hyperintense

10. What are other urologic applications of MRI?

- Staging of prostate cancer—MRI is the most accurate local staging examination, but it is not extensively used because it cannot assess microscopic capsular invasion
- Vascular imaging—Can be used as a screening test for renal artery stenosis and may be used as an alternative to duplex ultrasonography. Assessment is limited to the proximal 3 cm of the renal artery

BIBLIOGRAPHY

1. Goldfarb DA, Novick AC, Bretan PN, et al: Magnetic resonance imaging for assessment of vena caval tumor thrombi. A comparative study with vena cavography and CT scanning. J Urol 144:1100–1103, 1990.

2. Rackley R, Lorig R, Goldfarb DA, Kay R: Magnetic resonance imaging of pelvic tumors in pediatric patients. J Urol 151:449–452, 1994.
3. Rifkin MD, Zerhouni EA, Gatsonis CA, et al: Comparison of magnetic resonance imaging and ultrasonography in staging early prostate cancer. N Engl J Med 323:621–626, 1990.
4. Stark DD, Bradley WG: Magnetic Resonance Imaging, 3rd ed. St. Louis, Mosby, 1999.
5. Riccabona M, Simbruner RM, Ring E, et al: Feasibility of MR urography in neonates and infants with anomalies of the upper urinary tract. Eur Radiol 12:1442–1450, 2002.
6. Blandino A, Gaeta M, Minutoli F, et al: MR pyelography in 115 patients with a dilated renal collecting system. Acta Radiol 42:532–536, 2001.
7. Wallner K: MR imaging for prostate cancer staging: Beauty or beast? Int J Radiat Oncol Biol Phys 52: 886–887, 2002.
8. Weishaupt D, Debatin JF: Magnetic resonance: Evaluation of adrenal lesions. Curr Opin Urol 2:153–163, 1999.

8. RADIONUCLIDE STUDIES

Donald R. Bodner, M.D. and David A. Levy, M.D.

1. What is meant by the term *nuclear renogram?*

A nuclear renogram is the activity-vs.-time graph that is generated from the kidney after administration of a radionuclide. Studies are performed to document such factors as differential function of each kidney, renal perfusion, renal obstruction, and rejection.

2. Which radioactive nuclide is most commonly used in nuclear medicine?

Technetium (Tc) 99m is the most commonly used nuclide. It is ideal for examinations taking < 24 hours, because it has a half-life of 6 hours. The common agents used today for nuclear renograms include Tc 99m diethyltriamine pentaacetic acid (DTPA), Tc 99m Mag3, dimercaptosuccinic acid (DMSA), and 131 iodine (131-I) hippurate.

3. In an adult with suspected atherosclerotic vascular disease and renal insufficiency, which agent is most helpful in assessing renal blood flow?

DTPA is best used in a dynamic fashion for vascular imaging. Analysis is based on observation of the intensity and symmetry of kidney visualization. Peak activity in the kidney should be no more than 3 seconds after peak activity is noted in the aorta.

4. In a child with a history of pyelonephritis, what is the most useful agent in assessing renal parenchymal scarring?

DMSA provides detailed anatomic imaging, because it accumulates in the kidneys over several hours. Delayed views show better images of the renal cortex. DMSA is also helpful for interval imaging of the renal cortex.

5. What agents can be used in chronic renal failure?

123-I and 131-I hippurate are the recommended agents, because renal concentration may occur with as little as 3% of normal renal function. Technetium compounds may be preferred when renal vascular problems are suspected, and Mag3 may prove superior to hippurate.

6. When is Mag3 the preferred radionuclide?

Mag3 imaging sequence is similar to DTPA and is often used in the pediatric population, because considerably less uptake in the liver and spleen allows more accurate assessment of renal function.

7. When should Lasix (furosemide) be given during a Lasix renogram?

Lasix should be given when the suspected kidney has the peak number of counts of the radionuclide in the collecting system.

8. What is meant by a superscan noted on a bone scan of a patient with prostate cancer?

A superscan refers to extensive bony involvement of the axial skeleton, which results in intense uptake of the radionuclide in the bone and no uptake by the kidneys.

9. What other nuclear tests are available to the urologist?

Testicular blood flow studies may be performed to aid in the differential diagnosis of testicular torsion and epididymitis. Bone scans are used commonly in the work-up of metastatic disease of the prostate and other urologic malignancies. Metaiodobenzylguanidine (MIBG) is a tracer that identifies sympathetic activity and may be helpful in localizing ectopic pheochromocytomas. Positron emission tomography (PET scan) is used to image genitourinary malignancies

and shows promise in detecting their metastatic spread. PET scans, along with ProstaScint®
(capromab pendetide) imaging, show promise in the early detection and localization of prostate
cancer recurrence in the clinical setting of rising PSA after radical prostatectomy.

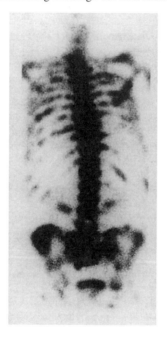

Positive bone scan in metastatic carcinoma of the prostate.

BIBLIOGRAPHY

1. Croft BY, Joyce JM, Parekh J, Teates CD: Nuclide studies. In Gillenwater JY, Grayhack JT, Howards SS,
   Duckett JW (eds): Adult and Pediatric Urology, 3rd ed. St. Louis, Mosby, 1996, pp 193–217.
2. Foreman J: The role of radionuclide studies in urologic patient management. Probl Urol 3:531–547, 1989.
3. Papanicolaou N: Urinary tract imaging and interpretation: Basic principles. In Walsh PC, Retik AB,
   Vaughan ED, Wein AJ (eds): Campbell's Urology, 7th ed. Philadelphia, W.B. Saunders, 1998,
   pp 170–260.
4. Rosenthal SA, Haseman MK, Polascik TJ: Utility of capromab pendetide (ProstaScint) imaging in the
   management of prostate cancer. Tech Urol 7:27–37, 2001.

9. RENAL MASS EVALUATION

Andrew C. Novick, M.D.

1. How are renal masses usually detected?

Radiographic evaluation for a renal mass may be prompted by suggestive symptoms such as abdominal or flank pain, hematuria, or a palpable flank mass upon physical examination. An increasing number of renal masses are currently being detected in asymptomatic patients who undergo a noninvasive abdominal imaging study, such as ultrasonography, computed tomography (CT), or magnetic resonance imaging (MRI), for an unrelated reason. More than 50% of all renal cell carcinomas are being detected incidentally in this manner.

2. What is the differential diagnosis of a renal mass in an adult?

- Benign renal cyst
- Abscess
- Hematoma
- Infarct
- Vascular malformation
- Benign mesenchymal tumor
- Renal pseudotumor
- Metastatic carcinoma
- Angiomyolipoma
- Oncocytoma
- Transitional cell carcinoma
- Renal cell carcinoma

3. Which tests are available for establishing the diagnosis of a renal mass?

The available radiographic imaging modalities for evaluating a renal mass include intravenous pyelography (IVP), ultrasonography, CT, MRI, and renal arteriography. Occasionally, percutaneous aspiration of a renal cyst or percutaneous biopsy of a solid renal mass may provide useful diagnostic information.

4. Compare the relative merits of IVP, ultrasonography, CT, and MRI in evaluating a renal mass.

IVP with or without nephrotomography can detect many renal masses but may not always distinguish solid from cystic lesions. IVP will also fail to demonstrate small anterior or posterior masses that do not distort the architecture of the kidney.

Ultrasonography is reliable in differentiating solid tissue from fluid and can reliably establish the diagnosis of a simple renal cyst. It can also allow the diagnosis of an angiomyolipoma by the characteristic increased echogenicity produced by fat.

CT scanning is the single most important radiographic test for delineating the nature of a renal mass. CT, with and without contrast administration, is recommended to take full advantage of the enhancement characteristic of highly vascular renal parenchymal tumors. Solid masses with areas of negative CT attenuation numbers (Hounsfield units) indicative of fat are diagnostic of angiomyolipoma. In approximately 10% of renal masses, CT is indeterminate and additional tests or surgical exploration is needed to establish a definitive diagnosis.

MRI is done with gadolinium injection to detect vascular parenchymal tumors, which will enhance. MRI offers no diagnostic advantage over ultrasound or CT in characterizing the nature of a renal mass. Because ultrasound and CT are considerably less expensive and easier to obtain, MRI is not recommended for primary evaluation of a renal mass. The major indication for MRI is in patients with azotemia in whom contrast administration is contraindicated.

5. What is the difference between a simple renal cyst and a complex renal cyst?

A **simple renal cyst** is a benign lesion and appears as a round, well-marginated mass on ultrasound or CT with a thin smooth wall. A simple renal cyst is anechoic on ultrasound and demonstrates a low density (<20 Hounsfield units) with no contrast enhancement on CT.

A **complex renal cyst** has one or more features that may be indicative of malignancy, such as internal septations, calcium in the cyst wall or septum, a high density or heterogeneous internal appearance, an irregular margin, or areas with contrast enhancement on CT scan. Complex cysts with thin septa or calcium in the cyst wall or septum are most likely benign; however, the other listed features are more suggestive of renal cell carcinoma.

6. What is a renal pseudotumor?

A renal pseudotumor is an area of normal renal parenchyma that gives the appearance of a solid renal mass. A renal pseudotumor may represent a hypertrophied column of Bertin, an area of segmental renal hypertrophy, or an unusually shaped kidney. The diagnosis can be established with a technetium dimercaptosuccinic acid (DMSA) renal scan, which will demonstrate increased uptake of isotope with a pseudotumor and decreased uptake of isotope with a cystic or solid renal mass.

7. What is the role of arteriography in the evaluation of a renal mass?

There are relatively few indications for arteriography during the diagnostic evaluation of a renal mass. Most renal cell carcinomas demonstrate neovascularity, whereas metastatic renal tumors and transitional cell carcinomas are relatively avascular. However 20%–25% of renal cell carcinomas are also avascular. Arteriography is also rarely indicated for surgical planning and has been replaced in this setting by three-dimensional volume-rendered CT scanning.

8. When should percutaneous aspiration of a renal cyst or percutaneous biopsy of a renal mass be performed?

Aspiration of fluid from a renal cyst that remains equivocal after CT scanning is occasionally helpful. The presence of abnormal cytology or blood in the aspirate is suggestive of malignancy and indicates a need for probable surgical exploration. **Percutaneous biopsy** of a solid renal mass is indicated when a metastatic lesion, abscess, or infected cyst is suspected. Routine biopsy of solid renal masses is not recommended owing to a high incidence of falsely negative findings in patients with renal cell carcinoma.

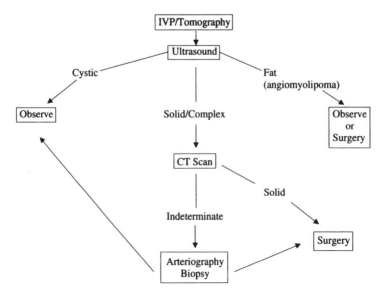

9. Outline the appropriate evaluation of an indeterminate renal mass observed on IVP in an asymptomatic patient.

For a mass demonstrated upon IVP, the next step is an ultrasound study. If this demonstrates a simple renal cyst, further evaluation is usually unnecessary. The demonstration of fat within a solid mass on ultrasound indicates an angiomyolipoma. Other solid or complex cystic masses require further evaluation with a CT scan. Contrast enhancement of a solid mass on CT scanning indicates renal cell carcinoma until proven otherwise, although approximately 10% of such masses may prove to be benign (an oncocytoma or adenoma). An indeterminate renal mass on a CT scan may **occasionally** be evaluated further with **MRI** or percutaneous biopsy. Using this approach, it is currently possible to establish the diagnosis of a renal **carcinoma** in most patients.

BIBLIOGRAPHY

1. Beldegrun A, deKernion JB: Renal tumors. In Walsh PC, Retik AB, Vaughn ED, Wein AJ (eds): Campbell's Urology, 7th ed. Philadelphia, W.B. Saunders, 1998.
2. Bosniak MA: Problems in the radiologic diagnosis of renal parenchymal tumors. Urol Clin North Am 20:217–230, 1993.
3. Levin E: Malignant renal parenchymal tumors in adults. In Pollack HM (ed): Clinical Urography. Philadelphia, W.B. Saunders, 1990.
4. Jennings SB, Linehan WM: Renal perirenal and ureteral neoplasms. In Gillenwater JY, Grayhack JT, Howards SS, Duckett JW (eds): Adult and Pediatric Urology. St. Louis, Mosby, 1996, pp 643–694.
5. Novick AC, Campbell SC: Renal tumors. In Walsh P, Wein A, Retik A, Vaughan D (eds): Campbell's Urology, 8th ed. Philadelphia, W.B. Saunders, 2002.

10. ABDOMINAL MASSES IN CHILDREN

Jeffrey S. Palmer, M.D. and Jack S. Elder, M.D.

1. In a newborn, what is the most common cause of an abdominal mass?
Hydronephrosis, usually secondary to a ureteropelvic junction obstruction.

2. What is the second most common cause of an abdominal mass in the neonate?
Multicystic kidney.

3. How common are tumors as causes for an abdominal mass in a neonate?
Tumors account for approximately 12% of neonatal abdominal masses.

4. What types of neoplasms occur in neonates that may result in an abdominal mass?
The most common tumors in the newborn include neuroblastoma, mesoblastic nephroma, and sacrococcygeal teratoma. Less common tumors include gastric teratoma, leiomyosarcoma, and hepatoma.

5. What is the most common malignancy in a newborn?
Neuroblastoma, which accounts for 50% of all neonatal malignant tumors.

6. Is neuroblastoma in a neonate associated with better or poorer prognosis compared with neuroblastoma in older children?
Survival is better. The majority have low-stage or stage IV-S disease, with a 70% overall survival rate.

7. Of solid renal tumors in neonates, how common is Wilms tumor?
Wilms tumor is extremely uncommon in the newborn. A solid renal tumor is much more likely to be a mesoblastic nephroma.

8. From 1 month to 1 year of age, what are the two most common causes of an abdominal mass?
Hydronephrosis accounts for 40% of abdominal masses and tumor for 40%.

9. In children > 1 year old, what is the most common cause of an abdominal mass?
Tumor.

10. In a neonate, what is the most common cause of hydronephrosis?
Ureteropelvic junction obstruction.

11. Name some other causes of hydronephrosis in the neonate.
Ureterovesical junction obstruction, ectopic ureterocele, posterior urethral valves, ectopic ureter, and vesicoureteral reflux are common causes.

12. In neonates, what proportion of abdominal masses is caused by genitourinary disorders?
Approximately 75% of abdominal masses are genitourinary in origin.

13. What is the initial radiologic examination of choice in children with an abdominal mass? What information does it provide?
Ultrasonography is the initial radiologic study. This test often identifies the organ from which the mass is originating and shows whether it is fluid-filled or solid.

14. If ultrasonography identifies hydronephrosis, what is the next test that should be performed?

A voiding cystourethrogram should be performed to determine whether there is vesicoureteral reflux. In addition, the study may show whether there is a ureterocele or, in a boy, posterior urethral valves.

15. At what age is neuroblastoma more common than Wilms tumor?

Neuroblastoma is more common in children $<$ 2 years of age, whereas Wilms tumor is more common in children $>$ 2 years of age.

16. What is aniridia? What is its significance?

Aniridia is developmental absence of most of the iris. Spontaneous aniridia is associated with Wilms tumor.

17. What is the significance of microcephaly?

Microcephaly is associated with posterior urethral valves and also occurs in Beckwith-Wiedemann syndrome.

18. In which syndrome is macroglossia common?

It is common in Beckwith-Wiedemann syndrome, in which Wilms tumor and hepatoblastoma are also common.

19. What is the significance of hemihypertrophy?

In children with hemihypertrophy, Wilms tumor is more common.

20. Webbing of the neck is a sign of what syndrome?

It is a sign of Turner's syndrome, in which a horseshoe kidney is the most common renal anomaly.

21. What is the significance of respiratory distress or pneumothorax in a neonate with an abdominal mass?

These conditions are commonly associated with severe obstructive renal disorders—most commonly, posterior urethral valves and urethral atresia.

22. What is the significance of bright pink or bluish subcutaneous nodules in the newborn?

They may indicate the presence of disseminated neuroblastoma.

23. What is the typical appearance of a multicystic kidney on ultrasonography?

This condition consists of multiple cysts of varying sizes without overlying renal parenchyma.

24. What is the significance of hypertension in a child with an abdominal mass?

It may be indicative of neuroblastoma, congenital mesoblastic nephroma, and less commonly, Wilms tumor, hydronephrosis, or multicystic kidney.

25. Describe the two types of polycystic kidneys. What are the ultrasound findings in each type?

Polycystic kidneys may be autosomal recessive or autosomal dominant. The autosomal recessive form, also termed *infantile,* is more common in neonates. In this type, ultrasound shows enlarged, severely echogenic kidneys due to numerous tiny cysts. In infants with autosomal dominant polycystic kidney disease (also termed *the adult form*), the kidneys are enlarged and contain multiple large cysts of varying sizes. In some cases, hepatic cysts also occur. Polycystic kidney disease and multicystic kidney are distinct entities.

26. What is the significance of hematuria in a newborn with an abdominal mass?

Hematuria may be indicative of renal vein thrombosis.

27. What is the cause of renal vein thrombosis in the neonate? Describe its diagnosis and treatment.

Renal vein thrombosis results from any condition that causes reduced intravascular volume or a hypercoagulable state, including dehydration (e.g., from diarrhea), infection, vascular endothelial damage, or a deficiency of antithrombin III, protein C, or protein S. In addition, offspring of diabetic mothers are at increased risk. In most cases, the condition is unilateral and the thrombus originates in the small intrarenal branches of the renal vein. Classic findings include a firm enlarging kidney, hematuria, and proteinuria in an ill neonate. Anemia results from hemolysis, hematuria, and the enlarging thrombus. Thrombocytopenia results from trapping of platelets in the thrombus. Ultrasound is used for diagnosis. Therapy includes supportive measures directed at the cause, including hydration, correction of electrolyte imbalance, and broad-spectrum antibiotics. If bilateral involvement is present or the vena cava is involved, heparin or thrombolytic therapy may be necessary. Occasionally, selective thrombolytic therapy is necessary.

28. What is the most likely diagnosis of an abdominal mass in a female neonate if there is also a bulging interlabial mass?

Hydrocolpos secondary to an imperforate hymen.

29. What is the significance of stippled calcification in a retroperitoneal solid mass?

Approximately 50% of patients with neuroblastoma have stippled calcification.

30. Which tumor is more likely to be fixed rather than mobile—neuroblastoma or Wilms tumor?

Neuroblastoma.

31. Which abdominal masses are most likely to be mobile?

Masses in the ovaries, mesentery, and intestine.

32. Name the two primary causes of masses arising from the female genital system.

Hydrocolpos and ovarian cysts.

33. How often are the kidneys palpable in the neonate?

Both kidneys are usually palpable in the neonate.

34. If a renal mass with multiple cysts is detected on ultrasound, there is contralateral vesicoureteral reflux, and a renal scan shows that the mass has no function, what is the most likely diagnosis?

Multicystic kidney.

35. If the mass is found to be in the anterior abdomen, what are the most likely diagnoses?

Duplication anomaly of the gastrointestinal tract, mesenteric cyst, and intestinal atresia.

BIBLIOGRAPHY

1. Cendron M, Elder JS, Duckett JW: Perinatal urology. In Gillenwater JY, Grayhack JT, Howards SS, Duckett JW (eds): Adult and Pediatric Urology, 3rd ed., vol. 3. St. Louis, Mosby, 1996, pp 2075–2169.
2. Diamond DA, Gosalbez R: Neonatal urologic emergencies. In Walsh PC, Retik AB, Vaughan ED Jr., Wein AJ (eds): Campbell's Urology, 7th ed. Philadelphia, W.B. Saunders, 1998, pp 1629–1654.
3. Selzman AA, Elder JS: Contralateral vesicoureteral reflux in children with a multicystic kidney. J Urol 153: 1252, 1995.

11. EVALUATION OF ACUTE SCROTAL SWELLING IN CHILDREN

Jonathan H. Ross, M.D.

1. List six causes of acute scrotal swelling in children.

Spermatic cord torsion (testicular torsion), torsion of the appendix testis, epididymo-orchitis, hernia, hydrocele, and testis tumor. The last three usually do not present acutely but may on occasion.

2. What are the physical findings suggestive of testicular torsion?

An extremely tender testis that is high-riding is typical of testicular torsion. The cremasteric reflex is often absent, the cord is thick or difficult to distinguish, and elevation of the testis offers no relief (as it may in epididymitis). Although these findings are typical or suggestive of testicular torsion, their absence does not exclude the possibility.

3. Explain the difference between intravaginal and extravaginal torsion.

Typically, testicular torsion is intravaginal—it occurs within the tunica vaginalis. Thus, on exposure of the testicle, the hydrocele sac (the tunica vaginalis) is opened and the torsed cord and testis are inside. In newborns, the tunica vaginalis is not adherent to the surrounding dartos fascia. Hence, the testis and processus vaginalis and tunica vaginalis can torse as a unit (extravaginal torsion). Because the tunica vaginalis becomes adherent to the dartos fascia within the first weeks of life, extravaginal torsion does not occur beyond the newborn period.

4. Do any anatomic features predispose to testicular torsion?

Yes (or I wouldn't have asked the question). The "bell-clapper deformity" results from a variation in the way in which the tunica vaginalis reflects on the testis. This anatomic variant can be detected on physical examination and predisposes to testicular torsion. In patients with a bell-clapper deformity, the testes have a horizontal lie with the long axis oriented in the anteroposterior direction. The variant is bilateral, explaining the risk of metachronous contralateral torsion in patients who have experienced a testicular torsion.

5. How is testicular torsion treated surgically?

Bilateral scrotal orchidopexy. Through a scrotal incision, the torsed testis is detorsed and, if viable, fixed to the scrotal wall at three points. Contralateral orchidopexy is also performed because of the high risk of metachronous contralateral torsion. Newer techniques use a subcutaneous pouch without sutures because of concern about possible suture reaction in the testis.

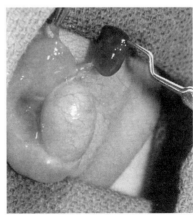

Intraoperative photograph demonstrating normal testicle and torsed appendix testis (at tip of forceps).

6. Does testicular torsion always present as a single acute event?

No. Patients with recurrent testicular pain and swelling who have a bell-clapper deformity may be suffering from intermittent torsion. In this condition, the testis torses, resulting in symptoms, but spontaneously detorses within a short time. In patients with a convincing history and the bell-clapper deformity, bilateral preemptive scrotal orchidopexy should be considered.

7. What is the "blue dot" sign?

A torsed appendix testis has a bluish hue when viewed through the scrotal skin. A "blue dot" at the upper pole of the testis on physical examination suggests the diagnosis. In the absence of a blue dot, the diagnosis may still be made if scrotal tenderness is isolated to a hard nodule at the upper pole of the testis in the absence of other findings suggesting spermatic cord torsion.

8. How is appendiceal torsion treated?

Nonsteroidal anti-inflammatory drugs (most commonly ibuprofen). The pain usually resolves within 1–2 weeks.

9. What laboratory test is essential in a patient with acute scrotal swelling?

Urinalysis. Significant pyuria is extremely suggestive of epididimitis.

10. What radiographic study should be obtained in a young boy with epidimymitis?

Renal ultrasound. Because an ectopic ureter in boys inserts into the wolffian duct structures (e.g., the seminal vesicle or vas), it may present with epididimitis. An ectopic ureter can be detected by hydroureteronephrosis on ultrasound.

11. Which radiographic studies can distinguish testicular torsion from other causes of scrotal swelling?

Radionuclide testicular scan and color-flow Doppler ultrasound. On a radionuclide scan, a torsed testis will appear photopenic. In contrast, epididymo-orchitis results in increased blood flow and, therefore, increased radionuclide. False-positive studies may result from abscess formation or an associated hydrocele. False-negative studies may occur due to scrotal wall hyperemia or, in old torsion, from the inflammatory response. Doppler ultrasonography will demonstrate an absence of blood flow to the testis, although because the intratesticular vessels are small, reliable detection may be difficult. Both studies are very operator dependent, and their availability differs among institutions. However, most centers favor Dopper ultrasound.

12. Name the definitive way to diagnosis testicular torsion.

Surgical exploration. Because time is essential, immediate exploration is indicated in any patient suspected of having testicular torsion. Waiting for a nuclear scan or ultrasound to confirm the diagnosis is inappropriate. Radiographic studies should be reserved for patients who are thought to have a low likelihood of testicular torsion. As with appendicitis, occasional negative explorations are to be expected and are far better than a delayed exploration in a boy who has a torsion.

13. How long before a torsed testicle is no longer salvageable?

Most testicles explored within 6 hours of the onset of symptoms are salvaged. Most testicles explored after 24 hours are not. However, the history is often unreliable. Therefore, the decision of whether to perform an orchidopexy or orchiectomy is based primarily on the appearance of the testis at exploration.

14. Pus in the scrotum of a young boy should suggest what diagnosis?

Appendicitis. Admittedly, this is a zebra, but it is important to realize that, particularly in infancy, the scrotum is the window to the peritoneum. In many newborns (especially premature infants), the processus vaginalis is patent. Thus, intraperitoneal processes can spread to the scrotum. Other examples are hydroceles in infants with ascites and hard scrotal masses due to dystrophic calcification in infants with meconium peritonitis.

BIBLIOGRAPHY

1. Bartsch G, Frank S, Marberger H, Mikuz G: Testicular torsion: Late results with special regard to fertility and endocrine function. J Urol 124:375–378, 1980.
2. Bartsch G, Mikuz G, Ennemoser O, Janetschek G: Testicular torsion. In Resnick MI, Kursh ED (eds): Current Therapy in Genitourinary Surgery. St. Louis, Mosby, 1992, pp 436–440.
3. Cass AS, Cass BP, Veeraraghaven K: Immediate exploration of the unilateral acute scrotum in young male subjects. J Urol 124:829–832, 1980.
4. Dresner M: Torsed appendage diagnosis and management: Blue dot sign. Urology 1:63–66, 1973.
5. Gislason T, Noronha RFX, Gregory JG: Acute epididymitis in boys: A 5-year retrospective study. J Urol 124:533–534, 1980.
6. Hadziselimovic F, Geneto R, Emmons LR: Increased apoptos is in the contralateral testes of patients with testicular torsion as a factor for infertility. J Urol 160:1158–1160, 1998.
7. Kass EJ, Stone KT, Cacciarelli AA, Mitchell B: Do all children with an acute scrotum require exploration? J Urol 150:667–669, 1993.
8. Kogan S, Hadziselimovic F, Howards SS, et al: Pediatric andrology. In Gillenwater JY, Grayhack JT, Howards SS, Duckett JW (eds): Adult and Pediatric Urology, 3rd ed. St. Louis, Mosby, 1996, pp 2634–2668.
9. Skoglund RW, McRoberts JW, Ragde H: Torsion of the testicular appendages: Presentation of 43 new cases and a collective review. J Urol 104:598–600, 1970.
10. Steinhardt GF, Boyarsky S, Mackey R: Testicular torsion: Pitfalls of color Doppler sonography. J Urol 150:461–462, 1993.

12. EVALUATION OF ACUTE RENAL FAILURE

Stuart M. Flechner, M.D.

1. What is acute renal failure?

Acute renal failure can be defined as any sudden decline in renal function. The degree of renal dysfunction is directly proportional to the decrease in the glomerular filtration rate (GFR) measured in mL/min.

2. How often does acute renal failure occur, and how is it different from chronic renal failure?

Up to 5% of all hospitalized patients and up to 20% of all patients treated in an intensive care unit experience some degree of acute renal failure. It is associated with increased mortality when it accompanies other potentially life-threatening conditions. Compared to chronic renal failure, acute renal failure is usually reversible and limited if the offending cause is identified, and proper treatment instituted. Acute renal failure can lead to permanent renal injury or chronic renal failure in certain circumstances. Currently, the most effective treatment of acute renal failure is primary prevention.

3. How does one know that a patient has acute renal failure?

When a sudden decline in renal function has occurred sufficient to raise the level of nitrogenous waste products in the blood above established laboratory control values. This may also be accompanied by (but not necessarily) a diminished urine output of < 30 mL/hr in an adult.

4. What is the most accurate test to determine if acute renal failure has occurred?

The most accurate measurement of renal function is the glomerular filtration rate. However, its determination can be cumbersome because it requires the use of agents that are removed from the circulation only by filtration at the glomerulus. The clearance of the sugar inulin and certain radioisotopes can be used to accurately measure the glomerular filtration rate.

5. What is the best clinical test to determine if acute renal failure has occurred?

The most useful test is the measurement of the clearance of creatinine in mL/min. Creatinine is an endogenous product of muscle catabolism produced at a fairly constant rate of about 1 mg/min in an average-size adult. The clearance of creatinine from the blood approximates the GFR, and can be measured on a timed basis such as over 12 or 24 hours. It is calculated by using the formula: UV/P, where U is the urinary concentration of creatinine, V is the rate of urine production over a timed interval, and P is the plasma blood concentration of creatinine. Approximately 80% of creatinine clearance is due to GFR and about 20% is due to renal tubular secretion of creatinine. Therefore, the result is not as precise as the clearance of an agent removed by GFR alone. Clinically, this becomes important only at low levels of renal function, when tubular secretion of creatinine may account for a relatively greater percentage of the creatinine clearance.

6. Does urine have to be collected for 24 hours?

Renal function can be monitored serially by determining the serum creatinine level alone. The relationship of serum creatinine to creatinine clearance (by inference to the GFR) follows a hyperbolic curve. A healthy adult with a serum creatinine of 1 mg/dl has a GFR of about 120 mL/min (Other examples: a creatinine of 2 mg/dl = a GFR of about 60 mL/min; a creatinine of 4 mg/dl = a GFR of about 30 mL/min). It is important to note that when the creatinine doubles from 1 to 2 mg/dl, about 50% of the renal function has been lost. This steep part of the curve often masks the degree of renal dysfunction present, because the creatinine may remain below 2 mg/dl.

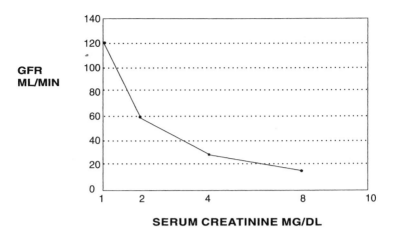

SERUM CREATININE MG/DL

7. Do other factors affect the serum creatinine?

Yes. Because creatinine is a product of muscle catabolism, large muscular individuals produce more creatinine than small individuals. Therefore, body size influences serum creatinine. The aging kidney also loses GFR, which results in a higher relative creatinine level.

These considerations led Cockroft and Gault to develop an equation to estimate creatinine clearance from clinical data.

$$\frac{creatinine}{clearance} = \frac{(140-age) \times weight\ (kg)}{serum\ creatinine\ (mg/dl)\ times\ 72}$$

Skeletal muscle injury may raise the serum creatinine while GFR remains constant. Certain drugs that interfere with filtration or tubular secretion such as cephalosporins, cimetidine, and trimethoprim can elevate the serum creatinine. However, a rising serum creatinine is rare in patients with normal kidney function and remains the best indicator of acute renal failure. In the complete absence of kidney function, the level rises about 1–2 mg/dl/day.

8. Is there a difference in creatinine clearance between males and females?

Yes. Because males manufacture more anabolic steroids than females, they generally have larger muscle mass; therefore, they produce more creatinine. For this reason, the Cockroft-Gault formula also incorporates a modifier of 0.85 for the calculation of creatinine clearance in females.

9. What other abnormalities are associated with acute renal failure?

Acute renal failure can result in several clinical signs and symptoms, such as hypertension, fluid overload, congestive heart failure, pericarditis, nausea, vomiting, weakness, lassitude, encephalopathy, and bleeding. In addition, a number of metabolic abnormalities result from the loss of GFR.

Most Frequent Blood Abnormalities in Acute Renal Failure

INCREASE	DECREASE
Serum creatinine	Serum bicarbonate (acidosis)
Blood urea nitrogen	Free calcium
Serum potassium	Red blood cell mass
Serum phosphorus	Platelet function
Serum magnesium	

10. What causes acute renal failure?

Amyriad of insults either alone or in combination can result in kidney dysfunction. For classification they are best thought of as **prerenal**—a decrease in the amount of blood delivered to the kidney; **renal**—a malfunction of the kidney parenchyma; and **postrenal**—obstruction to the flow of urine.

11. Which processes lead to prerenal azotemia?

These insults account for 50–70% of all cases of acute renal failure and produce decreased renal perfusion pressure, resulting in the constriction of the afferent arterioles. These events decrease glomerular capillary pressure and the formation of the glomerular filtrate. To compensate, the tubules avidly reabsorb salt and water, resulting in oliguria.

Prerenal azotemia results from a depletion in the extracellular fluid volume, decreased cardiac output, or direct renal vasoconstriction. Volume loss can result from dehydration, hemorrhage, over-diuresis, burns, diarrhea, sepsis, or sequestration such as crush injuries or pancreatitis. Cardiac output can drop from cardiomyopathy, arrhythmia, valvular disease, pericardial tamporade, coronary artery disease, or cardiogenic shock. Interestingly, volume overload leading to congestive heart failure will result in decreased renal perfusion as well.

Direct renal vasoconstriction can be precipitated by sepsis, liver disease, and drugs. Reversible prerenal azotemia can be caused by both angiotensin-converting enzyme (ACE) inhibitors and nonsteroidal anti-inflammatory delete agents, add drugs (NSAIDs). ACE inhibitors decrease levels of angiotensin II, resulting in lowered renal perfusion pressure, dilation of the efferent arteriole, and, therefore, lower glomerular capillary filtration pressure. Patients with preexisting renal artery stenosis are particularly susceptible. NSAIDs inhibit the enzyme cyclooxygenase, causing depletion of renal vasodilatory eicosanoids, resulting in afferent arteriolar constriction.

12. Which processes lead to renal azotemia?

These insults account for 20–30% of all cases of acute renal failure, the most common of which is acute tubular necrosis (ATN) (so named for the histopathologic finding of necrotic and regeneration renal tubules with intact basement membranes). Predisposing factors that result in acute tubular necrosis are prolonged prerenal azotemia, nephrotoxic drugs, and pigmenturia. Prolonged prerenal hypoperfusion is the most frequent event. Nephrotoxic drugs such as aminoglycoside antibiotics, iodinated radiographic contrast agents, cisplatinum, amphotericin B, and pentamidine are commonly given to hospitalized patients. Patients with diabetes or myeloma are especially susceptible. Pigmenturia caused by intravascular hemolysis or traumatic rhabdomyolysis can lead to acute tubular necrosis. This can be caused by simply lying too many hours on an operating room table with pressure applied to muscle groups (the flank position).

Others forms of renal azotemia can result from disorders of large and/or small renal blood vessels. These include thrombi, emboli, malignant hypertension, hemolytic uremic syndrome, and various forms of vasculitis. Acute glomerulonephritis and interstitial nephritis due to drug allergy or infection may result in acute renal failure.

13. Which processes lead to postrenal azotemia?

These insults are the least common causes of acute renal failure, accounting for < 10% of all cases. Obstructive uropathy can be caused by any process that blocks the flow of urine from the distal tubules to the end of the urethra. Within the kidney, stone crystals or myeloma proteins can obstruct urine flow. Above the bladder, obstruction to both renal collecting systems or ureters is required. Stones, tumors, clots, fungus balls, sloughed papillae, extrinsic cancerous lesions, fibrosis, or surgical injuries are the more common etiologies. Benign and malignant prostatic disease represent the major causes of obstruction below the bladder. Urethral strictures and phimosis can ultimately result in renal injury if severe.

14. How is the patient with acute renal failure diagnosed?

The most reliable way to distinguish among the various causes of prerenal, renal, and postrenal azotemia is to take a careful history and do a careful physical examination, highlighting recent clinical events and drug administration. Begin with a detailed review of the hospital record, focusing on the reasons for hospitalization and the therapy given. The most recent vital signs, daily weights, and serial intake and output recordings are essential. Bladder catheterization may be required in the anuric patient, and may be diagnostic of lower tract obstruction as well as provide urine for culture and sediment evaluation. Complete anuria is uncommon and usually signifies severe postrenal obstruction or bilateral vascular occlusion.

15. What should one look for in the history?

1. Which drugs, how frequently, and at what doses have they been given?

2. Does the patient describe irritative or obstructive voiding symptoms, hematuria, a history of stones, trauma, or previous episodes of acute renal failure?

3. Has there been a history of cardiac disease or those disorders that cause extracellular fluid volume loss (e.g., diarrhea, vomiting, liver disease, burns)?

4. Has the urinary tract or the abdominal vasculature been instrumented or operated upon?

5. Does the patient have rashes or fevers suggesting allergy?

6. Is there a history of cancer or use of chemotherapy?

The creation of a flow sheet noting timing of renal dysfunction and drugs given may be useful.

16. What should one look for on physical examination?

Prerenal causes may be entertained if volume depletion (negative intake/output or weight loss) is present. An orthostatic drop in blood pressure or rise in heart rate may be a clue. Has the patient exhibited a drop in mean blood pressure since admission? Cardiac dysfunction with signs and symptoms of congestive failure (pulmonary edema, peripheral edema, ventricular gallop, jugular venous distention) can also be suggestive. Flank pain, suprapubic distention, and incontinence can suggest obstructive causes. Harsh abdominal bruits or a palpable aortic aneurysm suggests vascular causes. Skin rashes or ecchymoses suggest vasculitis. In critically ill patients, the insertion of a Swan-Ganz catheter to assess intracardiac pressures may be necessary.

17. Is examination of the urine helpful?

Yes. Pyuria points to an infectious or inflammatory etiology, and hematuria suggests stones, trauma, or urinary tract tumors. Well-formed RBC casts are diagnostic of glomerulonephritis, and specific crystals (e.g., uric acid, cysteine) suggest urinary calculi. A large amount of urinary protein suggests glomerular injury. A urine specific gravity > 1.022 in an oliguric patient implies that the concentrating mechanism is intact.

A spot urine sodium can help to distinguish prerenal azotemia from acute tubular necrosis. In the prerenal state, the kidney avidly retains salt and water to compensate for decreased perfusion. This produces a sodium concentration generally < 30 mEq/L and a fractional sodium excretion $< 1\%$. Injured and regenerating tubules found in acute tubular necrosis are unable to reabsorb salt and water efficiently, resulting in concentrations above these levels. Spot urine chemistries usually are not helpful in cases of postrenal obstruction.

Culture of the urine can be diagnostic in cases of bacterial or fungal infection.

Urine Findings in Acute Renal Failure

CAUSES OF AZOTEMIA	URINE SEDIMENT	FRACTIONAL Na EXCRETION AND Na CONCENTRATION
Prerenal	Rare hyaline casts, usually normal	$<1\%$, <30 mEq/L
Renal		
Tubular necrosis	Tubular epithelial cells granular casts	$>1\%$, >30 mEq/L
Interstitial nephritis	Pyuria with white blood cell casts, eosinophils	Similar to tubular necrosis, nondiagnostic
Glomerulonephritis	Proteinuria, high molecular weight; RBCs and RBC casts	Similar to prerenal, non-diagnostic

(continued)

Urine Findings in Acute Renal Failure (Continued)

CAUSES OF AZOTEMIA	URINE SEDIMENT	FRACTIONAL Na EXCRETION AND Na CONCENTRATION
Vascular disorders	RBCs may be present	Similar to prerenal, non-diagnostic
Postrenal		
Stones	Crystals, fragments, hematuria, pyuria	Nondiagnostic
Tumors	Malignant cytology	Early disease may be similar to prerenal
Extrinsic compression	May be normal	Late disease may be similar to postrenal

18. Are blood tests helpful in making the diagnosis?

The hemogram can provide supportive information. Leukocytosis may be present in septic patients, and eosinophilia suggests an allergic interstitial disease. Abnormal RBC morphology and hemolysis can point to the hemolytic uremic syndrome (HUS). Low platelet counts suggest HUS or thrombotic thrombocytopenic purpura (TTP). Sickled RBCs are pathognomonic for sickle cell disease.

19. When are radiographic tests helpful?

If diminished renal perfusion is suspected, an **isotopic renal scan** can document the presence of renal blood flow as well as differences between the two kidneys. If more specific anatomic information is required, a **renal arteriogram** and/or a **renal venogram** will precisely define, e.g., stenoses, occluded segments, aneurysms of the renal vasculature. In cases where postrenal obstruction is suspected, an **excretory urogram** or an **ultrasound** examination of the kidneys is useful. Most cases of hydronephrosis can be determined by such tests. However, when the creatinine is elevated above 2.5 mg/dl, contrast agents can cause renal injury and retrograde contrast studies are required. More definitive anatomic information can be provided by a CT scan or MRI examination of the abdomen and pelvis. Recently, magnetic resonance angiography, with the use of gadolinium in lieu of iodinated contrast, has provided excellent delineation of the renal vasculature.

20. Is any one test more reliable in determining the cause of acute renal failure?

No. The history and physical examination should direct the clinician to one of several possibilities. If other methods are nondiagnostic, the renal biopsy (either percutaneous or open) can provide definitive information as to vascular, tubular, or glomerular pathology.

21. How is acute renal failure treated?

The key to effective treatment is making the correct diagnosis. Removal of an offending drug, restoring euvolemia, normalizing cardiac performance, and relieving obstruction are essential remedies. Nonoliguric renal failure is easier to manage than oliguric renal failure. Therefore, diuretics may be helpful. Ensuring adequate nutrition is also helpful. Other abnormalities such as hyperkalemia, hyperphosphatemia, acidosis, and anemia should also be corrected. Some have suggested that low doses of dopamine may improve renal perfusion. When obstruction cannot be promptly relieved, a percutaneous nephrostomy tube can temporarily relieve more distal obstruction and restore metabolic imbalance. Ultimately, if acute renal failure is severe and causing systemic metabolic toxicity, temporary renal replacement therapy with hemodialysis or peritoneal dialysis will be required.

22. How can acute renal failure be prevented?

This may not always be possible. However, certain measures can diminish renal injury if instituted promptly. Dehydration, especially in the elderly, is a universal problem. Replacement of fluids in cases of burns, trauma, surgery, lymphatic loss, and infection is essential. Likewise, inducing a diuresis with loop diuretics, volume expansion, and mannitol can be helpful in cases of pigmenturia, contrast agents, myeloma, crystalluria, and nephrotoxins. The use of known nephrotoxic drugs should be monitored with dose adjustments made as indicated by the level of renal function. Nephrotoxic agents should be avoided if possible in high-risk patients.

Risk Factors for Acute Renal Failure

1. Renal Hypoperfusion
   a. Volume depletion
   b. Low cardiac output states
   c. Systemic vasodilation
   d. Sepsis
2. Advanced age
3. Chronic diseases
   a. Cardiac diseases
   b. Renal insufficiency
   c. Liver disease
   d. Hypertension
   e. Peripheral vascular disease
   f. Diabetes mellitus
4. Exposure to multiple, potentially nephrotoxic drugs

BIBLIOGRAPHY

1. Davidman M, et al: Iatrogenic renal disease. Arch Intern Med 151:1809–1810, 1991.
2. Gurwitz JH, et al: Nonsteroidal anti-inflammatory drug associated azotemia in the very old. JAMA 264:471–473, 1990.
3. Hou SH, et al: Hospital acquired acute renal insufficiency: A prospective study. Am J Med 74:242–245, 1983.
4. Kaufman J, et al: Community acquired acute renal failure. Am J Kidney Dis 17:191–194, 1991.
5. Kaloyanides G: Acute renal failure. In Suki WN, Massay SG (eds): Therapy of Renal, Disease and Related Donors, 3rd ed. Boston, Kluwer Academic, 1998, pp 359–386.
6. Shusterman N, et al: Risk factors and outcome of hospital acquired acute renal failure. Am J Med 83: 65–68, 1987.
7. Piccinni P, Lieta E, Marafon S: Risk factors for **acute** renal failure in the intensive care unit. Contrib Nephrol 132:22–25, 2001.
8. Porter GA: Effects of contrast agents on renal function. Invest Radiol 28:51–55, 1993.
9. Perazella MA: **Acute** renal failure in HIV-infected patients: A brief review of common causes. Am J Med Sci. 319:385–391, 2000.
10. Sheridan AM, Bonventre JV: Pathophysiology of ischemic acute renal failure. Contrib Nephrol 132: 7–21, 2001.
11. Block CA. Manning HL: Prevention of acute renal failure the critically ill. Am J Resp Crit Care Med. 165:320–324, 2002.
12. Weldon BC, Monk TG: The patient at risk for **acute** renal failure. Recognition, prevention, and preoperative optimization. Anesth Clin North Am 18:705–717, 2000.
13. Pozzi Mucelli R, Bertolotto M, Quaia E: Imaging techniques in **acute** renal failure. Contrib Nephrol 132:76–91, 2001.
14. Albright RC Jr: **Acute** renal failure: A practical update. Mayo Clin Proc 76:67–74, 2001.

13. EVALUATION OF HYDRONEPHROSIS IN CHILDREN

Robert Kay, M.D.

1. Is hydronephrosis the same as upper tract obstruction?

No. Hydronephrosis, which is the dilatation of the urinary tract, may be seen with obstruction, vesicoureteric reflux, or nonobstructive uropathy such as megacalycosis.

2. In children, hydronephrosis is best detected by what test?

Without question, **screening ultrasound** is the best test to anatomically define the kidney. It is noninvasive, inexpensive, very accurate, and involves no radiation in determining the presence or absence of hydronephrosis. Other tests such as CT scan or MRI may detect hydronephrosis— even a bone scan done for different reasons may suggest hydronephrosis.

3. Can ultrasound determine the level of obstruction?

An experienced ultrasonographer can determine the level of obstruction. The presence of a dilated ureter suggests lower urinary tract obstruction. Conversely, if no ureter is seen, it is unlikely that the obstruction is beyond the ureteropelvic junction. Other tests, such as a renal scan or retrograde pyelogram, may be needed to confirm the initial suspicion.

4. How is a retrograde or antegrade pyelogram helpful in evaluating obstruction?

A retrograde or an antegrade pyelogram is the most definitive method to define the level of obstruction. In many cases, particularly in small infants, the combination of ultrasound and renal scan or an intravenous pyelogram may define the level of obstruction, obviating the need for invasive instrumentation. The disadvantage of a retrograde pyelogram, particularly in neonatal males, is urethral manipulation and the possibility of urethral injury. An antegrade pyelogram may be helpful in neonate males or in other unique situations where further radiologic delineation is needed, but it is an invasive procedure.

5. What is the best way to determine if obstruction is present?

If a cystogram has ruled out reflux, a provocative test may be used to assess the functional status of the kidney. If urine transport is impeded, then obstruction is present. This may be diagnosed by subjecting the kidney to an extreme diuresis and then examining the response by a diuretic renal scan or a diuretic intravenous pyelogram. The obstructed kidney also may be tested by a pressure perfusion test (Whitaker test) in which the collecting system of the kidney is percutaneously accessed and fluid is infused at constant rates and pelvic pressures are measured. An increase in pressure suggests the pressure of obstruction to the collecting system.

6. What is the normal washout in a kidney during a diuretic renal scan?

A normal kidney has a characteristic pattern in which there is initially an increase of the renal isotope as the kidney excretes the isotope into the collecting system followed by rapid clearance of the isotope. When measuring the clearance, the half-life of the renal isotope should be less than 10–15 minutes. If the half-life is greater than 20 minutes, obstruction is likely. Of course, these results must be correlated to the clinical state and other studies.

7. Can false-positive test results occur in the diuretic renal scan?

False-positive results may be seen due to either functional or technical reasons. If renal function is poor and cannot respond to a diuresis, a washout curve may not be seen. Technical factors include timing of administration of the diuretic and (material deleted -a full bladder and other) bladder abnormalities. The bladder needs to be catheterized to remove it as an interfering factor in analyzing the results of the study.

8. What leads to false-negative test results in the diuretic renal scan?

The test may be read as normal if the cursor is not over the area of concern. For example, if distal obstruction is present, the pelvis may appear to clear, but the ureter may be the problem and it needs to be monitored. Also, the test needs to be interpreted carefully in solitary kidneys and neonates.

9. Why was the pressure perfusion test developed?

Originally, the test was created to distinguish obstructed ureters from nonobstructed ureters in posterior urethral valve patients. Some patients with severe posterior urethral valves have severe hydroureteronephrosis which may persist following the ablation of the valves. The test was described by Whitaker in 1973 to confirm his hypothesis that most of these urinary systems were dilated but not obstructed.

10. What is the normal pressure of the urinary system?

Most kidneys have a pressure of 7 cm H_2O or less. The range of normal is up to 15 cm H_2O with perfusion.

11. At what perfusion rate is the Whitaker test done?

To stress the system to superphysiologic levels, a rate of at least 10 ml/min is used.

12. Obstruction is indicated by what pressure?

Intrarenal pressures > 22 cm H_2O are felt to represent obstruction. This is a subtracted pressure, with the bladder pressure eliminated.

13. Are other tests used in assessing the functional state of obstruction?

Real-time ultrasonography and color-flow Doppler with calculated vascular resistance.

14. If in utero hydronephrosis is noted, when should the kidney be evaluated?

A baby with in utero hydronephrosis should have an ultrasound on day 1 or 2. However, caution must be used in interpretation. Physiologic dilatation, rehydration, and a low urinary output secondary to low levels of neonatal glomerular filtration rate may give erroneous results. If the child is not seriously ill or if there is no evidence of urethral valves, the infant should be placed on prophylactic antibiotics and a repeat sonogram done at 1 month of age. At this time, the glomerular filtration rate will have reached normal levels, dehydration will have resolved, and the physiologic dilatation of the neonate may have disappeared. If hydronephrosis is still present, further evaluation with a voiding cystourethrogram and renal scan should be done.

15. What size of the renal pelvis in the newborn is considered abnormal?

The renal pelvis greater than 12 mm is usually indicative of significant dilatation and probable abnormalities.

BIBLIOGRAPHY

1. Chung S, Majd M, Rushton HG, Belman AB: Diuretic renography in the evaluation of neonatal hydronephrosis: Is it reliable? J Urol 150:765, 1993.
2. Dejter SW, Gibbons MD: The fate of infant kidneys with fetal hydronephrosis but initially normal postnatal sonography. J Urol 142:661, 1989.
3. Garcia-Pena BM, Keller MS, Schwartz DS, et al: The ultrasonographic differentiation of obstructive versus nonobstructive hydronephrosis in children: A multivariate scoring system. J Urol 158:560–565, 1997.

4. Homsy YL, Saad F, Laberge I, et al: Transitional hydronephrosis of the newborn and infant. J Urol 144: 579, 1990.
5. Kass EJ, Majd M, Belman AB: Comparison of the diuretic renogram and the pressure perfusion study in children. J Urol 134:92, 1985.
6. Koff SA, Thrall JH, Keyes JW: Diuretic radio-nuclei urography: A non-invasive method for evaluating nephroureteral obstruction. J Urol 122:451, 1979.
7. O'Reilly PH: Investigation of obstructive uropathy. In O'Reilly PH, George NJ, Weiss RM (eds): Diagnostic Techniques in Urology. Philadelphia, W. B. Saunders, 1990.
8. O'Reilly P, Aurell M, Britton K, et al: Consensus on diuresis renography for investigating the dilated upper urinary tract. Radionuclides in Nephrourology Group. Consensus Committee on Diuresis Renography. J Nucl Med 37:1772–1776, 1996.
9. Palmer JM, Lindfords KK, Ordorica RC, Marder DM: Diuretic Doppler sonography in postnatal hydronephrosis. J Urol 146;605, 1991.
10. Ross JH, Kay R, Knipper N, Streem SB: The absence of crossing vessels in association with ureteropelvic junction obstruction detected by prenatal ultrasonography. J Urol 160:973–975, 1998.
11. Ulman I, Jayanthi VR, Koff SA: The long term follow-up of newborns with severe unilateral hydronephrosis initially treated nonoperatively. J Urol 164:1101–1105, 2000.
12. Weiss RM: Obstructive uropathy: Pathophysiology and diagnosis. In Kelalis PP, King LR, Belman AB (eds): Clinical Pediatric Urology, 3rd ed. Philadelphia, W. B. Saunders, 1992, pp 664–682.
13. Whitaker RH: Methods of assessing obstruction in dilated ureters. Br J Urol 45:15, 1973.

14. IMPOTENCE

Drogo K. Montague, M.D. and Milton M. Lakin, M.D.

1. What is impotence?

Impotence (the preferred term is erectile dysfunction or ED) is the persistent inability to obtain or maintain a penile erection adequate for coitus.

2. How common is erectile dysfunction?

Material deleted: Erectile dysfunction affects approximately 20 million men in the United States. New material: Some degree of erectile dysfunction (mild, moderate, and severe combined) is present in more than 50% of men between the ages of 40 and 70.

3. Describe two types of erectile dysfunction.

Psychogenic erectile dysfunction occurs primarily for psychological reasons. **Organic erectile dysfunction** is secondary to organic disease. Whereas erectile dysfunction may be exclusively psychogenic in origin, organic erectile dysfunction is often associated with varying degrees of psychological factors.

4. How do the relative frequencies of psychogenic and organic erectile dysfunction vary with age?

The incidence of erectile dysfunction is relatively low in young men but progressively increases with age. In men under age 35, psychogenic erectile dysfunction is probably more common than organic erectile dysfunction. In contrast, in men over age 50, erectile dysfunction is more likely to be organic rather than psychogenic.

5. What are the organic causes of erectile dysfunction?

The term **IMPOTENCE** itself is a useful mnemonic*:

	Examples
I = Inflammatory	Prostatitis
M = Mechanical	Peyronie's disease
P = Postsurgical	Radical prostatectomy
O = Occlusive vascular	Atherosclerosis
T = Traumatic	Pelvic fracture
E = Endurance factors	Chronic renal failure
N = Neurogenic	Multiple sclerosis
C = Chemicals	Antihypertensive drugs
E = Endocrine	Diabetes mellitus

*Modified from Smith AD: Urol Clin North Am 8:83, 1981.

6. List the ten elements in the evaluation of a man with erectile dysfunction.

1. Sexual history
2. Medical history
3. Psychological evaluation
4. Physical examination
5. Blood studies
6. Nocturnal penile tumescence
7. Duplex ultrasonography
8. Cavernosometry
9. Cavernosography
10. Penile arteriography

7. Are any conditions likely to be confused with erectile dysfunction?

Men with premature ejaculation or hypoactive sexual desire (low libido) may be mistakenly thought to have problems obtaining or maintaining erections.

8. What is nocturnal penile tumescence (NPT)?

NPT is a test to help differentiate psychogenic from organic erectile dysfunction. Because penile rigidity and not just tumescence is required for coitus, NPT testing should record both penile tumescence and rigidity. With some exceptions, NPT in men with psychogenic erectile dysfunction is normal, whereas in men with organic erectile dysfunction, it is either absent or impaired.

9. How are vasoactive drugs used in the diagnostic evaluation of erectile dysfunction?

Vasoactive drugs such as papaverine, phentolamine, or prostaglandin E_1 promote cavernosal arterial dilatation and cavernosal smooth muscle relaxation. These drugs are injected into the penile corpora cavernosa at the time of duplex ultrasonography, cavernosometry, cavernosography, and penile arteriography to evaluate the arterial and veno-occlusive components of erectile function.

10. How is duplex ultrasonography used in the diagnostic evaluation of erectile dysfunction?

Duplex ultrasonography is used to evaluate the cavernosal arteries and thus the arterial inflow into the corpora cavernosa of the penis. After the intracavernosal injection of vasoactive drugs, a duplex ultrasound scanner images the cavernosal arteries and determines the velocity of blood flow through these vessels.

11. What are cavernosometry and cavernosography?

These tests also are performed after intracavernosal injection of vasoactive drug to evaluate the veno-occlusive mechanisms of the corpora cavernosa. Cavernosometry measures intracavernosal pressures while saline flow rates needed to obtain and maintain full erection are determined. In cavernosography, contrast is infused into the corpora cavernosa, and radiographic imaging is performed to document pathways of any venous leakage from the corpora.

12. List the treatments for erectile dysfunction.

1. Sex therapy	6. Penile prosthesis implantation
2. Medical therapy	7. Arterial revascularization
3. Vacuum erection devices	8. Penile venous ligation
4. Intracavernosal injection therapy	9. Combined therapy
5. Intraurethral pharmacotherapy	

13. What is sex therapy?

Sex therapy, which is most commonly used to treat psychogenic erectile dysfunction, involves treatment, whenever possible, for both the man and his sexual partner. Couple education and behavioral therapy are used in an attempt to reestablish normal sexual function.

14. How is medical therapy used in the treatment of erectile dysfunction?

1. **Withdrawal of offending medication.** When the onset of erectile dysfunction is associated with the administration of a new medication, it is appropriate, whenever possible, to select another drug with less potential to affect erectile function.

2. **Hormonal therapy.** Men with hypogonadism and erectile dysfunction may benefit from parenteral testosterone administration. Men with erectile dysfunction and hyperprolactinemia can usually be treated successfully with the oral medication bromocriptine. Significant hypogonadism or hyperprolactinemia in men with erectile dysfunction is, however, rather infrequent.

3. **Oral phosphodiesterase inhibitors.** Sildenafil citrate (Viagra) is a type 5 oral phosphodiesterase inhibitor that has proven effective in 30–80% of men with erectile dysfunction of diverse etiologies. Unlike other treatments for erectile dysfunction, sildenafil citrate administration does not produce an erection. Instead, when effective, it improves the quality and increases the duration of erections produced by sexual stimulation. This medication has no direct effect on li-

bido, orgasm, or ejaculation. The only contraindication to its use is men taking either short- or long-acting nitrates for coronary artery disease.

15. Describe how vacuum erection devices are used to treat erectile dysfunction.

Vacuum erection devices have three parts: an acrylic chamber that fits over the penis, a vacuum pump attached to this chamber, and an elastic constriction ring applied to the base of the chamber. The patient applies a water-soluble lubricant to his penis and to the inside of the opening to the chamber. He inserts his penis into the chamber and presses the chamber base against his body to create a tight seal. The pump is then used to create a vacuum inside the chamber, which results in an erection-like state. The constriction ring is transferred from the outside of the device to the base of the penis (to maintain the erection), the chamber is removed, and the patient has coitus.

16. What is intracavernosal injection therapy?

The injection of vasoactive drugs (papaverine, phentolamine, and prostaglandin E_1) is useful not only for the diagnosis of erectile dysfunction but also for its treatment. Men using this treatment are taught to inject these drugs into the corpora prior to coitus.

17. What is intraurethral pharmacotherapy?

Alprostadil, in the form of small suppository (MUSE), is placed in the distal urethra using an applicator system. Absorption is from the urethra directly into the corporeal bodies; thus, the medication is delivered directly to the erection chambers, eliminating the need for injection. Transfer of medication from the urethra to the corporeal bodies, however, is not as efficient as it is with injection therapy, making this a less effective therapy.

18. What is a penile prosthesis?

Penile prostheses are devices that are surgically implanted into the corpora to produce an erection-like state. The two types of penile prostheses are:

1. **Nonhydraulic penile prostheses** are paired rod-like devices that are implanted into the corpora cavernosa to create a permanent penile rigidity, which enables the recipient to have coitus.

2. **Hydraulic (inflatable) penile prostheses** consist of paired penile cylinders, a pump, and a fluid reservoir. An erection is created by pumping fluid from the reservoir to the cylinders. Penile flaccidity is achieved by activating a release mechanism that returns cylinder fluid to the reservoir.

19. How successful is penile arterial revascularization?

Various procedures have been developed to treat erectile dysfunction secondary to arterial insufficiency. In young men with traumatic arterial occlusion, the procedures are successful in approximately 70% of cases. In older men with atherosclerotic arterial disease, they are much less successful and seldom performed.

20. How successful is penile venous ligation surgery?

Penile venous ligation surgery was formerly used to treat erectile dysfunction resulting from impairment of the corporeal-venous occlusive mechanism. Short-term (1–3 years) success rates generally ranged from 50–60%; however, recurrent erectile dysfunction commonly occurred in a relatively short time after surgery, and such procedures, for the most part, are no longer being performed.

21. What is combined therapy?

Combined sex therapy and medical or surgical treatment of organic erectile dysfunction. By using couple sex therapy to provide education and reduce performance anxiety while medical or surgical treatment is used to correct or compensate for organic factors, it is often possible to achieve optimal treatment results.

BIBLIOGRAPHY

1. Carson CC: Implantation of semi-rigid rod penile prostheses. Urol Clin North Am 1:61–70, 1993.
2. Feldman HA, Goldstein I, Hatzichristou DG, Krane RJ, McKinlay JB: Impotence and its medical and psychological correlates: Results of the Massachusetts Male Aging Study. J Urol 151:54–61, 1994.
3. Fuchs AM, Mehringer CM, Rajfer J: Anatomy of penile venous drainage in potent and impotent men during cavernosography. J Urol 141:1353–1365, 1989.
4. Goldstein I, Lue TF, Padma-Nathan H, et al, for the Sildenafil Study Group: Oral sildenafil in the treatment of erectile dysfunction. N Engl J Med 338:1397–1404, 1998.
5. Hatzichristou D, Goldstein I: Penile microvascular arterial bypass surgery. Atlas Urol Clinic North Am 1:39–60, 1993.
6. Jarow JP, Pugh VW, Routh WD, Dyer RB: Comparison of penile duplex ultrasonography to pudendal arteriography. Invest Radiol 28:806–810, 1993.
7. Lakin MM, Montague DK: Surgical treatment of the patient with erectile dysfunction: Clinical evaluation and diagnostic techniques. Atlas Urol Clin North Am 1:9–19, 1993.
8. Lakin MM, Montague DK, Vanderbrug-Medendorp S, et al: Intracavernous injection therapy: Analysis of results and complications. J Urol 143:1138–1141, 1990.
9. Lewis RW: Venous surgery in the patient with erectile dysfunction. Atlas Urol Clin North Am 1:21–38, 1993.
10. Lowe MA, Schwartz AN, Berger RE: Controlled trial of infusion cavernosometry in impotent and potent men. J Urol 146:758–783, 1991.
11. Morale A, Condra M, Reid K: The role of nocturnal penile tumescence monitoring in the diagnosis of impotence: A review. J Urol 143:441–445, 1990.
12. Mulcahy JJ: Implantation of hydraulic penile prostheses. Atlas Urol Clin North Am 1:71–92, 1993.
13. Padma-Nathan H, Hellstrom WJG, Kaiser FE, et al, for the Medicated Urethral System for Erection (MUSE) Study Group: Treatment of men with erectile dysfunction with transurethral alprostadil. N Engl J Med 336:1–7, 1997.
14. Salvatore FT, Sharman GM, Hellstrom WJG: Vacuum constriction devices and the clinical urologist: An informed selection. Urology 38:323–327, 1991.
15. Virag R, Shoukry K, Floresco J, et al: Intracavernous self-injection of vasoactive drugs in the treatment of impotence: Eight-year experience in 615 cases. J Urol 145:287–293, 1991.

15. INFERTILITY

Allen D. Seftel, M.D.

1. Define infertility.
Infertility is the inability of a couple to conceive after 1 year of unprotected intercourse.

2. Which partner usually is the cause of the infertility?
Roughly 50% of infertility is due to male factor problems and roughly 50% to female issues.

3. What is the normal semen analysis?
The semen analysis is usually the first objective test sought to evaluate the male partner of the infertile couple. The semen analysis is the cornerstone of the evaluation of the infertile male. Recently, data have been put forward that define the "subfertile male." Subfertility is defined as follows: A sperm concentration of less than 13.5 times 10^6 (13.5 million sperm) per mL of semen, motility less than 32% of the sperm, and less than 9% of sperm with normal morphology (Kruger).

4. What are the causes of subfertility in the male?
Male factor infertility can be divided up into several categories. The most common identifiable cause of male factor infertility is the **varicocele**. Although present in approximately 15% of the total population, the varicocele is found in approximately 40% of infertile men. Other causes of male factor infertility include **nonobstructive azoospermia.** This is most often due to testicular failure, wherein the male has either sertoli-only syndrome (germ cell aplasia) or maturation arrest, in which spermatogonia are present but do not fully mature. **Obstructive azoospermia** implies obstruction to the egress of mature sperm from the testicle to the external urethral meatus. Congenital absence of the vas deferens (seen in virtually all cases of cystic fibrosis; also associated with the heterozygous form of cystic fibrosis, wherein the patient is heterozygous for the cystic fibrosis mutation) is a congenital cause as well. Acquired causes are usually noted to be obstruction of the vas deferens at the level of the epididymis due to infection, or obstruction at the level of the ejaculatory ducts due to a prostatic cyst. A low sperm count is known as **oligospermia;** poor motility of sperm is known as **asthenospermia;** and poor morphology may exist as well. Low count, motility, or morphology may exist individually or in combination. **Low semen volume** is also a possible cause of male factor infertility. **Prostatitis,** an infection of inflammation of the prostate, or various **ejaculatory problems** can be the causes of infertility in the male as well.

5. What is a varicocele?
A varicocele is a dilated vein or set of veins in the pampiniform plexus in the spermatic cord.

6. How does a varicocele cause infertility?
It is believed that the varicocele does not permit efficient blood flow out of the scrotum. Testicles that sit in the scrotum are approximately 2°C below body temperature and depend on an efficient inflow and outflow system to maintain that temperature. Just as in an automobile's cooling system, the coolant must circulate to maintain the temperature and prevent overheating. If there is stagnation of blood due to an inefficient mechanism (e.g., varicose vein), then there may be pooling of blood, an increase in temperature, and an adverse effect on spermatogenesis.

Specifically, the varicocele most commonly causes a "stress" pattern on semen analysis, characterized by a low sperm count (20,000,000 sperm/mL), low sperm motility (50% motile sperm), and a low sperm morphology (15% normal forms using strict criteria developed by Kruger et al.).

7. Are there common characteristics of men with varicoceles?

Most frequently, varicoceles are asymptomatic. On occasion, a varicocele can be painful or can present as a heaviness or fullness in the scrotal area. A large and easily identified varicocele by visual inspection in called grade 3. Grade 2 varicoceles are appreciated by physical examination, but may not be identified by visual inspection. Grade 1 varicoceles, often referred to as subclinical varicoceles, are not readily identifiable by visual inspection but are seen during physical examination.

8. How does one identify a varicocele?

Examine the patient in a warm room in the standing position. Grade 3 varicoceles are easily identifiable. Grade 1 and 2 varicoceles are identified by placing your right hand on the patient's left spermatic cord and asking the patient to perform a Valsalva maneuver. With the increased abdominal pressure, there may be a rush of blood through this venous plexus (a grade 2 vericocele). If this rush of blood is not felt, then an office Doppler can be used to detect the rush of blood. If the rush of blood is heard only with the Doppler, then it is a grade 1 varicocele. A similar procedure is carried out on the right.

9. Are varicoceles unilateral or bilateral?

Historically, varicoceles have been thought to occur most commonly on the left side. However, now they are often found to be bilateral. An exclusively right-sided varicocele is unusual. The new onset of a varicocele mandates evaluation of the kidneys because this may be the first presenting sign of a kidney tumor.

10. How is a varicocele managed?

Historically, they have been repaired surgically by various approaches.

1. **Inguinal approach.** The inguinal canal is opened similar to a hernia repair, and the varicose veins are ligated or excised in that portion of the inguinal canal.

2. **Retroperitoneal approach.** An incision is made near the anterior superior iliac spine, the muscles are retracted, and the veins are ligated as they exit the internal ring.

3. **Subinguinal approach.** A small incision is made inferior to the external ring and the veins are ligated at that site.

4. **Laparoscopic approach.** Through laparoscopic techniques, the veins are ligated high in the retroperitoneum.

5. **Interventional radiologic approach.** In a minimally invasive technique, the veins are embolized by access through the femoral vein, the vein is cannulated in the retrograde fashion, and then it is embolized by either coils or other embolization material.

11. How successful is varicocele ligation?

Approximately 95% of surgical cases are successful, meaning that varicocele does not recur. Seventy percent of men who have a successful repair will have an improvement in sperm parameters and usually a marked increase in sperm count and sperm motility. There is controversy as to whether correlation of a varicocele will correct the morphology.

12. What are the other common causes of male factor infertility?

Obstructive azoopsermia is blockage of egress of sperm from the testis to the outside world. If congenital, then aspiration of sperm from either the testicle or the epididymis is required. These sperm are then used in conjunction with in vitro fertilization for pregnancy. Oligospermia and low motility or morphology, not associated with a varicocele, are often congenital issues. Occasionally, partial obstruction of the vas deferens may cause the abnormalities.

OTHER POTENTIAL CAUSES

Hypogonadotropic hypogonadism is a deficiency of the luteinizing (LH) and follicle-stimulating hormones (FSH), which are important in testosterone and sperm production, respectively.

This disorder is manifested by low LH, FSH, and serum testosterone levels. These patients may have severely low sperm counts or may be totally azoospermic.

Uncommon causes of male factor infertility include occupational exposure or other medical syndromes such as Noonan's or Klinefelter's syndrome.

Genetic causes have recently gained attention as possible causes of male factor infertility; examination of the Y chromosome is of particular interest.

13. What are the causes of obstructive azoospermia?

Obstructive azoospermia can be congenital or acquired. Acquired causes include epididymitis or occur post vasectomy. Congenital causes include congenital absence of the vas deferens in which sperm production is normal but egress of sperm to the outside world is blocked. In many cases, the male is a carrier for one of the cystic fibrosis gene mutations. The male is not homozygous, in which case he would not have the fulminant form of cystic fibrosis. In cases of cystic fibrosis, the male usually does have the fulminant form of cystic fibrosis. Men with cystic fibrosis do have absent vasa. However, sperm production is normal in such individuals. Nonetheless, genetic counseling is clearly indicated: All children will be carriers and if the female partner is a carrier, there is a significant possibility of passing along fulminant cystic fibrosis to the children. The causes of severe oligospermia as well as nonobstructive azoospermia most likely have a genetic basis.

14. How are these men treated?

Treatment of men with hormonal disorders is usually hormonal replacement therapy. Men with obstructive azoospermia can either undergo microscopic testicular, epididymal, or vasal sperm aspiration, or, if a previous vasectomy has been done, or there is evidence of epididymal obstruction, undergo vasovasostomy (vas reconstruction). Patients with nonobstructive azoospermia or severe oligospermia also can undergo testicular biopsy and sperm extraction or epididymal sperm extraction and achieve fertilization via in vitro fertilization combined with intracytoplasmic sperm injection. Genetic counseling is clearly indicated in men with congenital absence of the vas deferens who may have one or more of the cystic fibrosis gene mutations. A man with nonobstructive azoospermia may have mutations of the Y chromosome and other chromosomes as well.

15. Does testicular cancer cause infertility?

Men who have testicular cancer who undergo radiation therapy to the abdomen after orchiectomy or retroperitoneal lymph node resection or who have chemotherapy for their malignancy may have impairment of sperm production as a consequence. It is imperative that men with testicular cancer bank sperm prior to the orchiectomy and other adjuvant therapies. In addition, these men may be subfertile before therapy.

16. Can any infectious diseases cause infertility?

Prostatitis and other urinary tract infections may predispose to male factor infertility by unknown mechanisms. Treating the prostatitis may result in pregnancy. Other systemic infectious diseases, such as tuberculosis, may cause vasal or epididymal obstruction.

17. What systemic diseases affect fertility?

Leukemia and lymphomas may involve testicular tissue and be associated with male factor infertility. Any type of chemotherapy given systemically for any malignancy may impair spermatogenesis. Thus, any young man facing chemotherapy should be counseled about banking sperm for future use.

18. What is the cardinal sign of testicular failure?

The FSH is usually elevated 1–2 and often 3 times above normal. On examination, the patient usually has smaller than normal testicles, or less commonly, overtly small testicles. Some of

the newer techniques are able to find sperm on rare occasions in men with nonobstructive azoospermia, and many men are now undergoing testis biopsy looking for pockets of sperm. The
sperm is then used in conjunction with cytoplasmic sperm injection for pregnancy.

19. How does the physician treat ejaculatory failure?

Most commonly, this is due to either spinal cord injury or diabetes. In such cases one can try
vibratory ejaculation, in which a small hand-held vibration device is placed again the glans penis
and a sperm sample is obtained and used for either intrauterine insemination or in vitro fertilization. If this is not successful, an electroejaculation procedure is performed in which a probe is
placed into the rectum and current is generated allowing for semen to be produced and used to get
a sperm specimen. In men with ejaculatory failure due to medicines known to inhibit ejaculation,
such as many antidepressants, the initial goal is to try to remove the offending agent, which in
many cases is not possible because of the underlying primary pathology, such as depression.
Rarely, ejaculatory failure can be psychogenic, and a session with a sex therapist is often helpful.
Electroejaculation can be used in refractory cases.

20. How is retrograde ejaculation treated?

Retrograde ejaculation means that sperm, instead of being propulsed outside the body, head
back into the bladder because the bladder neck is not closing properly. This is due to spinal cord
injury, diabetes, or previous surgery on the bladder neck. In such cases the initial goal is to restore closure of the bladder neck by using an oral adrenergic drug such as pseudofed. If this is not
successful, the patient is asked to ejaculate. The first voided sample after ejaculation, which contains the retrograde ejaculated sperm, is processed for either intrauterine insemination or in vitro
fertilization.

21. How is low semen volume treated?

If an isolated abnormality, without any prostatic obstruction, usually the couple will undergo
intrauterine insemination with the male partner's sperm, after a series of preparatory washes to
remove any impurities. If there is a blockage at the level of the prostate, then transurethral resection of the prostatic utricle or cyst is warranted.

22. Are there other causes of male factor infertility?

Certainly there are many environmental and work-related toxins that may contribute to male
factor infertility. Often is quite difficult to have people change careers or remove themselves from
environmental exposure. This is especially true for professional young men who have devoted a
significant amount of time and energy toward establishing themselves in their careers.

23. Are there any future issues concerning male factor infertility?

Recent evidence shows that sperm counts are declining universally. Although controversial,
it is thought that this may be due to the widespread use of contraceptives and estrogens in American society. This is a subject of great debate.

Other issues of concern include the fact that many men are now taking steroid supplements
and other vitamin supplements that may contain steroids, which have a negative impact on sperm
production. Thus, it is important to ask patients about medications to determine if any of them may
affect fertility. Finally, reproductive technologies may predispose to low-birth-weight infants,
given greater impetus to finding better and more effective therapies for male factor infertility.

BIBLIOGRAPHY

1. Anguiano A, Oates RD, Amos JA: Congenital bilateral absence of the vas deferens: A primarily genital
   form of cystic fibrosis. JAMA 267:1994–1997, 1994.
2. Lipschultz LI (ed): Male infertility. Urol Clin North Am 21(3):1994.
3. Lipschultz LI, Howards SS (eds): Infertility in the Male. New York, Churchill Livingstone, 1991.

4. Palermo GD, Colombero LT, Hariprashad JJ, et al: Chromosome analysis of epididymal and testicular sperm in azoospermic patients undergoing ICSI. Hum Reprod 17:570–575, 2002.
5. Pryor JL, Kent-First M, Muallem A, Van Bergen AH, Nolten WE, Meisner L, Roberts KP: Microdeletions in the Y chromosome of infertile men. N Engl J Med 336:534–539, 1997.
6. Lynn A, Koehler KE, Judis L, Chan ER, Cherry JP, Schwartz S, Seftel A, Hunt PA, Hassold TJ: Covariation of synaptonemal complex length and mammalian meiotic exchange rates. Science 296:2222–2225, 2002.
7. Sharlip ID, Jarow JP, Belker AM, Lipshultz LI, Sigman M, Thomas AJ, Schlegel PN, Howards SS, Nehra A, Damewood MD, Overstreet JW, Sadovsky R: Best practice policies for male infertility. Fertil Steril 77:873–882, 2002.
8. Guzik DS, Overstreet JW: Sperm morphology, motility and concentration in fertile and non fertile men N Engl J Med 345:1388–1393, 2001.
9. Schieve LA, Meikle SF, Ferre C, Peterson HB, Jeng G, Wilcox LS: Low and very low birth weight in infants conceived with use of assisted reproductive technology. N Engl J Med 346:731–737, 2002.
10. Schoor RA, Elhanbly SM, Niederberger C: The pathophysiology of varicocele-associated male infertility. Curr Urol Rep 2:432–436, 2001.
11. Pavlovich CP, King P, Goldstein M, Schlegel PN: Evidence of a treatable endocrinopathy in infertile men. J Urol 165:837–841, 2001.
12. Goldstein M, Li PS, Matthews GJ: Microsurgical vasovasostomy: The microdot technique of precision suture placement. J Urol 159:188–190, 1998.

16. NEUROGENIC BLADDER

Donald R. Bodner, M.D.

1. What is the role of the autonomic nervous system in micturition?

The autonomic nervous system consists of the parasympathetic and sympathetic nervous systems. The parasympathetic innervation to the bladder originates in the S2–S4 nerve roots and travels via the pelvic nerve or nervi erigentes. These nerve fibers stimulate the cholinergic fibers in the bladder and are responsible for bladder contraction, which produces bladder emptying. The sympathetic innervation to the bladder originates in the thoracolumbar portion of the spinal cord (T10–L2) and richly supplies the bladder neck and proximal urethra. Stimulation of the sympathetic nervous system causes contraction of the alpha fibers in the bladder neck, which closes the bladder neck and relaxes the bladder body, resulting in urinary storage.

2. What is the role of the somatic nervous system in micturition?

The somatic nervous sytem provides voluntary control to the striated muscle of the external urinary sphincter. Voluntary relaxation of the external sphincter is required to initiate the sacral reflex arc and micturition. The striated sphincter is also responsible for voluntarily stopping the urinary stream.

3. What is the role of the brainstem in normal micturition?

The micturition control center is located in the brainstem. Inhibitory signals are sent from the brainstem when micturition is not appropriate. Typically, stretch receptors from the bladder send signals to the spinal cord when the bladder is full. Were it not for inhibitory signals from the brainstem, urinary urge incontinence would occur, as in patients who suffer a stroke.

4. At what vertebral level does the spinal cord end in the adult?

In the adult the spinal cord ends between the L1 and L2 vertebral levels. Thus a severe injury, such as a burst fracture to the L1 or L2 vertebral body that causes spinal cord injury, may injure the cauda equina or the S2–S4 nerve roots, resulting in a lower motor neuron injury and a flaccid bladder.

5. What is meant by spinal shock?

Spinal shock is a loss of muscle reflexes below the level of spinal cord injury that may last for a period of hours to several months or longer after injury. The bladder initially may have low pressure and no detrusor contraction; then, like the muscles of the lower extremity, it may become spastic.

6. How do the bladder and sphincter function after a complete spinal cord injury above the level of the sacral reflex arc?

With filling of the bladder, stretch receptors send signals to the spinal cord that the bladder is distended, and reflex contractions of the bladder occur. The striated sphincter may become spastic and contract instead of relaxing as the detrusor contracts, thus resulting in bladder outlet obstruction (detrusor-sphincter dyssynergia). This obstruction prevents effective bladder emptying and results in high-pressure voiding with residual urine. Over time, this condition may result in hydronephrosis, vesicoureteral reflux, and eventually renal failure, if not treated.

7. What type of bladder dysfunction is seen in diabetes?

Typically, one thinks of a sensory neurogenic bladder in diabetes. Individuals with long-standing diabetes may not sense that the bladder is full. Persons without diabetes report the first sensation to void on a cystometrogram at approximately 125 mL and become quite uncomfortable at 400–500 mL. Diabetics may not sense that the bladder is full until quite large volumes have accumulated. Treatment consists of timed voiding. Patients must go to the bathroom to void every 3–4 hours by their watch. They are instructed to double-void to ensure that the bladder is empty. If this approach is not effective, treatment consists of intermittent self-catheterization.

8. What urologic manifestations are seen in multiple sclerosis?

Multiple sclerosis is unique in that the voiding problems change with time as the disease changes. The most common finding is uninhibited bladder contractions. Bladder-sphincter dyssynergia also may be seen.

9. What are the urologic manifestations of stroke?

Patients who have had strokes may experience acute urinary retention, and after recuperation the typical finding is urinary urge incontinence. Patients void with a normal bladder pressure, bladder-sphincter synergy, and low postvoid residuals. The pathology in stroke is the loss of inhibitory signals from the brainstem. Treatment consists of anticholinergic medication.

10. What are urodynamics and what are their role in the diagnosis and management of neurogenic bladder?

Urodynamics are a group of tests designed to study the bladder and the outlet (bladder neck and external sphincter mechanism) during bladder storage and bladder emptying. These tests consist of cystometrics, urinary flowmetry, external urinary sphincter electromyography, and urethral pressure profiles, and can be performed while observing the bladder and bladder outlet with fluoroscopy (or ultrasonography) in video-urodynamics. Urodynamics are important in identifying those individuals at risk for developing upper tract problems such as vesicoureteral reflux and hydronephrosis. Urodynamics confirm the clinical problem and suggest appropriate treatment.

11. What is the most consistent urodynamic finding in patients with neurogenic voiding dysfunction secondary to disc disease?

Detrusor areflexia is the most consistent urodynamic finding in patients with neurogenic voiding dysfunction secondary to disc disease. Most disc protrusions compress the spinal cord at the L4–L5 or L5–S1 disc spaces. Patients generally complain of low back pain with radiation along the path of the involved nerve and difficulty with voiding or urinary retention.

12. What is characteristic of cauda equina syndrome?

Cauda equina syndrome is characterized by the acute onset of urinary retention and loss of perineal sensation, often accompanied by severe low back pain. Spinal cord compression by disc disease or other pathology requires neurosurgical consultation for emergent decompression.

13. What is autonomic dysreflexia? How is it treated?

Autonomic dysreflexia is unopposed sympathetic discharge in patients with spinal cord injury at the level of T6 or above. With distention of the bladder or bowel or a painful stimulus to the lower extremity, autonomic dysreflexia may be triggered. The patient experiences headache, sweating, and piloerection. The patient is noted to be hypertensive and bradycardic. Treatment consists of eliminating the noxious stimuli (such as draining the bladder) and placing the patient in a sitting position. If the blood pressure does not come down, medications such as nifedipine or nitroprusside should be used. Untreated autonomic dysreflexia may result in cerebral vascular accidents.

14. What are the goals in the treatment of the neurogenic bladder?

The goals are to maintain kidney function, to prevent infection, and, if possible, to achieve continence. Clean, intermittent catheterization with selective use of the anticholinergic medication to lower bladder pressure and to prevent uninhibited bladder contraction is a mainstay of treatment.

BIBLIOGRAPHY

1. De Groat WC: Anatomy and physiology of the lower urinary tract. Urol Clin North Am 20:383–401, 1993.
2. Steers WD, Barrett DM, Wein AJ: Voiding function: Diagnosis, classification and management. In Gillenwater JY, Grayhack JT, Howards SS, Duckett JW (eds): Adult and Pediatric Urology, 3rd ed. St.
   Louis, Mosby, 1996, pp 1220–1325.
3. Wein AJ: Pathophysiology and categorization of voiding dysfunction. In Walsh PC, Retik AB, Vaughan
   ED, Wein AJ (eds): Campbell's Urology, 7th ed. Philadelphia, W.B. Saunders, 1998, pp 917–926.
4. Linsenmeyer TA, Culkin D: APS recommendations for the urologic evaluation of patients with spinal cord
   injury. J Spinal Cord Med 22:139–142, 1999.
5. Fowler CJ: Bladder afferents and their role in the overactive bladder. Urology 59(5 suppl 1):37–42, 2002.

II. Benign and Malignant Tumors of the Genitourinary Tract

17. RENAL CELL CARCINOMA

Andrew C. Novick, M.D.

1. What is the prevalence of renal cell carcinoma (RCC)?

In the United States, approximately 30,000 new cases of RCC are detected each year. RCC accounts for 3% of all adult malignancies and 85% of all primary malignant renal tumors.

2. What is the etiology of RCC?

The etiology of RCC is unknown; cigarette smoking is the only known risk factor. There is an increased incidence of RCC in patients with von Hippel-Lindau disease, horseshoe kidneys, adult polycystic kidney disease, and acquired renal cystic disease from uremia.

3. What is the staging system for patients with RCC?

There are two primary staging systems for renal cell carcinoma. The **Robson system** is simple and easy to use; however, the staging categories do not always relate directly to prognosis; for example, stage 3 disease includes isolated renal vein involvement, which carries a good prognosis, as well as lymph node involvement, which is associated with poor survival. The **tumor-node metastasis** (TNM) system is more detailed in classifying the extent of tumor involvement.

4. What are the signs and symptoms of RCC?

The most common presenting signs and symptoms of RCC are gross or microscopic hematuria, abdominal or flank pain, and a palpable abdominal mass. These findings will be present in 10–15% of patients. Patients with metastatic disease may present with symptoms of lung or bone metastasis, such as dyspnea, cough, or bone pain. RCC may also be associated with several paraneoplastic syndromes such as erythrocytosis, hypercalcemia, hypertension, and nonmetastatic hepatic dysfunction. A majority of RCCs are currently being detected in asymptomatic patients.

5. What is the appropriate evaluation for patients with suspected RCC?

The diagnostic evaluation of a renal mass is reviewed in chapter 9. When this evaluation is indicative of a renal cell carcinoma, additional studies are necessary for clinical staging of the tumor and in preparation for surgery. Routine clinical staging studies include a history and physical examination, complete blood count, renal and hepatic function tests, urinalysis, chest x-ray, and a CT scan of the abdomen. A radionuclide bone scan is indicated in patients with bone pain or an elevated serum alkaline phosphatase level. When abdominal CT scanning suggests inferior vena caval involvement, additional imaging is necessary to establish both the presence and complete extent of vena caval involvement. This can be accomplished with either MRI or a contrast inferior venacavogram. Renal arteriography is indicated in patients undergoing a complicated partial nephrectomy and in patients with a known vena caval tumor thrombus; in the latter group, if arteriography demonstrates an arterialized tumor thrombus, preoperative angioinfarction can facilitate surgical extraction of the thrombus.

Staging of Renal Cell Carcinoma

	ROBSON STAGE	TNM STAGE
Small tumor, minimal distortion	I	T1
Large tumor, renal distortion	I	T2
Perirenal fat involvement	II	T3a
Renal vein involvement	IIIa	T3b
Infradiaphragmatic vena caval involvement	IIIa	T3c
Invading adjacent structures	IVa	T4a
Superior vena caval involvement	IIIa	T4b
No nodes involved	I, II	N0
Single node involvement	IIIb	N1
Multiple nodes involved	IIIb	N2
Fixed nodes involved	IIIb	N3
Distant metastases	IVb	M1

6. What is the treatment for a localized unilateral RCC?

Surgical excision is the only curative form of treatment for RCC. **Radical nephrectomy** is the treatment of choice for patients with a localized unilateral RCC and a normal functioning opposite kidney. Radical nephrectomy involves removal of the entire kidney outside Gerota's fascia. The adrenal gland must also be removed if the upper portion of the kidney is involved with malignancy. The benefit of performing a regional lymphadenectomy is controversial. Radical nephrectomy can be performed with minimally invasive laparoscopic surgery for localized tumors < 8 cm in size. A traditional open surgical approach is indicated for larger tumors. The 5-year survival rate following radical nephrectomy for Robson stage 1 RCC is 80–85%.

This rate is reduced in the presence of perinephric fat involvement (70–75%), renal vein involvement (50–60%), vena caval involvement (40–50%), extension to regional lymph nodes (5–20%), invasion of adjacent organs (0–5%), and distant metastases (0–5%).

7. When should a nephron-sparing operation (partial nephrectomy) be done for localized RCC?

Nephron-sparing surgery is indicated in patients with localized RCC present bilaterally or in a solitary kidney, because radical nephrectomy would necessitate immediate renal replacement therapy. In recent years, the indications for nephron-sparing surgery have expanded to include other patients in whom preservation of renal function is clinically relevant. Examples include patients with unilateral RCC and a functioning but impaired contralateral kidney or patients with unilateral RCC and a contralateral kidney whose function is potentially threatened by a concomitant urologic or systemic disorder. For patients with low-stage RCC, the long-term results of nephron-sparing surgery are comparable to those of radical nephrectomy. Therefore, nephron-sparing surgery is now also being done in selected patients with a single, small (4 cm) unilateral RCC and a normal contralateral kidney. The major disadvantage of this approach is the risk of postoperative local tumor recurrence, which occurs in 4–6% of patients. Recently, energy ablative techniques such as cryoablation and radiofrequency ablation are being used for nephron-sparing treatment of some small renal cell carcinomas; however, these approaches are considered investigational.

8. What is the approach to RCC involving the inferior vena cava (IVC)?

For patients with nonmetastatic RCC and IVC involvement, 5-year survival rates of 47–68% have been reported following complete surgical excision. The presence of lymph node or distant metastases in such cases carries a dismal prognosis that is not appreciably altered by radical surgical extirpation. Surgery has a palliative role in some patients with metastasis who experience severe disability from intractable edema, ascites, cardiac dysfunction, or associated local symptoms such as abdominal pain or hematuria.

When performing radical nephrectomy with removal of an IVC thrombus, it is essential to obtain control of the IVC above the thrombus to prevent intraoperative embolization of a tumor fragment. When the thrombus extends above the diaphragm, a combined thoracic and abdominal surgical approach is necessary. In such cases, adjunctive cardiopulmonary bypass with deep hypothermic circulatory arrest allows extensive IVC thrombi to be completely and safely removed.

9. What are the indications for nephrectomy in patients with metastatic RCC?

Nephrectomy has a palliative role in some patients with metastatic RCC who experience severe disability from associated local symptoms, although some patients in this category can be managed with percutaneous renal angioinfarction. In patients with RCC and a solitary resectable metastasis, surgical excision of the primary and metastatic lesion is warranted based on reported 5-year survival rates of 30–35%. Many biologic response modifier protocols to treat patients with metastatic RCC currently require removal of the primary tumor before systemic therapy is initiated.

10. How frequently do metastases occur in RCC? How are they treated?

Approximately one-third of patients with RCC will have metastatic disease at the time of diagnosis, and an additional 30–50% will develop metastatic disease within 5 years. Currently, approximately 12,000 patient deaths occur per year from metastatic RCC in the United States.

Until recently, the treatment for metastatic RCC was relatively ineffective. Various hormonal and cytotoxic chemotherapeutic agents, used individually or in combination, have yielded response rates of < 15%. RCC is not sensitive to radiation therapy, although this modality can provide palliation for patients with symptomatic metastatic lesions. More recently, immunotherapy with biologic response modifiers, such as interferon-α and interleukin-2, are being evaluated in this setting. Although some immunotherapy protocols have demonstrated considerable promise with response rates as high as 30–40%, this form of therapy is investigational and requires further evaluation.

BIBLIOGRAPHY

1. Butler B, Novick AC, Miller D, et al: Management of small unilateral renal cell carcinomas: Radical versus nephron-sparing surgery. Urology 45:34–40, 1995.
2. Fergany A, Hafez K, Novick AC: Long-term results of nephron-sparing surgery for localized renal cell carcinoma. J Urol 163:442–445, 2000.
3. Figlin RA, Abi-Aad AS, Belldegrun A, deKernion JB: The role of interferon and interleukin-2 on the immunotherapeutic approach to renal cell carcinoma. Semin Oncol 18 (5 suppl 7):102–107, 1991.
4. Glazer A, Novick AC: Long-term follow-up after surgical treatment for renal cell carcinoma extending into the right atrium. J Urol 155:448–450, 1996.
5. Gill I, Novick AC, Soble J: Laparoscopic renal cryoablation: Initial clinical series. Urology 52:543–551, 1998.
6. Gill IS, Schweizer D, Hobart M, et al: Retroperitoneal laparoscopic radical nephrectomy: The Cleveland Clinic experience. J Urol 163:1665–1670, 2000.
7. Guinan P, Sobin L, Algaba F, et al: TNM staging of renal cell carcinoma. Cancer 80:992–993, 1997.
8. Licht M, Novick AC: Nephron-sparing surgery for renal cell carcinoma. J Urol 149:1–7, 1993.
9. Novick AC, Kaye M, Cosgrove DM, et al: Experience with cardiopulmonary bypass and deep hypothermic circulatory arrest in the management of retroperitoneal tumors with large vena caval thrombi. Ann Surg 212:472–476, 1990.
10. Novick AC, Campbell SC: Renal tumors. In Walsh P, Wein A, Retik A, Vaughan D: Campbell's Urology, 8th ed. Philadelphia, W.B. Saunders, 2002.
11. Rackley R, Novick AC, Klein E, et al: The impact of adjuvant nephrectomy on multimodality treatment of metastatic renal cell carcinoma. J Urol 152:1399–1403, 1994.
12. Robertson CN, Marston WM, Pass HI, et al: Preparative cytoreductive surgery in patients with metastatic renal cell carcinoma treated with adoptive immunotherapy with interleukin-2 or interleukin-2 plus lymphokine activated killer cells. J Urol 144:614–617, 1990.
13. Robson CJ, Churchill BM, Anderson W: The results of radical nephrectomy for renal cell carcinoma. J Urol 101:297–301, 1969.
14. Skinner DB, Colvin RB, Vermillion CD, et al: Diagnosis and management of renal carcinoma: A clinical and pathologic study of 309 cases. Cancer 28:1165–1177, 1971.

15. Skinner DG, Pritchett TR, Lieskovsky G, et al: Vena caval involvement by renal cell carcinoma: Surgical resection provides meaningful long-term survival. Ann Surg 210:387–392, 1989.
16. Thompson IM, Peek M: Improvement in survival of patients with renal cell carcinoma: The role of serendipitiously detected tumor. J Urol 140:487–490, 1988.
17. Tolia BM, Whitmore WF Jr: Solitary metastasis from renal cell carcinoma. J Urol 114:836–838, 1975.
18. Tosaka A, Ohya K, Yamada K, et al: Incidence and properties of renal masses and asymptomatic renal cell carcinoma detected by abdominal ultrasonography. J Urol 144:1097–1099, 1990.

18. PHEOCHROMOCYTOMA

David A. Goldfarb, M.D.

1. What is a pheochromocytoma?

Pheochromocytoma is a tumor derived from chromaffin cells that is associated with pathologic secretion of catecholamines (norepinephrine and epinephrine).

2. Where are they located?

About 90% are located in the adrenal gland; 10% may be extra-adrenal. Most extra-adrenal pheochromocytomas are associated with sympathetic ganglia in the retroperitoneum, but tumors may be found anywhere in the midline in association with the sympathetic chain from the bladder to the base of the skull. Extra-adrenal tumors are often called paragangliomas.

3. Who gets pheochromocytoma?

Most occur in middle-aged adults, but 10% occur in children, in whom they are more likely to be multiple or extra-adrenal. Ten percent occur in patients with multiple endocrine neoplasia (MEN) syndrome.

4. What syndromes are associated with pheochromocytoma?

- MEN (type 2) is composed of pheochromocytoma (often bilateral) in combination with medullary thyroid cancer and hyperparathyroidism.
- MEN (type 3) is pheochromocytoma (often bilateral) in combination with medullary thyroid cancer, mucosal neuromas, thickened corneal nerves, alimentary tract ganglioneuromatosis, and marfanoid habitus.
- Neurofibromatosis
- von Hippel-Lindau disease

5. What is the rule of 10%?

Ten percent of tumors are:
Extra-adrenal
Malignant
Associated with MEN syndromes
Bilateral
Pediatric

6. What are the symptoms?

The symptoms are those of excessive catecholamine secretion and include the classic triad of headaches, sweating, and palpitations. Pheochromocytoma, however, can present with various nonspecific symptoms, including tremors, nausea, dyspnea, fatigue, dizziness, and chest or abdominal pain. An increasing number of patients are being diagnosed without any symptoms other than the incidental finding of an adrenal mass on x-ray evaluation for an unrelated complaint.

7. What are the physical findings?

The most common physical finding is hypertension, which may be sustained or paroxysmal. Orthostatic hypotension may occur. Other signs of catecholamine excess include tachycardia, tremor, lean body habitus, and Raynaud's phenomenon. A mass may be noted in the abdomen. There may be signs of a familial syndrome.

8. Who should be evaluated?

Priority for evaluation should be given to patients with:

- Headaches, sweating, and palpitations
- Incidental adrenal mass
- Hypertensive crisis with surgery, anesthesia, or parturition
- Family history of pheochromocytoma

9. How is pheochromocytoma diagnosed?

The diagnosis is based on the finding of excessive catecholamines or their metabolics in blood and/or urine. Resting plasma catecholamines are measured first. Values >2000 pg/ml confirm the diagnosis and values <500 pg/ml are normal. Values between 500 and 2000 pg/ml are equivocal, and further evaluation with urinary tests or pharmacologic tests is needed. A 24-hour urine collection for metanephrines is the most accurate of the urinary tests. Other 24-hour urine tests that may show elevated results include vanillylmandelic acid and urinary free catecholamines. To optimize the identification of patients with pheochromocytoma, both plasma and urine testing is recommended.

10. What is pharmacologic testing?

In the hypertensive patient with equivocal plasma catecholamine levels, the clonidine suppression test helps to differentiate between pheochromocytoma and essential hypertension. Clonidine suppresses plasma catecholamines to <500 pg/ml in essential hypertension, but has no effect in pheochromocytoma. In patients with equivocal plasma catecholamines and mild hypertension, the glucagon stimulation test is used as a provocative test. It will result in an increase in catecholamines in patients with pheochromocytoma, but not with other causes of hypertension. The glucagon stimulation test has the risk of causing severe hypertension but can be performed while patients are on certain antihypertensive medications (calcium channel blockers).

11. How are pheochromocytomas localized?

1. **CT scan of the abdomen or pelvis** is the most common test for localization. It is an excellent initial examination because 97% of tumors are located below the diaphragm and 90% are intra-adrenal.

2. **Magnetic resonance imaging** (MRI) has the advantage of improved soft tissue characterization. Pheochromocytoma has a characteristically high signal intensity on the T2-weighted images. MRI has an improved sensitivity for the identification of multifocal and extra-adrenal disease.

3. **Metaiodobenzylguanidine** (MIBG) is a radiopharmaceutical analog of guanethidine that accumulates in pheochromocytomas. Although the sensitivity of MIBG is lower than that of MRI, MIBG scintigraphy can image the whole body. It is useful in cases in which localization is difficult. It can also confirm that an adrenal mass seen on CT is a pheochromocytoma.

12. Describe the preoperative regimen.

The goal of preoperative management is to prevent cardiovascular morbidity due to severe hypertension. The standard medical preparation has been to treat patients with the noncompetitive α-adrenergic blocker, phenoxybenzamine, for 4 weeks before surgery. The newer α-blocking agents, such as prazosin, terazosin, and doxazosin may also be used, as well as various calcium channel blockers. Occasionally, β-blocking drugs are used to control cardiac arrhythmias. In these cases, α-blockade should be in place first to avoid a paradoxical hypertensive crisis. In addition to medications, many of these patients are volume depleted and require vigorous intravenous hydration the day before surgery.

13. What is the surgical management?

All patients should be maintained with arterial and central venous catheters for hemodynamic monitoring. Rapidly acting vasoactive agents, such as nitroprusside, nitroglycerin, and phentolamine, should be readily available to deal with cardiovascular lability. Close communication between surgical and anesthetic teams is necessary.

The operative approach depends on the location and size of the tumors. Historically, a transperitoneal approach (subcostal incision) has been used with complete abdominal exploration to identify any new tumors that have escaped radiologic detection.

Recently, this traditional surgical approach has been challenged in light of the increased accuracy of contemporary imaging techniques (CT, MRI, MIBG). Recent reports also show that laparoscopic adrenalectomy for pheochromocytoma is safe and has become an established standard. Tumors < 5 cm are most appropriate for a laparoscopic approach. For larger tumors a subcostal (chevron) incision or thoracoabdominal incision can be used. For surgeons not comfortable with advanced laparoscopic techniques, an extraperitoneal (flank or posterior) incision can be used.

14. What is the postoperative management?

Hypotension is a common problem, due to the release from catecholamine-induced vasoconstriction. It should be managed primarily by volume repletion, not vasoconstrictors. Hypoglycemia is occasionally observed and blood glucose should be routinely monitored.

15. What about follow-up?

These patients can develop recurrent or metastatic disease. Blood pressure should be monitored yearly. Repeat biochemical evaluation should be conducted in patients in whom hypertension persists after surgery or recurs at some point in follow-up.

BIBLIOGRAPHY

1. Bravo EL: Pheochromocytoma: New concepts and future trends. Kidney Int 40:544–556, 1991.
2. Greene JP, Gray AT: New perspectives in pheochromocytoma. Urol Clin North Am 16:487–503, 1989.
3. Manger WM, Gifford RW: Pheochromocytoma: Current diagnosis and management. Cleve Clin J Med 60:365–378, 1993.
4. Sheps SG, Jiang NS, Klee GG, vanHeerden JA: Recent developments in the diagnosis and treatment of pheochromocytoma. Mayo Clin Proc 65:88–95, 1990.
5. Ulchaker JC, Goldfarb DA, Bravo EL, Novick AC: Successful outcomes in pheochromocytoma in the modern era. J Urol 161:764–767, 1999.
6. Kinney MAO, Narr BJ, Warner, MA: Perioperative management of pheochromocytoma. J. Cardiothorac Vasc Anesth 16:359–369, 2002.

19. PRIMARY ALDOSTERONISM

David A. Goldfarb, M.D.

1. Define primary aldosteronism.
It is a secondary cause of hypertension characterized by excessive and unregulated secretion of aldosterone.

2. What are its causes?
An adrenal cortical adenoma is present in 60% to 80% of cases, whereas bilateral adrenal hyperplasia is responsible for 20% to 40% of cases. This distinction is important because adenomas respond to surgery, whereas hyperplasia is treated medically.

3. What are the signs and symptoms?
Hypertension is a central feature of the disease. Other symptoms are nonspecific and may include polyuria, nocturia, proximal muscle weakness, and headaches (bitemporal).

4. List the biochemical features of primary aldosteronism.
1. Hypokalemia
2. High plasma aldosterone
3. Low plasma renin activity
4. Metabolic alkalosis

5. Who should be screened for the disease?
Hypertensive patients with:
- Spontaneous hypokalemia (serum $K+$ < 3.5 mEq/L)
- Moderately severe hypokalemia after conventional diuretic therapy (serum $K+$ < 3.0 mEq/L)
- Refractory hypertension

6. How do you screen for primary aldosteronism?
1. **Hypokalemia** occurs with inappropriate kaliuresis (24-hr urine $K+$ > 30 mEq, serum $K+$ < 3.5 mEq/L).

2. **Plasma renin activity** (PRA) is usually low (<1.0 ng/mL/hr), although there is a large overlap with levels seen in essential hypertension. A PRA <3.0 ng/mL/hr after 4 hours of upright posture suggests primary aldosteronism.

3. **Plasma aldosterone** (PA) is physiologically quite variable and is neither sensitive nor specific for the disease. However, a PA/PRA ratio >20 suggests primary aldosternoism.

If several of these features are identified in a hypertensive patient, confirmatory testing should be pursued.

7. How is the diagnosis confirmed?
The best way to confirm the diagnosis of primary aldosteronism is to demonstrate nonsuppressible aldosterone secretion during prolonged salt repletion. This can be accomplished in the outpatient setting by adding 10–12 gm of sodium chloride to the patient's diet for 5–7 days. Then, a 24-hour urine collection for aldosterone and sodium should be obtained. A urinary sodium >250 mEq suggests adequate salt repletion. Urinary aldosterone >14 μg/24 hours indicates primary aldosteronism.

8. What are the localization procedures?
Computed tomographic (CT) scan of the adrenals should be the first imaging study, as it can identify 90% of adenomas. Sometimes the adenomas are small (<1.0 cm) and beyond the resolution of CT. Bilaterally enlarged adrenals suggest hyperplasia.

Scintigraphy with radiolabeled iodocholesterol (NP59) is a noninvasive test to differentiate between adenoma and hyperplasia. Unilateral concentration of NP59 suggests adenoma, whereas symmetric activity suggests hyperplasia.

Adrenal vein sampling for aldosterone can be performed if the results of CT or NP59 scintigraphy are ambiguous. This is the *most accurate* localization technique. An ipsilateral/contralateral aldosterone concentration ratio of >10:1 implies the presence of an adenoma.

9. Are there any biochemical clues to differentiate adenoma from hyperplasia?

Severe spontaneous hypokalemia (<3.0 mEq/L), plasma 18-OH-corticosterone >100 mg/dl, and anomalous postural decrease in plasma aldosterone are associated with adenoma (but are not present in all cases).

10. What are the indications for surgery?

A patient with biochemical evidence of primary aldosteronism and a unilateral adenoma.

11. Which patients are treated medically?

Those with bilateral hyperplasia or patients with adenoma who are unsuitable surgical candidates.

12. What surgical approach should be used?

Since adenomas are small, laparoscopic adrenalectomy has emerged as the surgical approach of choice. In experienced hands, this is safe and convalescence is rapid. Newer needlescopic techniques have been developed that even further diminish morbidity. In the absence of a skilled laparoscopist the posterior or flank approach can be used.

13. What medications are used to treat primary aldosteronism?

Spironolactone, because it is a potassium-sparing diuretic. Triamterene or amiloride may also be used.

14. Can these tumors be malignant?

Adrenal cortical carcinoma causing only primary aldosteronism is rare, accounting for <1% of these cancers.

BIBLIOGRAPHY

1. Bravo EL: Primary aldosteronism. Urol Clin North Am 16:481–486, 1989.
2. Bravo EL: Primary aldosteronism: New approaches to diagnosis and management. Cleveland Clin J Med 60:379–386, 1993.
3. Geisinger MA, Zelch MG, Bravo EL, et al: Primary hyperaldosteronism: Comparison of CT, adrenal venography and venous sampling. AJR 141:299–302, 1983.
4. Novick AC: Surgery for primary hyperaldosteronism. Urol Clin North Am 16:535–545, 1989.
5. Novick AC, Straffon RA, Kaylor W, Bravo EL: Posterior transthoracic approach for adrenal surgery. J Urol 141:254–256, 1989.
6. Young WF, Hogan MJ, Klee GG, et al. Primary aldosteronism: Diagnosis and treatment. Mayo Clin Proc 65:96–110, 1990.
7. Gill IS: Needlescopic adrenalectomy—the initial series: Comparison with conventional adrenalectomy. Urology 52:180–186, 1998.
8. Doppman JL, Gill JR Jr, Miller DL, et al: Distinction between hyperaldosteronism due to bilateral hyperplasia and unilateral aldosteronoma: Reliability of CT. Radiology 184:599–600, 1997.
9. Rossi H, Kim A, Prinz RA: Primary hyperaldosteronism in the era of laparoscopic adrenalectomy. Am Surg 68:253–256, 2002.
10. Bravo EL: Medical management of primary hyperaldosteronism. Curr Hypertens Rep 3:406–409, 2001.

20. ADRENAL CORTICAL ADENOMA AND CARCINOMA

Andrew C. Novick, M.D.

1. Which clinical syndromes may be caused by a functioning adrenal cortical adenoma or carcinoma?

Adrenal cortical adenomas and carcinomas may be nonfunctioning or functioning. The term *functioning* refers to metabolically active tumors that produce excessive amounts of adrenal cortical hormones. The most common clinical syndromes associated with a functioning adrenal cortical **adenoma** are primary hyperaldosteronism or Cushing's syndrome. The most common clinical syndrome associated with a functioning adrenal cortical **carcinoma** is Cushing's syndrome; however, many patients also have evidence of virilization. Feminization occasionally occurs in men with an adrenal cortical carcinoma, whereas aldosterone-secreting adrenal cortical carcinomas are rare.

2. What is Cushing's syndrome?

Cushing's syndrome is caused by excessive adrenal secretion of corticosteroid with a resulting characteristic clinical presentation of truncal obesity, buffalo hump, virilization in the female, impotence or gynecomastia in the male, increased bruising and striae, hypertension, osteoporosis, peripheral extremity muscle wasting, and variable mental aberrations. Cushing's syndrome may be due to a pituitary adenoma (Cushing's disease, 70%), an ectopic ACTH-producing tumor (10%), or a primary adrenal cortical tumor (20%).

3. Which biochemical tests are most useful in determining that Cushing's syndrome is due to a primary adrenal tumor?

In all cases of Cushing's syndrome, the plasma cortisol level is elevated with loss of normal diurnal variation. In patients with true Cushing's disease due to a pituitary adenoma, the plasma cortisol level is suppressed by administration of exogenous dexamethasone. Cases of Cushing's syndrome that do not suppress with dexamethasone have either an independently functioning adrenal cortical tumor or an extra-adrenal ACTH-producing tumor; the differentiation between these two conditions is made by measurement of the plasma ACTH, which is high in the latter and low in the former.

4. Which radiographic imaging tests are indicated in patients with a suspected adrenal cortical adenoma or carcinoma?

Most adrenal cortical adenomas and carcinomas can be detected with a noninvasive imaging study such as **CT, MRI,** or **ultrasonography.** These imaging modalities can demonstrate masses as small as 1 cm within the adrenal gland and also detect tumor spread into adjacent organs, regional lymph nodes, or the inferior vena cava.

Arteriography adds little diagnostic information to the above studies and is of value primarily in delineating the vascular supply of a large tumor in preparation for surgery. Intravenous pyelography and adrenal venography are no longer useful screening or diagnostic studies in patients with a suspected adrenal cortical adenoma or carcinoma.

5. In patients with Cushing's syndrome due to a primary adrenal tumor, how can one determine if the underlying lesion is an adenoma or carcinoma?

In patients with Cushing's syndrome due to a primary adrenal tumor, the underlying pathology may be a benign adenoma or an adrenal cortical carcinoma. An adrenal adenoma is more likely when the size of the lesion is < 6 cm, when pure Cushing's syndrome is present, and when the lesion yields a low signal intensity upon the T2-weighted image of a magnetic resonance scan. Features favoring an adrenal cortical carcinoma includes size > 6 cm, a mixed hormonal pattern (i.e., Cushing's and virilization or feminization), markedly elevated urinary 17-ketosteroids, and a hyperintense signal from the mass upon the T2-weighted image of a magnetic resonance scan.

6. What is the treatment for Cushing's disease?

The primary treatment for Cushing's disease of pituitary origin is **transsphenoidal hypophysectomy,** which is currently successful in approximately 80–90% of patients. The remaining 10–20% in whom this form of treatment is ineffective require bilateral surgical adrenalectomy with subsequent corticosteroid replacement therapy.

7. What is the treatment for Cushing's syndrome due to a primary adrenal cortical tumor?

Surgical adrenalectomy is indicated for Cushing's syndrome due to a primary adrenal tumor. Small adenomas may be removed laparoscopically. Adrenal lesions that are large or potentially malignant are removed through a surgical transabdominal incision.

8. How common is adrenal cortical carcinoma?

Adrenal cortical carcinoma is an uncommon malignancy, occurring with a frequency of 1–2 cases/million population/year.

9. What is the clinical presentation of patients with an adrenal cortical carcinoma?

Approximately 50% of adrenal cortical carcinoma patients are functioning with symptoms related to excessive adrenal cortical steroid production. The remaining 50% are nonfunctioning tumors and these patients present with nonspecific symptoms such as abdominal pain, abdominal mass, fatigue, and weight loss. More than half of patients with adrenal cortical carcinoma have regional or distant tumor spread when the diagnosis is established. This is presumably due to the large number of patients with nonfunctioning tumors as well as the anatomic location of the adrenal gland deep within the retroperitoneum, which renders it inaccessible to physical examination.

10. What treatment options are available for patients with an adrenal cortical carcinoma?

Currently, **complete surgical excision** is the only effective form of therapy for patients with adrenal cortical carcinoma. Such tumors are not sensitive to radiation therapy, and the results with cytotoxic chemotherapy have been disappointing. Some studies have suggested that survival of patients with metastatic adrenal cortical carcinoma can be prolonged with surgical adrenalectomy followed by adjuvant administration of mitotane (o, p'-DDD).

11. How successful is treatment for adrenal cortical carcinoma?

The prognosis for patients with adrenal cortical carcinoma is relatively poor. In a large series of 82 patients with adrenal cortical carcinoma from the Cleveland Clinic, the overall 3- and 5-year survival rates were 37.5% and 25.1%, respectively. The only factor influencing patient survival was the presence of localized (i.e., surgically resectable) disease at initial diagnosis; in these patients, the 3- and 5-year survival rates after excision were 57% and 43.9%, respectively. The 5-year survival rates for patients with regional or metastatic disease were 12.5% and 5.5%, respectively. In patients with regional or metastatic disease, no difference in survival was found among those who received mitotane, cytotoxic chemotherapy, radiation therapy, or none of these treatment methods.

BIBLIOGRAPHY

1. Bellegrun A, Hussain S, Seltzer SE, et al: Incidentally discovered mass of the adrenal gland. Surg Gynecol Obstet 163:203–208, 1986.

2. Bodie B, Novick AC, et al: Cleveland Clinic experience with adrenal cortical carcinoma. J Urol 141: 257–260, 1989.
3. Brown D, Schumacher OP: Adjuvant therapy, o, p'-DDD in the treatment of metastatic adrenocortical carcinoma. Clin Res 27:626A, 1979.
4. Daitch JA, Goldfarb D, Novick AC: Cleveland Clinic experience with adrenal Cushing's syndrome. J Urol 158:2051–2055, 1997.
5. Gill I, Soble J, Sung G, et al: Needlescopic adrenalectomy—The initial series: Comparison with conventional laparoscopic adrenalectomy. Urology 52:180–186, 1998.
6. Gold EM: The Cushing's syndrome: Changing views of diagnosis and treatment. Ann Intern Med 90:829, 1979.
7. Guz BV, Straffon R, Novick AC: Operative approaches to the adrenal gland. Urol Clin North Am 16: 527–534, 1989.
8. Lipsett MB, Hertz R, Ross GT: Clinical and pathophysiologic aspects of adrenocortical carcinoma. Am J Med 35:374, 1963.
9. Mitty HA, Cohen BA: Adrenal imaging. Urol Clin North Am 12:771–785, 1985.
10. Nader S, Hickey RC, Sellin RV, Samaan NA: Adrenal cortical carcinoma: A study of 77 cases. Cancer 52:707–711, 1983.
11. Novick AC, Libertino J (eds): Adrenal Surgery. Urol Clin North Am 16(Aug):1989.

21. TRANSITIONAL CELL CARCINOMA OF THE RENAL PELVIS

Andrew C. Novick, M.D.

1. How common is transitional cell carcinoma (TCC) of the renal pelvis?

TCC of the renal pelvis comprises 5–7% of all renal malignancies, and the incidence of bilaterality is 2–4%. Renal pelvic TCC comprises only 3–4% of all urothelial malignancies. Approximately 30–50% of patients with renal pelvic TCC subsequently develop TCC of the bladder.

2. What signs and symptoms are caused by renal pelvic TCC?

Gross hematuria is the most common presenting symptom and is seen in 70–90% of patients. **Flank pain** may result from ureteral obstruction caused by the tumor or associated blood clots. **Irritative voiding symptoms** are present in 5–10% of patients. **Systemic symptoms** of anorexia, weight loss, and weakness are uncommon and are usually associated with metastatic disease. Approximately 10% of patients will present with a **flank mass** due to hydronephrosis or a large tumor.

3. How is the diagnosis of renal pelvic TCC established?

The standard diagnostic regimen for renal pelvic TCC is radiographic evaluation with intravenous pyelography (IVP) and retrograde pyelography, ureteroscopy, and, occasionally, selective upper urinary tract cytology studies. If retrograde pyelography is not possible (as in patients with an existing urinary diversion), percutaneous nephrostomy with antegrade pyelography can provide radiographic access to the involved kidney. Occasionally, angiography is indicated to differentiate renal cell carcinoma, which is typically hypervascular, from an invasive TCC, which has a characteristic pruned-tree appearance as a result of encasement of vessels.

When a filling defect is seen upon IVP or retrograde pyelography, ultrasonography can distinguish a tumor from a calculus. A thin-cut computed tomography (CT) scan obtained with and without intravenous contrast can also make the distinction. When the diagnosis remains in doubt following the above studies, ureteropyeloscopy with or without biopsy of the renal pelvis can establish the diagnosis with a high degree of accuracy.

4. What is the staging system for TCC of the renal pelvis?

The staging of renal pelvic TCC is analogous to that of bladder TCC and is determined by the presence of invasion through the thin muscle wall of the renal pelvis, or extension into surrounding structures. The criteria for TNM stages are essentially those of bladder TCC, except that T2 and T3a (superficial and deep muscle invasion) cannot be differentiated in the thin muscle layer of the collecting system. Tumor grade and stage correlate closely with survival.

Staging of Renal Pelvic TCC

	BATATA SYSTEM	TNM SYSTEM
Confined to mucosa	O	T_aT_{is}
Invasion of lamina propria	A	T1
Invasion of muscularis	B	T2
Extension into fat or renal parenchyma	C	T3
Spread to adjacent organs	D	T4
Lymph node spread	D	N1
Distant metastases	D	M1

5. What is the treatment for localized renal pelvic TCC?

In patients with localized unilateral renal pelvic TCC and a normal-functioning opposite kidney, **nephroureterectomy** is the treatment of choice for several reasons: the multifocal nature of renal pelvic TCC, the high attendant risk of ipsilateral recurrence, the low incidence of contralateral renal involvement, and the anatomically thin wall of the renal pelvis that may favor local invasion and metastatic spread at an early stage. For patients with low-grade noninvasive renal pelvic TCC, the 5-year survival rate following nephroureterectomy is 75–90%.

6. When is conservative or nephron-sparing surgery indicated?

A conservative surgical approach for localized renal pelvic TCC is indicated in selected patients with malignancy present bilaterally or in a solitary kidney or in patients with two kidneys but marginal renal function. The available nephron-sparing surgical options in these patients include partial nephrectomy, open pyelotomy with tumor excision and fulguration, percutaneous endoscopic tumor resection, or ureteropyeloscopic resection. Following a nephron-sparing procedure, a topical chemotherapeutic agent, such as BCG, may be instilled directly into the renal pelvis as an added measure toward preventing tumor recurrence.

7. How should patients with metastatic disease be managed?

Patients with metastatic renal pelvic TCC should receive cisplatin-based chemotherapy analogous to patients with metastatic bladder TCC. The involved kidney is removed if significant associated local symptoms are present or if there is a complete response to chemotherapy. Radiation therapy is generally not effective.

BIBLIOGRAPHY

1. Batata M, Grabstald H: Upper urinary tract urothelial tumors. Urol Clin North Am 3:79–86, 1976.
2. Guz BV, Streem S, Novick AC, et al: Role of percutaneous nephrostomy in patients with upper tract transitional cell carcinoma. Urology 37:331–336, 1991.
3. Huffman JL, Bagky D, Lyon E, et al: Endoscopic diagnosis and treatment of upper tract urothelial tumors: A preliminary report. Cancer 55:1422–1428, 1985.
4. Messing EM, Catalona WJ: Urothelial tumors of the urinary tract. In Walsh PC, Retik AB, Vaughan ED Jr, Wein AJ (eds): Campbell's Urology, 7th ed. Philadelphia, W.B. Saunders, 1998, pp 2327–2409.
5. Smith AD, et al: Percutaneous management of renal pelvic tumors: A treatment option in selected cases. J Urol 137:383, 1986.
6. Streem S, Pontes E, Novick AC, et al: Ureteropyeloscopy in the evaluation of upper tract filling defects. J Urol 136:383–385, 1986.
7. Studer UE, et al: Percutaneous BCG perfusion of the upper urinary tract of carcinoma in situ. J Urol 142: 975–977, 1989.
8. Vasavada SP, Streem SB, Novick AC: Definitive tumor resection and percutaneous BCG for management of renal pelvic transitional cell carcinoma in solitary kidneys. Urology 45:381–386, 1995.
9. Zeigelbaum M, Novick AC, Streem SB, et al: Conservation surgery for transitional cell carcinoma of the renal pelvis. J Urol 138:1146–1149, 1987.

22. WILMS TUMOR

Jeffrey S. Palmer, M.D. and Jack S. Elder, M.D.

1. Who is Wilms tumor named after?

The tumor is named after Max Wilms, who characterized the tumor in 1899, although Rance first described it in 1914.

2. What percentage of all solid malignancies does Wilms tumor represent?

Wilms tumor accounts for approximately 8% of all solid childhood malignancies. Wilms tumor represents > 80% of all genitourinary cancers in children < 15 years old.

3. What is the typical age of patients with Wilms tumor?

More than 90% of all Wilms tumor cases are noted before age 7, with a peak incidence between ages 3 and 4.

4. Describe the major pathologic event thought to account for the development of Wilms tumor.

Wilms tumor arises from abnormal proliferation of metanephric blastema without differentiation into glomeruli and tubules. The majority of Wilms tumors are thought be nonhereditary. Patients with bilateral or familial tumors and tumors associated with aniridia or genitourinary anomalies present at a younger age and their tumors are thought to be hereditary in origin.

5. What are the microscopic characteristics of Wilms tumor?

The tumor is triphasic, consisting of a blastemal component ("nephrogenic" cells with a tubuloglomerular pattern), a stromal component, and an epithelial component, which may contain mature tubules or be primitive in appearance.

6. The Wilms tumor suppressor gene has been localized to which chromosome?

The short arm of the eleventh chromosome (11p13).

7. How do patients with Wilms tumor typically present?

More than 90% of patients with Wilms tumor have a palpable smooth abdominal or flank mass, 33% have abdominal pain, and 30–50% exhibit microscopic or gross hematuria. Approximately 50% are hypertensive.

8. What is the differential diagnosis of a childhood abdominal mass?

Renal masses	Nonrenal causes
Wilms tumor	Mesenteric and choledochal cysts
Multicystic dysplastic kidney	Intestinal duplication cysts
Hydronephrosis	Splenomegaly
Polycystic kidney	Neuroblastoma
Congenital mesoblastic nephroma	Rhabdomyosarcoma
	Lymphoma
	Hepatoblastoma

9. Name some common anomalies associated with Wilms tumor.

Approximately 15% of patients with Wilms tumor will exhibit associated anomalies, including hemihypertrophy, Beckwith-Wiedemann syndrome, aniridia, musculoskeletal anomalies, neurofibromatosis, and a wide spectrum of genitourinary anomalies such as hypospadias, cryptorchidism, renal duplication, ectopia, and fusion anomalies.

10. What is the WAGR syndrome?

The WAGR syndrome consists of **W**ilms tumor, **A**niridia, **G**enitourinary anomalies, and mental **R**etardation.

11. What is the Beckwith-Wiedemann syndrome?

Beckwith-Wiedemann syndrome consists of visceromegaly involving the adrenal cortex, kidney, liver, pancreas, and gonads. Other findings include hemihypertrophy, omphalocele, mental retardation, microcephaly, and macroglossia. Neoplasm develops in approximately 10% of cases.

12. Describe the role of imaging studies in the diagnosis of Wilms tumor.

Ultrasound shows that the abdominal mass is solid and arising from the kidney. It also allows one to image the renal vein and inferior vena cava to assess whether a tumor thrombus is present. An intravenous pyelogram (IVP) or CT scan should be obtained to image the contralateral kidney and assess renal function. A chest x-ray or CT scan of the chest should be done to check for pulmonary metastases. The roles of MRI and MR angiography have yet to be determined.

13. What does nonvisualization of the kidney on IVP suggest?

Nonvisualization suggests complete obstruction of the collecting system (renal pelvis or ureter) with tumor, severe obstruction of the renal vein, or massive parenchymal replacement of the kidney with tumor. Approximately 10% of Wilms tumors are not visualized.

14. What are the unfavorable pathologic subtypes of Wilms tumor?

Recognition of unfavorable histologic features has allowed clinicians to identify an important prognostic factor. Although unfavorable subtypes account for only 10% of Wilms tumors, they are responsible for 60% of tumor deaths. Unfavorable subtypes include anaplastic tumor, rhabdoid tumor, and clear cell sarcoma. The rhabdoid tumor is the most lethal, and many consider this variant to be a sarcoma not of metanephric origin. These tumors tend to metastasize to the brain. Clear cell sarcoma ("bone metastasizing renal tumor of childhood") also is thought to be a separate tumor from Wilms tumor.

15. Name the favorable types of Wilms tumor.

Favorable tumors include any lesions that do not contain unfavorable elements. Specific favorable subtypes include multilocular cyst, congenital mesoblastic nephroma, and rhabdomyosarcoma tumor (not rhabdoid tumor).

16. Describe a congenital mesoblastic nephroma.

Congenital mesoblastic nephroma is a renal tumor that presents in early infancy. This tumor often has a male predilection. Grossly, it is a massive, firm tumor that contains interlacing bundles of whitish tissue resembling a leiomyoma. When completely excised, it has a benign course and no further treatment is necessary.

17. What are nephrogenic rests? Nephroblastomatosis? What is their relationship to Wilms tumor?

Wilms tumor is not congenital. It has been speculated that precursors of Wilms tumor are present that undergo transformation in the two-step process of tumor induction. It has been postulated that nephrogenic elements that persist beyond the end of nephrogenesis at 36 weeks might be these precursors. These lesions have been found in 1% of infant autopsies and 30–40% of kidneys containing a Wilms tumor.

Nephrogenic rests are abnormally persistent nephrogenic cells that can be induced to form a Wilms tumor. Nephrogenic rests have been subdivided into perilobar (peripheral) and intralobar (central) rests. Perilobar rests are often smooth and well defined, with a distribution at the lobar periphery. Intralobar rests, on the contrary, are irregular, usually single, and are distributed randomly throughout the renal lobe. Perilobar rests often contain predominantly blastemal cells early, whereas intralobar rests often are composed primarily of stromal cells. Perilobar nephrogenic rests are identified in 17% of Wilms tumors and intralobar rests in 22% of Wilms tumors.

Nephroblastomatosis refers to a diffuse pattern of nephrogenic rests or their derivatives.

18. How is Wilms tumor staged?

National Wilms Tumor Staging System

Stage I:	Tumor limited to kidney and completely excised. The surface of the renal capsule is intact. Tumor was not ruptured before or during removal. There is no residual tumor apparent beyond the margins of resection.
Stage II:	Tumor extends beyond the kidney but is completely removed. There is regional extension of the tumor, i.e., penetration through the outer surface of the renal capsule into perirenal soft tissue. Vessels outside the kidney substance are infiltrated or contain tumor thrombus. The tumor may have undergone biopsy or there has been local spillage of tumor confined to the flank. There is no residual tumor apparent at or beyond the margins of excision.
Stage III:	Residual nonhematogenous tumor confined to abdomen.
	Any one or more of the following occur:
	a. Lymph nodes on biopsy are found to be involved in the hilus, the periaortic chains, or beyond.
	b. There has been diffuse peritoneal contamination by tumor, such as by spillage or tumor beyond the flank before or during surgery, or by tumor growth that has penetrated through the peritoneal surface.
	c. Implants are found on the peritoneal surfaces.
	d. The tumor extends beyond the surgical margins either microscopically or grossly.
	e. The tumor is not completely resectable because of local infiltration into vital structures.
Stage IV:	Hematogenous metastases. Deposits beyond stage III, e.g., lung, liver, bone, and brain.
Stage V:	Bilateral renal involvement at diagnosis. An attempt should be made to stage each side according to the above criteria on the basis of extent of disease before biopsy.

19. What are the most important prognostic determinants in children with Wilms tumor?
Histopathology (favorable or unfavorable) and tumor stage.

20. What are the most common sites of metastasis for Wilms tumor?
The lungs are the most common metastatic site for Wilms tumor. The liver is the second most common site, followed by bone and brain.

21. Describe the preferred initial surgical approach to Wilms tumor.
All patients should be explored through a transverse supraumbilical transperitoneal incision. The contralateral (normal) kidney is mobilized and inspected carefully to be absolutely certain that it is not involved. Any suspicious area should be biopsied. If the normal kidney contains Wilms tumor, the patient should be managed as a stage V (bilateral Wilms tumor) patient. Next, resectability of the tumor is determined.

Important points to stress include gentle handling of the tumor to avoid spillage of tumor cells. NWTS-III patients with intraoperative tumor spill had a > sixfold increase in abdominal relapse. The adrenal gland is taken with the kidney if the tumor involves the upper pole. A lymph node sampling is important for staging, but formal lymph node dissection does not improve survival.

22. What if the tumor is unresectable?
Preoperative chemotherapy should be administered followed by renal exploration.

23. Which chemotherapeutic agents are most effective in children with Wilms tumor?
Actinomycin D, vincristine, and doxorubicin.

24. What is the role of radiation therapy in Wilms tumor?
The first National Wilms Tumor Study (NWTS-I) showed that there was no survival advantage for routine radiotherapy in patients who were given actinomycin D for at least 15 months. NWTS-III showed that radiation therapy conferred no additional benefit in patients with stage II tumors either. In stage III, 1000 cGy is as effective as higher doses. If the lungs or liver is involved, those areas should be radiated also.

25. What are the treatment plans following radical nephrectomy in children with Wilms tumor?

Stage I:	Actinomycin D plus vincristine for 18–24 weeks.
Stage II:	Actinomycin D plus vincristine for 18–65 weeks.
Stage III:	Actinomycin D, vincristine, and doxorubicin for 24–65 weeks plus radiation therapy. Half of these patients (stages I–III) receive their chemotherapy in a pulsed/intensive manner.
Stage IV:	Radiation therapy plus actinomycin D, vincristine, and doxorubicin for 65 weeks.

26. What is the role of pulse-intensive chemotherapy in Wilms tumor?
Treatment with 6 months of pulse-intensive chemotherapy is as effective as 15 months of standard chemotherapy in Stages II, III, and IV with favorable histology (data from NWTS-IV).

27. What is the initial treatment in a child with suspected Wilms tumor who presents with pulmonary metastases?
If the tumor is resectable, radical nephrectomy.

28. What is the survival for children with stages I, II, III, and IV Wilms tumor with favorable histology following treatment by the NWTS protocol?
I: 97%; II: 92%; III: 84%; IV: 83% (data from NWTS-III).

29. What is the survival for children with stages I–III, unfavorable histology, and stage IV, unfavorable histology?
I–III, unfavorable histology: 68%; IV, unfavorable histology: 55%.

30. Describe some common toxicities associated with Wilms tumor therapy.
As a result of the chemotherapeutic effect on the bone marrow, hematologic toxicity occurs relatively frequently. Similarly, hepatic toxicity frequently occurs as a result of the liver's inclusion in the radiotherapy field and from chemotherapeutic agents. Renal effects of radiation often cause azotemia, microhematuria, and chronic nephritis. Late orthopedic complications have been reported in as many as 30% of patients receiving radiation therapy, and are most severe with children under 2 years of age treated with high-dose radiation therapy. Vertebral hypoplasia and scoliosis are the most common complications. Myocardial damage may result from doxorubicin. Ovarian failure may result following radiation therapy.

31. What is the incidence of secondary neoplasms following treatment for Wilms tumor?
Approximately 17% of patients develop a secondary neoplasm following radiotherapy, with a peak incidence 15–19 years following diagnosis.

32. What is the approximate incidence of bilateral Wilms tumor?
It is 5%, synchronous accounting for 4% and metachronous for 1%.

33. What is the optimal therapy for bilateral Wilms tumor?
Previously bilateral Wilms tumor was managed with a primary surgical approach, whereby a nephrectomy was performed in the more involved kidney and, if feasible, a contralateral partial

nephrectomy was performed. Recently the preferred approach has been to perform an initial biopsy, to confirm the diagnosis, to determine whether the tumor is favorable or unfavorable, and to start chemotherapy. Surgical exploration with definitive tumor resection is performed after significant reduction in the tumor burden has occurred. Overall, patients with bilateral Wilms tumor necessitate close follow-up, as late recurrences have been documented.

BIBLIOGRAPHY

1. Banner MP, Pollack HM, Chatten J, Witzleben C: Multilocular renal cysts: Radiologic-pathologic correlation. AJR 136:239, 1981.
2. Beckwith JB, Palmer NF: Histopathology and prognosis of Wilms tumor. Cancer 41:1937, 1978.
3. Beckwith JB, D'Angio GJ: Anaplastic Wilms tumor: Clinical and pathological studies. J Clin Oncol 3:513–520, 1985.
4. Blute ML, Kelalis PP, Offord KP, et al: Bilateral Wilms tumor. J Urol 138:968–973, 1987.
5. D'Angio GJ, Breslow W, Beckwith JB, Evans A, et al: Treatment of Wilms tumor: Results of the Third National Wilms Tumor Study. Cancer 64:349–360, 1989.
6. D'Angio GJ, Evans AE, Breslow N, et al: The treatment of Wilms tumor: Results of the National Wilms Tumor Study. Cancer 38:633, 1976a.
7. D'Angio GJ, Evans AE, Breslow N, et al: The treatment of Wilms tumor: Results of the Second National Wilms Tumor Study. Cancer 47:2302–2311, 1981.
8. D'Angio GJ, Evans AE, Breslow N, et al: Results of the Third National Wilms Tumor Study (NWTS-3): A preliminary report [Abstract 723]. Proc Am Assoc Cancer Res 25:183, 1984.
9. D'Angio GJ, Tefft M, Breslow N, et al: Radiation therapy of Wilms tumor: Results according to dose, field, post-operative timing and histology. Int J Radiat Oncol Biol Phys 4:769–780, 1978.
10. de Lorimier AA, Belzer FO, Kountz SL, Kushner JO: Treatment of bilateral Wilms tumor. Am J Surg 122:275, 1971.
11. Green DM, Norkool P, Breslow NE, et al: Severe hepatic toxicity after treatment with vincristine and dactinomycin using single-dose or divided dose schedules: A report from the National Wilms Tumor Study. J Clin Oncol 8:1525–1530, 1990.
12. Green DM, Breslow NE, Beckwith JB, et al: Effect of duration of treatment on treatment outcome and cost of treatment for Wilms' tumor: A report from the National Wilms' Tumor Study Group. J Clin Oncol 16:3744–3751, 1998.
13. Jones B: Metachronous bilateral Wilms tumor. Am J Clin Oncol 5:545, 1982.
14. Keating MA, D'Angio GJ: Wilms tumor update: Current issues in management. Dialogues Pediatr Urol 11:1–8, 1988.
15. Pendergrass TW: Congenital anomalies in children with Wilms tumor. Cancer 37:403, 1976.
16. Ritchey ML, Haase GM, Shochat S: Current management of Wilms tumor. Semin Surg Oncol 9:502–509, 1993.
17. Snyder HM III, D'Angio GJ, Evan AE, et al: Pediatric oncology. In Walsh PC, Retik AB, Vaughan ED Jr, Wein AJ (eds): Campbell's Urology, 7th ed. Philadelphia, W.B. Saunders, 1998, p 2210.
18. Sotelo-Avila C, Gonzales-Crussi F, deMello D, et al: Renal and extrarenal rhabdoid tumors in children: A clinicopathologic study of 14 patients. Semin Diagn Pathol 3:151, 1986.
19. Zuppan C, Beckwith JB, Luckey D: Anaplasia in unilateral Wilms tumor: A report from the National Wilms Tumor Study Pathology Center. Hum Pathol 19:1199–1209, 1988.

23. NEUROBLASTOMA

Jonathan H. Ross, M.D.

1. How common is neuroblastoma?

Neuroblastoma is the most common extracranial solid tumor of childhood, with an annual incidence of approximately 1/100,000 children. The median age at diagnosis is 22 months, and 80% of children are diagnosed at < 4 years of age.

2. Where in the body do neuroblastomas occur?

These tumors are of neural crest cell origin and can occur anywhere in the neuroectodermal chain. Approximately 50% arise in the adrenal medulla, and most of the others occur along the sympathetic chain in the abdomen or mediastinum.

3. Describe the histologic appearance.

Neuroblastomas are one of the "small blue tumors of childhood." They occur in sheets or lobules of cells. Pseudorosettes of one or two layers of neuroblasts surrounding pink material (neuropil) are a characteristic feature seen in approximately 30% of cases.

4. Are ganglioneuroblastomas a type of neuroblastoma?

Sort of. Ganglioneuroma is a benign tumor that occurs most commonly in young adults. It is composed of mature neural elements (as opposed to neuroblasts). Ganglioneuroblastomas are tumors composed of neuroblastic elements and benign foci of ganglioneuroma. The relative preponderance of these elements occurs in a spectrum from tumors closely resembling ganglioneuromas to those that are nearly indistinguishable from neuroblastoma. Although the relative amount of neuroblastic tissue in a given tumor probably affects the prognosis, the presence of any immature elements makes the tumor potentially malignant.

5. How do neuroblastomas present?

Neuroblastomas may present with various symptoms due to the primary lesion or metastases. Unlike patients with Wilms tumor, patients with neuroblastoma often have systemic findings at the time of presentation. The most common presenting signs and symptoms are fever, abdominal pain or distension, abdominal mass, weight loss, anemia, bone pain, and/or proptosis and periorbital ecchymoses (due to retro-orbital metastases). Neuroblastomas may also present on prenatal ultrasonography.

6. How is neuroblastoma staged?

Although there is no universally accepted staging system for neuroblastoma, several factors seem to be most important, including the local extent of tumor beyond the organ of origin or across the midline, the completeness of surgical resection, the status of regional lymph nodes, and the presence and specific location of metastatic deposits. The international staging system suggested by Broeder et al. and used by the Children's Cancer Study Group is shown here.

Staging System for Neuroblastoma

Stage 1	Tumor confined to organ of origin with grossly complete excision
Stage 2A	Unilateral tumor with gross residual after resection
Stage 2B	Unilateral tumor with positive ipsilateral lymph nodes
Stage 3	Tumor crossing the midline or positive contralateral lymph nodes
Stage 4	Metastatic disease beyond regional lymph nodes
Stage 4S	Unilateral tumor with or without positive ipsilateral lymph nodes with metastatic disease limited to the liver, skin, and/or bone marrow

7. What is the significance of stage 4S disease?

Stage 4S reflects a unique expression of metastatic neuroblastoma. Patients are generally < 1 year of age and have relatively localized primary tumors, as well as metastases limited to the liver, skin, and bone marrow. These tumors have a tendency to resolve with little or no treatment. The survival rate for these patients in one study was 77%, compared with 6% for those with standard stage 4 disease.

8. Describe the appropriate radiographic work-up of the primary tumor in a patient with neuroblastoma.

Ultrasound is the most frequent first study in the evaluation of a child with an abdominal mass.

Either **computed tomography** (CT) or **magnetic resonance imaging** (MRI) is obtained to further characterize and stage the lesion. Both studies will detect extension beyond the midline and hepatic involvement. However, MRI better displays the relationship of the tumor to the great vessels and is able to detect intraspinal extension without invasive myelography. The latter capability is more important for neuroblastomas arising in the sympathetic chain than it is for adrenal neuroblastomas. CT offers the advantage of detecting calcification in most neuroblastomas. Because calcification is rare in Wilms tumor, this capability may be particularly important for large suprarenal tumors for which the organ of origin is uncertain.

9. Describe the metastatic evaluation.

The most common metastatic sites at presentation are regional and distant lymph nodes, bone marrow, cortical bone, liver, and skin. Preoperative radiographic evaluation of **lymphatic spread** is inaccurate. Because lymphatic involvement will ultimately be detected at surgical exploration, invasive studies, such as lymphangiography, are not routinely performed. **Bone marrow metastases** are best detected by aspiration biopsy and trephine biopsy at two sites—usually both iliac crests. Immunostaining of aspirates with monoclonal antibody has further improved the sensitivity of this technique. Bony metastates are evaluated by ^{99}Tc-MDP (technetium 99 methylene diphosphate) bone scan and a conventional skeletal survey. **Liver metastates** are detected on the MRI or CT scan used to evaluate the primary tumor. **Lung metastases** are uncommon, and a chest x-ray is adequate for detecting pulmonary involvement.

10. Why are urinary catecholamine metabolites measured?

In addition to radiographic evaluation, all patients undergo a 24-hour urine collection for measurement of catecholamine metabolites. Urinary homovanillic acid (HMA) and/or vanillylmandelic acid (VMA) levels are elevated in more than 90% of patients with neuroblastoma. The diagnosis of neuroblastoma is confirmed either by histologic evaluation of a tumor biopsy or by a positive bone marrow in conjunction with elevated urinary HMA and VMA levels.

11. What is an MIBG scan?

Metaiodobenzylguanidine (MIBG) is an amine precursor that is concentrated in neuroblastomas and other neuroendocrine tumors. MIBG scans are very sensitive for detecting neuroblastomas. They also may be helpful occasionally in distinguishing a neuroblastoma from a Wilms tumor or in detecting residual or recurrent disease.

12. List three biochemical markers of prognostic significance in neuroblastoma.

The urinary ratio of VMA/HMA, serum ferritin, and serum neuron-specific enolase. In disseminated disease, there is an inverse relation between the VMA/HMA ratio and survival. Elevated levels of ferritin and neuron-specific enolase are associated with a poor prognosis.

13. The amplification of which oncogene is associated with a poor prognosis?

The N-*myc* oncogene. A strong correlation has been found between amplification of this oncogene and poor outcome. In a study of 89 patients, 18-month progression-free survival was 70%, 30%, and 5% for patients whose tumors had 1, 3–10, and > 10 N-*myc* copies, respectively.

14. How is treatment selected for patients with neuroblastoma?
Many different treatment protocols are available for children with neuroblastoma. Treatment is generally based on a risk assessment that considers tumor stage, grade, and biochemical and genetic risk factors. Patients with low-stage favorable tumors may be treated with surgical excision alone. Patients with higher risk tumors require adjuvant multiagent chemotherapy and sometimes radiotherapy as well. Patients with very aggressive tumors are candidates for newer modalities, such as autologous bone marrow transplantation.

15. How are patients with stage 4S disease treated?
Patients with 4S disease generally do well without treatment. Patients who are good surgical risks should undergo an initial exploration to ensure that the stage assignment is correct (e.g., to ensure negative contralateral lymph nodes). The primary tumor is resected only if this can be accomplished safely. Patients are treated with low-dose irradiation and oral cyclophosphamide if massive liver involvement is present.

16. What is the general outlook for patients with neuroblastoma?
Unfortunately, despite intense research, adjunctive measures have had little impact on patient survival. Children with favorable tumors (a minority) do well without treatment beyond surgical excision, and those with unfavorable tumors do poorly despite the addition of radiation or chemotherapy.

17. Can neuroblastomas regress spontaneously?
Yes. The evidence for this comes from two sources. First, autopsy studies reveal an incidence of "neuroblastoma in situ" in fetuses and infants that is 40 times the incidence of clinically apparent neuroblastoma. Presumably, most "neuroblastomas in situ" regress. However, recent evidence suggests that what has previously been referred to as "neuroblastoma in situ" may represent a normal stage in adrenal development and may not have any direct relation to neuroblastoma itself. The second line of evidence supporting spontaneous regression comes from the behavior of stage 4S tumors. Clearly, many of these tumors become inactive despite incomplete surgical extirpation.

BIBLIOGRAPHY

1. Alexander F: Neuroblastoma. Urol Clin North Am 27:383–392, 2000.
2. Ater JL, Gradner KL, Foxhall LE, et al: Neuroblastoma screening in the United States: Results of the Texas Outreach Program for neuroblastoma screening. Cancer 82:1593–1602, 1998.
3. Brodeur GM, Nakagawara A: Molecular basis of clinical heterogeneity in neuroblastoma. Am J Pediatr Hematol Oncol 14:111–116, 1992.
4. Brodeur G, Seeger R, Barrett A, et al: International criteria for diagnosis, staging, and response to treatment in patients with neuroblastoma. J Clin Oncol 6:1874–1881, 1998.
5. Evans AE, Baum E, Chard R: Do infants with stage IV-S neuroblastoma need treatment? Arch Dis Child 56:271–274, 1981.
6. Johnson FL, Goldman S: Role of autotransplantation in neuroblastoma. Hematol Oncol Clin North Am 7:647–662, 1993.
7. Joshi VV, Cantor AB, Brodeur GM, et al: Correlation between morphologic and other prognostic markers of neuroblastoma: A study of histologic grade, DNA index, N-*myc* gene copy number, and lactic dehydrogenase in patients in the Pediatric Oncology Group. Cancer 71:3173–3181, 1993.
8. Look AT, Hayes FA, Shuster JJ, et al: Clinical relevance of tumor cell ploidy and N-*myc* gene amplification in childhood neuroblastoma: A Pediatric Oncology Group study. J Clin Oncol 9:581–591, 1991.
9. Pizzo PA, Poplack DG, Horowitz ME, et al: Solid tumors of childhood. In DeVita VT Jr., Hellman S, Rosenberg SA (eds): Cancer: Principles and Practice of Oncology. Philadelphia, J.B. Lippincott, 1993, pp 1738–1791.
10. Seeger RC, Brodeur GM, Sather H, et al: Association of multiple copies of the N-*myc* oncogene with rapid progression of neuroblastomas. N Engl J Med 313:1111–1116, 1985.

24. BENIGN TUMORS OF THE KIDNEY

Craig D. Zippe, MD

1. What CT criteria differentiate benign simple cysts from potentially malignant "complex" cysts ?

Renal cysts may be categorized by CT criteria known as **the Bosniak classification.**

Type I: seen on CT or ultrasound; require no further management.

Type II: may have a few internal septations, thin peripheral calcifications, or an attenuation value >20 Hounsfield units ((HUs) on CT. These minimally complex cysts are usually sequelae from prior hemorrhage or infection and are almost always benign. However, Bosniak type II cysts do have an incidence of carcinoma of 10–15%.

Type III: may have internal debris, thick walls or septations, or irregular calcifications. Because 40–50% of Bosniak type III cysts are malignant, they are managed surgically by either radical or partial nephrectomy.

Type IV: these lesions are complex cystic masses with enhancing nodular elements and are considered renal cell carcinoma until proven otherwise, with the incidence of cancer approaching 90%.

2. What is the most common benign renal lesion?

A **simple cyst** may be single or multiple, unilateral or bilateral, and can range from a few millimeters to several centimeters in diameter. Most simple cysts are found incidentally on abdominal ultrasound or renal imaging studies, are symptomatic, and require no treatment. Occasionally, large cysts may cause pain or obstruction of the collecting system and require excision or laparoscopic marsupialization.

3. What are the radiologic characteristics of simple cysts?

On **renal ultrasound,** simple cysts are smooth-walled, anechoic, are demarcated from surrounding parenchyma, and often exhibit posterior acoustic shadowing. On **intravenous urography,** cysts usually show a mass effect and may distort the renal outline or collecting system. On **computed tomography** (CT), cysts are thin-walled, sharply demarcated, and fluid-filled with a tissue attenuation similar to water. On **angiography,** simple cysts are vascular.

4. What is a renal cortical adenoma?

Renal cortical adenomas are small (<3 cm), asymptomatic solid tumors that are commonly encountered at autopsy or found incidentally. These adenomas comprise uniform clear and acidophilic cells with uniform histology. Although considered benign tumors histologically, renal cortical adenomas represent a premalignant early stage of renal carcinoma growth.

5. Can a renal cortical adenoma be distinguished clinically from a small renal cell carcinoma?

No. In clinical practice, these lesions are indistinguishable. Both adenomas and small renal cell carcinomas appear radiographically as solid tumors. Because small renal cell carcinomas (<3 cm) can metastasize, all solid lesions should be considered malignant. The diagnosis of adenoma is therefore based solely on pathologic examination. Molecular and cytogenetic studies suggest that adenomas of papillary histology are characterized by a loss of the Y chromosome and trisomy of chromosomes 7 and 17, as compared with renal cell carcinoma, which is characterized by a deletion of the short arm of chromosome 3.

6. Describe the gross and histologic appearance of renal oncocytoma.

On gross examination, oncocytomas vary considerably in size and have ranged from 0.3–20 cm in diameter. Classically, they are well circumscribed and have a mahogany-brown surface. The larger tumors may contain a central stellate fibrotic scar. Hemorrhage is uncommon, and cystic change is rare. Histologically, they have a homogeneous appearance, composed of uniform polygonal cells with a moderate amount of eosinophilic, granular cytoplasm. Mitoses are rare. Electron microscopy demonstrates an abundance of mitochondria, which are responsible for the characteristic eosinophilic cytoplasm. Oncocytomas are believed to arise from proximal convoluted tubules and show no tendency to invade surrounding structures or metastasize.

7. Can renal oncocytoma be distinguished clinically or radiographically from renal cell carcinoma?

No. Although increasingly diagnosed as incidental radiographic findings, both tumors may present with hematuria or other symptoms and appear radiographically as solid mass lesions that distort the renal contour and/or collecting system. Although the appearance of a central stellate scar on CT or a spoke-wheel pattern of tumor vessels on angiography is suggestive of oncocytoma, such patterns are rare (<10%) and nonspecific. Both oncocytoma and renal cell carcinoma can be multicentric in the same kidney (5–10%) or bilateral (3–5%) at presentation. Both show a predilection for males (2:1) with mean ages in the sixth decade at presentation. Oncocytoma can occur simultaneously with renal cell carcinoma in the same or contralateral kidney in up to one third of cases. The main clinical difference in presentation is the incidence of the two lesions: <5% of renal neoplasms are renal oncocytomas, but renal cell carcinoma accounts for 95% of all solid renal masses.

8. Can renal oncocytoma be distinguished pathologically from renal cell carcinoma?

Yes. True oncocytomas are low grade, have a homogeneous organoid histologic appearance, have diploid DNA histograms, lack expressions of HLA A, B, and C antigens, and are characterized by loss of the Y chromosome and translocations involving the long arm of chromosome 11. It should be emphasized that many renal cell carcinomas may contain variable "oncocytic" features on histologic examination that may be misleading if the tumor is not adequately sampled. However, the histologic appearance of (1) necrosis or hemorrhage, (2) clear cell foci, (3) prominent papillary patterns, or (4) nuclear atypia or mitoses confirms a diagnosis of renal cell carcinoma. The frequent coexistence of "oncocytic" histology with renal cell carcinoma in the same or opposite kidney limits the preoperative use of percutaneous needle biopsy of solid renal masses to establish the diagnosis of oncocytoma.

9. How is renal oncocytoma treated?

Surgical excision, by open/laparoscopic partial or radical nephrectomy.

10. Describe the gross and histologic appearance of angiomyolipoma (or renal hamartoma).

Grossly, angiomyolipomas are unencapsulated, yellow-to-gray in appearance, and may extend into the collecting system or perirenal fat. These tumors arise from mesenchymal tissue and are composed of variable amounts of abnormal blood vessels (*angio-*), smooth muscle (*myo-*), and mature fat (*lipoma*). The smooth muscle cells are benign in appearance and are arranged in sheets and bundles. The blood vessels are thick with muscular walls and lack elastic lamellae. The vascularity, rigidity, and tortuosity of the blood vessels predispose them to hemorrhage.

11. Describe the radiologic appearance of renal angiomyolipoma.

The radiologic appearance of these lesions is determined by their proportion of fat content. By ultrasonography, they appear as highly well-circumscribed but not encapsulated, echogenic, and hyperechoic renal masses. Although ultrasound may be suggestive of angiomyolipoma, a CT scan is recommended to confirm the presence of fat, renal cell carcinoma, or both. On CT, angiomyolipomas appear as heterogeneous solid tumors that can achieve massive size. The CT hallmark of such tumors is the presence of fat density within the tumor, which usually appears black on CT and measures -10 to -30 HUs. Negative HU or attenuation numbers normally confirm the diagnosis of angiomyolipoma and rule out renal cell carcinoma. Wilms tumor, oncocytomas, liposarcomas, and large renal cell cancers involving perirenal fat, however, can occasionally contain fat. The presence of calcification on CT is rare in angiomyolipoma and prompts further evaluation. In 25% of cases, the tumors may be confused with malignancy because of extension outside of the renal capsule. Occasionally, lymph node involvement occurs, but deaths from these "metastases" have never been reported and no systemic dissemination following nodal involvement has been documented.

12. What is the incidence and clinical presentation of angiomyolipoma?

Angiomyolipomas account for only 0.3% of all renal neoplasms and present sporadically (80% of patients) or in association with tuberous sclerosis (20%). Sporadic angiomyolipomas are more commonly unilateral, right-sided lesions (two-thirds of cases), occur almost exclusively in adult females (5:1 ratio), and are usually smaller and less frequently bilateral than those seen with tuberous sclerosis. Alternatively, 40–80% of patients with tuberous sclerosis develop renal angiomyolipomas. Patients with tuberous sclerosis (an autosomal dominant disorder) are characterized by mental retardation, epilepsy, and adenoma sebaceum, and may have coincident renal cell carcinoma with the angiomyolipoma. In addition to the kidneys, angiomyolipomas (hamartomas) may be found in the brain, eye, heart, lung, and bone. Because of the high incidence and potential morbidity of renal hamartomas, all patients with tuberous sclerosis should be screened with renal ultrasonography or CT.

13. Are there are other differences in the presentation of patients with renal hamartomas of tuberous sclerosis versus those with sporadic angiomyolipomas?

The angiomyolipomas of tuberous sclerosis occur at a younger age, are bilateral in 80% of cases, and tend to be larger at the time of diagnosis. The symptomatic presentations and histologic appearances are similar. Although increasingly diagnosed incidentally, both types occur with similar symptoms, including abdominal or flank pain, palpable mass, intratumoral hemorrhage, hematuria, anemia, and hypertension.

14. How is angiomyolipoma treated?

The treatment of angiomyolipoma depends on the tumor size and the presence of symptoms. Nearly 80% of tumors < 4 cm in diameter are usually asymptomatic, whereas 80% of tumors >4 cm are symptomatic. Solitary asymptomatic lesions <4 cm may be observed with yearly CT or ultrasound. Larger asymptomatic tumors may be similarly observed, but CT scans or sonograms need to be performed every 6 months. Any lesion that is symptomatic or showing progressive growth on follow-up studies should be embolized or excised surgically with a partial nephrectomy. Since the diagnosis of angiomylipoma can usually be suspected preoperatively and is rarely associated with renal cell carcinoma, a nephron-sparing surgical procedure is indicated. Delaying treatment until a spontaneous rupture occurs or until there is a large intratumoral hemorrhage often will necessitate a radical nephrectomy.

15. Are the angiomyolipomas associated with tuberous sclerosis treated differently?

The nephron-sparing approach is particularly important in patients with tuberous sclerosis, in whom both kidneys may be affected by multiple tumors. In these cases, surgery should be delayed until tumors reach >4 cm or are associated with significant symptoms.

16. What other benign tumors affect the kidneys?

Fibromas, lipomas, myomas, lymphangiomas, and **hemangiomas** occur rarely, arising from the renal capsule or other stromal elements of the kidney. Radiographically, these can be large solid masses and treatment is surgical excision. Because of the uncertainty of clinical diagnosis, the true benign potential of such tumors is usually not established until they are removed surgically and examined histologically.

17. What rare benign renal tumor can cause hypertension in a young patient?

A **juxtaglomerular tumor.** This functional tumor causes a syndrome of hypertension, elevated serum renin, and hyperaldosteronism due to a renin-secreting tumor of the juxtaglomerular cells. Tumors are usually small (<3 cm), not routinely detected radiographically, located in the cortex, and curable by surgery. The diagnosis of a juxtaglomerular tumor is made by selective renal vein sampling, with an extremely high differential renal vein:renin ratio.

BIBLIOGRAPHY

1. Bennington JL: Renal adenoma. World J Urol 5:6, 2987.
2. Bonavita JA, Pollack HM, Banner MP: Renal oncocytoma: Further observation and literature review. Urol Radiol 2:229–232, 1981.
3. Bosniak M: The current radiological approach to renal cysts. Radiology 158:1–10, 1986.
4. Bosniak MA, Megibow AJ, Hulnick DH: CT diagnosis of renal angiomyolipoma: The importance of detecting small amounts of fat. AJR 151:497–501, 1988.
5. Licht MR, Novick AC, Tubbs RR, et al: Renal oncocytoma: Clinical and biological correlates. J Urol 150:1380–1383, 1993.
6. Maatman TJ, Novick AC, Tancino BF, et al: Renal oncocytoma: A diagnostic and therapeutic dilemma. J Urol 132:878–880, 1984.
7. Meloni A, Bridge J, Sandbert AA: Reviews on chromosome studies in urological tumors. I. Renal tumors. J Urol 148:253–265, 1992.
8. Murphy GP, Mostofi FK: Histological assessment and clinical prognosis of renal adenoma. J Urol 103: 31–36, 1970.
9. Oesterling J, Fishman EK, Goldman SM, Marshall FF: The management of renal angiomyolipomas. J. Urol 125:1121–1125, 1992.
10. Quinn MJ, Hartman DS, Friedman A, et al: Renal oncocytoma: New observations. Radiology 153:49–52, 1984.
11. Siegel CL, McFarland EG, Brink JA, et al: CT of cystic renal masses: Analysis of diagnostic performance and interobserver variation. AJR 169:813, 1997.
12. Steiner MS, Goldman SM, Fishman EK, Marshall FF: The natural history of renal angiomyolipoma. J Urol 150:1782–1786, 1993.
13. Stillwell TJ, Gomez MR, Kelalis PP: Renal lesions in tuberous sclerosis. J Urol 138:477–481, 1987.
14. Wegryn JD, Resnick MI: Angiomyolipoma: Diagnosis and conservative management. Contemp Urol 10: 55–61, 1998.
15. Weiss MA, Mills SE. Genitourinary Tract Pathology. St. Louis, Mosby-Wolfe, 1992.
16. Wills JS: Management of small renal neoplasms and angiomyolipoma: A growing problem. Radiology 197:583–586, 1995.

25. RETROPERITONEAL TUMORS

Elroy D. Kursh, M.D.

1. How common are primary retroperitoneal tumors?

They are rare. In a large series from the United States, retroperitoneal tumors represented 0.16–0.2% of all malignancies. Of all the soft tissue sarcomas, about 15% are retroperitoneal in origin.

2. What are the pathologic types of primary retroperitoneal tumors?

There are numerous varieties of retroperitoneal neoplasms. Malignant tumors are more common than benign lesions, accounting for 70–80%. Liposarcoma predominates, followed by leiomyosarcoma, fibrosarcoma, and neurogenic sarcoma. Malignant fibrous histiocytomas are being diagnosed with increased frequency due to a better understanding of the histopathology of this lesion and subsequent reclassification of many tumors previously diagnosed as pleomorphic variants of the above-mentioned neoplasms.

3. Describe the signs and symptoms of a retroperitoneal tumor.

The most common early signs of a retroperitoneal tumor are the insidious development of abdominal enlargement and weight loss, which may be associated with diffuse and often vague abdominal pain and fever. Because of their location in the retroperitoneum, the tumors may become large or even mammoth before they are noticed. Various other symptoms may be associated with retroperitoneal tumors, such as nausea or vomiting, obstipation, leg edema, flank pain, dysuria, urgency, and hematuria; back pain may occur later in the course of disease from compression or invasion of adjacent organs. Oddly, the patient rarely notes an increase in abdominal girth despite the frequent large size of the mass, which is usually palpable and represents the most constant physical finding, occurring in about 75% of patients.

4. How is the diagnosis of primary retroperitoneal tumor established?

Radiographic examination confirms the presence of a retroperitoneal mass. Contrast-enhanced computed tomography (CT) and magnetic resonance (MR) imaging have become the most reliable means of determining the size and consistency of the tumor and the relationship of the neoplasm to contiguous retroperitoneal and intraperitoneal structures.

5. Are any other diagnostic studies indicated?

Because nephrectomy is often required to completely excise the neoplasm (in about 20% of cases), excretory urography may be indicated to assess the status of the involved and opposite kidney if abdominal CT and/or MR imaging does not yield satisfactory information. Varying degrees of hydronephrosis may be present, and displacement of the kidney is not uncommon. If the patient has symptoms referable to the intestinal tract or the CT scan suggests possible involvement, barium contrast studies of the gastrointestinal tract are indicated. If there is questionable involvement of the vena cava or aorta, MR imaging should be performed because this study provides superior resolution of the great vessels. MR imaging is also superior in assessing invasion of contiguous structures, particularly in assessing possible muscle involvement. Venography may be indicated if the MR image does not provide satisfactory resolution of the vena cava. Three-dimensional CT is an excellent relatively new imaging study to define the relationship of the mass to contiguous structures, particularly in relation to surgical planning. Staging of retroperitoneal sarcomas includes evaluation of the liver and lungs because these are the primary sites of metastasis in approximately 40–50% of those that metastasize; most, however, recur locally before developing metastasis.

6. What is the treatment of primary retroperitoneal tumors?

The only effective treatment is **surgical removal** of the mass. Bowel preparation is indicated preoperatively because complete excision may require bowel resection in up to 20% of cases. Adequate exposure is achieved through an abdominal transperitoneal route and, if possible, excision of the tumor is done well outside the tumor "pseudocapsule." Excision of adjacent organs, such as the kidney, is performed concurrently if it is necessary to widely remove all gross tumor; it has been demonstrated that if this maneuver provides complete resection, long-term survival is comparable to patients with complete resection without adjacent organ removal. Unfortunately, complete excision is feasible in only about 50–75% of cases. If complete extirpation of the tumor is feasible, it is preferable to avoid open biopsy because of the risk of implanting the tumor and causing diffuse peritoneal sarcomatosis. If all gross tumor cannot be removed, partial resection should be reserved for patients with significant symptoms that can be palliated by surgery because recent data do not show a survival advantage for those patients undergoing incomplete resection compared with no resection at all (median survival, 18 months). Involvement of the large vessels, spinal cord, or nerve plexus clearly renders a patient's tumor unresectable. Modern aggressive surgery has led to a reported increased resectability rate of 80–85% in recent reviews of patients presenting with primary disease.

7. What is the prognosis of a primary retroperitoneal tumor?

In the past, 5-year survival figures have been dismal, ranging from 5–20%. Reported 5-year survival rates continue to improve to >50% with more aggressive surgical resection and improved perioperative care. A recent review of a large clinical experience with a median follow-up of 28 months (range, 1 to 172 months) revealed a median survival of patients who underwent complete resection of 103 months. The median survival was 72 months for patients with primary disease compared with 28 months for those with local recurrence and 10 months for those with metastasis. Survival, therefore, is significantly dependent on both the ability of the surgeon to completely resect the tumor and histologic grade, but it has been shown that tumor size does not influence the outcome, which differs from soft tissue sarcoma of the extremity.

8. Is any other therapy indicated for primary retroperitoneal tumor?

Because of the success of radiotherapy in soft tissue sarcomas of the extremities, some have advised adjuvant radiation following surgical removal of retroperitoneal sarcomas, but its exact role remains unclear. In the past, the ability to deliver large enough doses of radiation therapy was limited owing to toxicity of adjacent intraperitoneal organs, particularly the small bowel. Innovative methods to escalate the dosage of adjuvant radiation therapy above 55 Gy and to reduce the local recurrence rate are being attempted more often by using intraoperative radiation therapy, brachytherapy, and small bowel exclusion devices, in addition to preoperative and/or postoperative external beam radiotherapy. Postoperative radiation therapy is generally attempted if the tumor cannot be completely resected or pathology reveals positive margins. The role of adjuvant chemotherapy in the treatment of retroperitoneal sarcomas, except for embryonal rhabdomyosarcoma, is unknown because randomized studies have not been published, but it is being attempted more often. Patients with incomplete initial resection who are <50 years old and who have high-grade tumors are candidates for investigational adjuvant therapy such as intraperitoneal chemotherapy or experimental immunotherapy.

9. How should patients be followed after a primary surgical extirpation?

Retroperitoneal sarcomas lend themselves to repeat attempts at removal because of their tendency to recur locally and their slow growth. Therefore, follow-up CT scans of the abdomen are indicated. Scans are obtained every 4–6 months for an arbitrary period of 3 years postoperatively, and then yearly thereafter for up to 10 or more years because late recurrence is common (some estimate that it may exceed 70% in patients who have undergone complete surgical resection), and the median time to local recurrence was longer than 5 years in a recent review. If recurrent tumor is noted, repeat surgical excision is worthwhile and may even provide a cure; a definite survival advantage has been demonstrated in patients undergoing multiple resections.

BIBLIOGRAPHY

1. Heslin MJ, Lewis JJ, Nadler E, et al: Prognostic factors associated with long-term survival for retroperitoneal sarcoma: Implications for management. J Clin Oncol 15:2832–2839, 1997.
2. Lewis JJ, Leung D, Woodruff JM, et al: Retroperitoneal soft-tissue sarcoma: Analysis of 500 patients treated and followed at a single institution. Ann Surg 228:355–365, 1998.
3. Mahajan A: The contemporary role of the use of radiation therapy in the management of sarcoma. Surg Oncol Clin North Am 9:503–524, 2000.
4. McGinn CJ: The role of radiation therapy in resectable retroperitoneal sarcomas. Surg Oncol 9:61–65, 2000.
5. Wyndham TC, Pearson AS, Skibber JM, et al: Significance and management of local recurrences and limited metastatic disease in the abdomen. Surg Clin North Am 80:761–774, 2000.

26. URETERAL TUMORS

Stevan B. Streem, M.D.

1. How do patients with ureteral tumors present?
The most frequent symptoms are hematuria or flank pain associated with obstruction. However, because ureteral tumors are generally slow-growing, the obstruction can be insidious and is often painless.

2. Are ureteral tumors usually benign or malignant?
Benign tumors of the ureter are the exception, although pediatric patients in particular may have fibroepithelial polyps. The vast majority of ureteral tumors are urothelial in origin, and almost all of these are transitional cell carcinoma (TCC). Squamous cell carcinoma of the ureter is extremely rare but may occur in association with chronic inflammation or infection.

3. Are the risk factors for TCC of the ureter the same as for TCC of the bladder?
The environmental carcinogens associated with TCC of the bladder appear to place the patient at increased risk for upper tract TCC. In addition, specific risk factors for upper tract TCC have been described and include analgesic abuse, papillary necrosis, and Balkan nephropathy. Cigarette smoking places the entire urothelium at increased risk for TCC.

4. Does a history of TCC of the bladder place the patient at increased risk for ureteral tumors?
Yes. TCC represents urothelial "field change," a disease characterized by a tendency to polychronotopism (multiple recurrences in time and space). The incidence of upper tract disease in patients with TCC of the bladder is approximately 3%.

5. Are all parts of the ureter affected with equal frequency?
No. The risk for ureteral TCC increases progressively from the rarely affected proximal ureter to the more frequently involved distal ureter.

6. How is the diagnosis of a ureteral tumor made?
Generally, a patient with hematuria will undergo an intravenous pyelogram (IVP) that reveals a filling defect of the ureter or obstruction. A retrograde study is then often done for better radiographic definition. A tumor is suggested by a persistent intraluminal filling defect.

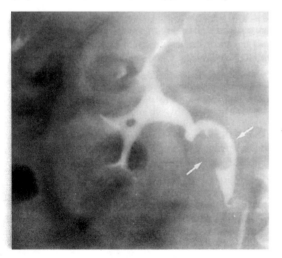

Retrograde pyelogram reveals a proximal ureteral "filling defect" (*arrows*) in a patient with painless hematuria (subsequently proven to be TCC).

7. What radiographic studies can be done to differentiate the radiographic appearance of a tumor from a benign problem such as a lucent calculus?

Calculi can be distinguished from ureteral tumors by ultrasound or CT. Of these two options, CT is the more sensitive.

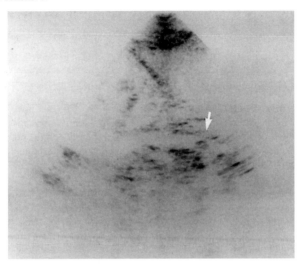

This patient had left-sided obstruction to the level of a proximal ureteral filling defect by intravenous urography. Ultrasound clearly reveals the problem to be a calculus in the proximal ureter ("defect" is highly echogenic and casts acoustic shadows. This is consistent with a calculus, presumably uric acid).

8. Is urine cytology helpful?

A voided cytology has a relatively high false-negative rate for ureteral tumors. Cytologic accuracy may be improved by examination of urine obtained selectively from the involved side at the time of cystoscopy and retrograde studies. Brushing the lesion for cytologic examination also may be done at that time.

9. What is the single most accurate way of diagnosing a ureteral tumor?

If the diagnosis remains in doubt, upper tract endoscopy with semi-rigid or flexible ureteroscopes offers a high degree of reliability in diagnosis. During ureteroscopy, biopsies may be obtained to help with preoperative grading and even staging of the tumor.

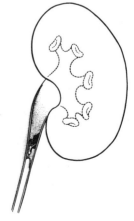

Diagrammatic representation of transureteroscopic biopsy of a ureteral tumor.

10. What is the staging classification for ureteral tumors?

Staging is analogous to that for TCC of the bladder:

Staging System for Ureteral Tumors

UICC	JEWITT	PATHOLOGY
pTa	0	Confined to mucosa
pT_1	A	Confined to lamina propia
$pT_2'pT_3a$	$B_1.B_2$	Confined to muscularis
$pT_{3b}'pT_4'N1$	C'D	Periureteral tissue or lymph node involvement

11. What is the best treatment for a ureteral tumor?

Because TCC of the ureter can be multifocal, standard definitive treatment (assuming the contralateral kidney is normal) is a nephroureterectomy during which the entire kidney, ureter, and a cuff of the bladder are removed. If the tumor is limited to the distal ureter, a distal ureterectomy with reimplantation is also acceptable and, in fact, is generally preferred.

12. What about removing just part of the ureter if the tumor is in the proximal or mid-ureter?

The risk of ipsilateral recurrence is highest when the ureter is left below the level of the tumor. However, segmental ureterectomy can almost always be justified in the presence of a functionally solitary kidney, significant contralateral renal disease, or bilateral upper tract TCC. Indications for segmental ureterectomy in the presence of a normal contralateral kidney are controversial, although some urologists feel segmental ureterectomy is justifiable if the tumor is unifocal, low-grade, and low-stage.

13. What roles do radiation and chemotherapy have in ureteral carcinoma?

Radiation therapy has marginal proven benefit for upper tract TCC. However, for invasive disease, combination chemotherapy protocols analogous to those for invasive TCC of the bladder may be beneficial.

BIBLIOGRAPHY

1. Albarran MJ, 1902, cited by Melicow MM and Findlay HV: Primary benign tumors of the ureter: Review of literature and report of a case. Surg Gynecol Obstet 54:680, 1932.
2. Babaian RJ: Primary carcinoma of the upper urinary tract urothelium: An overview. In Crawford ED, Pas S (eds): Current Genitourinary Cancer Surgery. Philadelphia, Lea and Febiger, 1990.
3. Babaian RJ, Johnson DE: Primary carcinoma of the ureter. J Urol 123:357, 1980.
4. Babaian RJ, Johnson DE, Chan RC: Combination nephroureterectomy and postoperative radiotherapy for infiltrative ureteral carcinoma. Int J Radiat Oncol Biol Phys 6:1229, 1980.
5. Batata MA, et al: Primary carcinoma of the ureter: A prognostic study. Cancer 35:1626, 1975.
6. Hendin BN, Streem SB, Levin HS, et al: Impact of diagnostic ureteroscopy on long-term survival in patients with upper tract transitional cell carcinoma. J Urol 161:783, 1999.
7. Huffman JL, Bagley DH, Lyon ES, et al: Endoscopic diagnosis and treatment of the upper tract urothelial tumors. Cancer 55:1422, 1985.
8. Keeley FX Jr, Bibbo M, Bagley DH: Ureteroscopic treatment and surveillance of upper urinary tract transitional cell carcinoma. J Urol 157:1560, 1997.
9. Keeley FX Jr, Kulp DA, Bibbo M, et al: Diagnostic accuracy of ureteroscopic biopsy in upper tract transitional cell carcinoma. J Urol 157:33, 1997.
10. McCoy JG, Honda H, Reznicek M, et al: Computerized tomography for detection and staging of localized and pathologically defined upper tract urothelial tumors. J Urol 146:1500, 1991.
11. Schmauz R , Cole P: Epidemiology of cancer of the renal pelvis and ureter. I.N.C.I. 523:1431, 1974.
12. Streem SB, Pontes JE, Novick AC, et al: Ureteropyeloscopy in the evaluation of upper tract filling defects. J Urol 136:383, 1986.
13. Vest SA: Conservative surgery in certain benign tumors of the ureter. J Urol 53:97, 1945.
14. Zincke H, et al: Significance of urinary cytology in the early detection of transitional cell cancer of the upper urinary tract. J Urol 116:781, 1976.

27. TRANSITIONAL CELL CARCINOMA OF THE BLADDER

William A. Larchian, M.D.

1. What is the incidence of transitional cell carcinoma (TCC) of the bladder?

About 55,500 new cases of bladder TCC were diagnosed in the United States in 2001, occurring in a 3:1 male-to-female ratio. TCC is the fourth most common cancer in men and eighth most common in women. Worldwide, TCC accounts for 250,000 new diagnoses of bladder cancer and 120,000 deaths annually.

2. What risk factors are associated with bladder TCC?

- Age (peak incidence in seventh decade)
- Occupational exposure to aniline dyes and aromatic amines
- Cigarette smoking (four times increased risk)
- Phenacetin abuse
- Treatment with cyclophosphamide

3. Describe the histologic appearance of normal bladder urothelium.

Normal bladder is lined by transitional cell epithelium that varies from 3–7 cells in thickness. The basal layer rests on a lamina propria basement membrane and is covered by several layers of intermediate cells, with the most superficial layer composed of flat "umbrella" cells. The lamina propria contains a discontinuous muscularis mucosa and is rich in lymphatics. The muscularis propria lies deep to the lamina propria.

4. What proliferative lesions in bladder urothelium can be confused with TCC?

1. Epithelial hyperplasia
2. Atypical hyperplasia
3. Inverted papilloma
4. Cystitis cystica
5. von Brunn's nests
6. Cystitis glandularis
7. Nephrogenic adenoma
8. Squamous metaplasia

5. What is the significance of epithelial and atypical hyperplasia?

Epithelial hyperplasia is a benign proliferation of urothelium in response to inflammation or irritation. **Atypical hyperplasia** is characterized by an increased number of cell layers *and* nuclear atypia with derangement of the umbrella layer. Atypical hyperplasia is preneoplastic.

6. Describe von Brunn's nests and their significance.

von Brunn's nests are islands of benign-appearing urothelium residing in the submucosa and resulting from inward proliferation of the basal cell layer. They are a normal variant of urothelial histology.

7. What are cystitis cystica and cystitis glandularis?

Both are variants of von Brunn's nests with additional histologic changes. In **cystitis cystica,** the center of the nest is filled with liquefied material and appears more cyst-like than glandular. In **cystitis glandularis,** the transitional epithelium has undergone glandular metaplasia, and the cells appear columnar with mucin-containing cytoplasm. Cystitis glandularis may appear as a papillary lesion, is often associated with pelvic lipomatosis, and may give rise to adenocarcinoma.

8. Describe inverted papilloma and nephrogenic adenoma and explain their significance.

Both inverted papilloma and nephrogenic adenoma are benign lesions that occur in response to trauma or infection. **Inverted papilloma** is a submucosal proliferative lesion that typically occurs on the trigone and vesical neck and is covered by normal urothelium. **Nephrogenic adenoma** appears raised or papillary and histologically resembles primitive renal collecting tubules.

9. What is squamous metaplasia?

Squamous metaplasia is a benign proliferative and metaplastic lesion in which normal urothelium is replaced by nonkeratinized squamous epithelium. It appears most commonly as whitish plaques on the trigone in women.

10. Bladder cancer most frequently occurs as what histologic type?

Transitional cell carcinoma accounts for > 90% of all bladder cancers. Other histologic subtypes arising from urothelium include adenocarcinoma, squamous carcinoma, and urachal carcinoma.

11. Which nonurothelial tumors occur in the bladder?

- Small cell carcinoma
- Lymphoma
- Sarcoma (typically leiomyosarcoma)
- Pheochromocytoma
- Carcinosarcoma
- Metastatic tumors

12. Explain the staging system for TCC.

TCC is divided into noninvasive ("superficial") and invasive forms. Noninvasive tumors may appear papillary or flat and do not invade the muscularis propria. Papillary tumors are frondular or more solid-appearing exophytic tumors that project into the bladder lumen. Flat tumors are usually carcinoma-in-situ (CIS), which appears as an erythematous velvety patch comprising high-grade TCC.

Invasive tumors demonstrate invasion into muscularis propria, are usually solid, and exhibit a sessile growth pattern. Papillary tumors that invade the lamina propria are sometimes called "superficially invasive."

Staging System for TCC

STAGE	DEFINITION
Superficial tumors	
Ta	Confined to mucosa
T1	Invasion into lamina propria
TIS	Intraepithelial CIS
Invasive tumors	
T2	Invasion into superficial muscularis propria
T3a	Invasion into deep muscularis propria
T3b	Invasion through muscle into perivesical fat
T4	Invasion into adjacent organs

13. How is TCC graded histologically?

Most systems assign grade based on the degree of cellular anaplasia, although there is no universally accepted scheme. Normal urothelium exhibits a very regular pattern of base-to-surface cellular maturation and polarity. TCC exhibits progressive degrees of disturbance in this orderly array and is graded accordingly. Distinction is usually made between well, moderately, and poorly differentiated tumors which correspond to low, medium, or high grades. Most CIS is considered high grade, although some systems include lower grades.

14. Explain the difference between bladder papilloma and well-differentiated TCC.

Some pathologists distinguish these as separate entities. A **papilloma,** sometimes referred to as a grade 0 tumor, is a papillary lesion with a thin fibrovascular core covered with normal urothelium. A **well-differentiated papillary TCC** is a grade 1 papillary tumor with a thickened urothelium exhibiting mild anaplasia and pleomorphism.

15. What cytogenetic abnormalities have been obeserved in TCC?

Abnormalities (gains, losses, or rearrangements) of chromosomes 3, 5, 7, 9, and 11 are observed with increased frequency in TCC. Trisomy 7 and deletions of all or part of chromosomes 9 and 11p occur most commonly. In addition, defects in the P450 cytochrome oxidase system have been identified in the induction of neoplastic tranformation.

16. What is meant by "field change"?

The common occurrence of multifocal TCC, the high frequency of recurrent tumors at new sites, and the occasional occurrence of concurrent or asynchronous upper tract TCC have suggested that the entire urothelium has a propensity to develop tumors. Presumably this is due to diffuse genetic instability or urothelium that leads to multiple tumor clones. However, some evidence suggests that at least some tumors are derived from a single (monoclonal) source that gives rise to multifocal tumors by implantation, pagetoid spread, or lymphatic spread.

17. How does bladder cancer present?

The most frequent presenting symptom is painless hematuria, especially for noninvasive tumors. Irritative symptoms, including frequency, urgency, and dysuria, are also common and suggest diffuse CIS or invasive cancer. Other symptoms can include flank pain due to ureteral obstruction, pelvic mass, or those due to metastatic disease.

18. What is the natural history of noninvasive TCC? Invasive TCC?

Approximately 70–75% of TCC are superficial, noninvasive tumors at presentation, and most low-grade tumors are destined to remain so. However, most patients, depending upon tumor size, grade, focality, ploidy, and other factors, are prone to multiple recurrences over time and in other bladder sites. About 10–15% of noninvasive tumors, usually those of higher grade and with documented invasion of the lamina propria, progress to muscle invasion.

Most invasive tumors are invasive at the time of diagnosis, and about one-half have occult metastatic disease. Untreated invasive disease predictably results in patient death within about 2 years.

19. What prognostic factors predict an aggressive potential for noninvasive tumors?

Tumor grade*	Ploidy
Tumor stage*	Frequency of recurrence
Presence of CIS*	Marker chromosomes
Lymphatic invasion	Expression of Lewis X antigen
Size	Epidermal growth factor receptor expression
Multifocality	Expression of p53
	Loss of expression of the Rb protein

*Most important prognostic factors.

20. Describe the clinical features of CIS.

CIS may be asymptomatic or produce irritative urinary symptoms (urgency, frequency, bladder pain) that are often confused with prostatism, infection, interstitial cystitis, or neurogenic bladder. CIS occurs more commonly in men and may occur alone or in association with noninvasive papillary or invasive TCC. Symptomatic CIS is typically due to diffuse urothelial involvement. When associated with other tumors, CIS is usually more focal and may surround the base of a high-grade papillary tumor. The occurrence of CIS in conjunction with papillary tumors indicates a higher likelihood of recurrence and progression to invasive disease. Urinary cytology is almost universally positive in the presence of CIS because of tumor cell slough from the basement membrane of the lamina propria.

21. How should patients with suspected TCC be evaluated?

Patients should have a urinary cytology, bimanual examination under anesthesia, diagnostic cystoscopy with tumor biopsy or resection, and an upper tract imaging study. In some patients, biopsy of the prostatic urethra is also indicated. Flow cytometric and quantitative fluorescent image analysis to detect aneuploid stem lines in bladder wash specimens is still investigative.

22. Should random areas of normal-appearing mucosa be biopsied at resection of noninvasive tumors?

This is controversial. Some urologists believe that the detection of occult dysplasia or focal CIS by this method adds prognostic information and influences treatment decisions. Several studies have shown, however, that routine use of random biopsies is not helpful. A disadvantage of random biopsies is the potential for tumor implantation at the biopsy sites.

23. What is the ideal imaging study in evaluating patients with TCC?

The ideal study should evaluate renal function, test for the presence of renal parenchymal abnormalities, and visualize the upper tract urothelium. This is best achieved with an intravenous urogram, although renal ultrasound and retrograde pyelograms yield similar information but without functional details. A CT scan of the abdomen and pelvis is not indicated in patients with noninvasive tumors because of the low likelihood of extravesical disease. MRI is not capable of distinguishing the depth of tumor invasion. In patients with invasive tumors, a CT scan of the abdomen and pelvis is helpful in determining tumor extent and the presence of macroscopically enlarged lymph nodes, but a "negative" scan does not rule out the presence of microscopic lymphatic metastasis.

24. What markers in voided urine help in the detection of TCC?

Bladder tumor antigen (BTA) detects substances released from the extracellular matrix in the presence of bladder cancer. Unfortunately, BTA does not appear to have sufficient sensitivity to detect most low-grade malignancies. NMP22 is derived from nuclear matrix protein mitotic apparatus. The sensitivity of NMP22 for low-grade disease appears to be better than that of BTA or urine cytology, approximately 70%. Telomerase is a ribonucleoprotein enzyme responsible for the production of DNA sequences that protect the ends of chromosomes from mutation during replication. Interpretation of telomerase levels in voided urine has an overall sensitivity of 80% in detecting urothelial malignancies.

25. How are noninvasive tumors managed?

TCC is initially managed by transurethral resection. In patients with low-grade (1 or 2) Ta tumors, cystoscopy at regular intervals and with repeat resection or fulguration as necessary is usually adequate. In patients with multiple and frequent recurrences and those with grade 3 or T1 tumors at presentation, intravesical immunotherapy or chemotherapy is generally employed.

26. What is the recommended regimen for surveillance cystoscopy following resection of noninvasive TCC?

Historical practice has been to do cystoscopy at 3-month intervals for the first 2 years, then every 6 months for 1–2 years, then yearly, although recent evidence suggests that low-grade tumors can be safely followed with urinary cytology and less frequent cystoscopy.

27. What are the most effective intravesical agents for treating noninvasive TCC?

Immunotherapy with bacille Calmette-Guérin (BCG) is the most active agent for most patients with noninvasive tumors. Recently, studies using a combination of BCG with interferon-α have shown significant response rates for patients who failed BCG alone. Mitomycin C is the most active chemotherapeutic agent. Doxorubicin, Epodyl, and thiotepa are also used occasionally.

28. How is CIS treated?

Because the natural history of CIS is variable, some patients have an indolent course of multiple recurrences without progression, whereas others progress soon after diagnosis and develop metastatic disease despite early therapy. Current first-line treatment for diffuse CIS is intravesical immunotherapy with BCG, which produces complete responses in up to 70% of patients. Treatment of refractory or recurrent CIS after BCG therapy is still evolving, with some advocating repeat BCG instillation, second-line therapy with another intravesical agent such as mitomycin C or interferon-α, or radical cystectomy. Patients with CIS who fail two courses of intravesical therapy are at high risk for progressive cancer and should undergo cystectomy.

29. What are the goals of intravesical immunotherapy or chemotherapy?

It depends on the stage and grade of the tumor:

STAGE	GOAL
Multiple recurrent low-grade Ta	Prevent or reduce rate of recurrences
Grade 3 and T1	Prevent recurrences and progression to muscle invasion
Diffuse CIS	Eradicate established tumor

30. What are the side effects of BCG?

Local symptoms of bladder irritability are most prominent. Mild systemic symptoms with low-grade fever and myalgias are also common. High or persistent fever (> 24–48 hr) and/or more severe systemic symptoms require early antituberculous therapy. Several deaths have been attributed to systemic "BCGosis," usually occurring after intravesical administration following traumatic urethral catheterization.

31. Do lasers have a role in the treatment of TCC?

The Nd:YAG laser is an alternative to fulguration of recurrent low-grade noninvasive tumors with the potential advantages of outpatient use without anesthesia, a low risk of infield recurrence, and lower risk of tumor implantation. However, use of the laser without resection or biopsy provides no pathologic or prognostic information and should be restricted to patients with recurrent tumors who are judged to be at low risk of progression.

Photodynamic therapy with a systemic photosensitizer and argon-dye laser is an experimental approach for treating BCG-refractory diffuse CIS and for prophylaxis against recurrent papillary tumors. This method is cumbersome owing to cutaneous photosensitivity, uncertainties about light dosimetry, and the development of severe bladder contractures.

32. What is the risk of developing an upper tract TCC after diagnosis of bladder TCC?

Approximately 5%. The frequency with which repeat upper tract screening studies (urogram or retrograde pyelograms) need to be performed has never been adequately defined. Historical practice has been to perform them at yearly intervals.

33. What is the risk of developing bladder TCC after diagnosis of an upper tract TCC?

Approximately 40–70%. All patients with upper tract TCC require cystoscopy at the time of diagnosis and at routine intervals thereafter.

34. How is muscle-invasive TCC (stage T2 or greater) treated?

Usually by radical cystectomy. Unfortunately, up to 50% of patients have occult systemic metastasis at the time of presentation and are not cured by cystectomy alone.

35. What are the commonest sites of metastasis from invasive TCC?

1. **Lymphatic metastases:** pelvic lymph nodes, including the obturator nodes, external iliac nodes, paravesical nodes, and common iliac nodes.

2. **Hematogenous metastases:** liver, lung, bone, adrenal, and bowel.

36. What is meant by "radical" rather than "simple" cystectomy?

In men, radical cystectomy implies bilateral pelvic lymphadenectomy and wide excision of the bladder and prostate, including the urachal remnant, overlying peritoneum, and vascular pedicles. In selected cases, nerve-sparing cystoprostatectomy with a more limited dissection of the posterior vesical pedicles is indicated and does not compromise cancer control. In women, radical cystectomy implies anterior pelvic exenteration, including the uterus, fallopian tubes, ovaries, anterior vaginal wall, and complete removal of the urethra.

37. What is the incidence of unsuspected TCC of the prostate in men undergoing radical cystectomy for invasive tumors?

As high as 45% in one series. The presence of prostatic TCC is best evaluated by deep transurethral and transrectal prostatic biopsies before cystectomy. These should be routinely performed in all candidates for orthotopic bladder replacement to the urethra.

38. How frequently does urethral TCC recur after cystectomy? Should all men have a prophylactic urethrectomy?

Clinical recurrence occurs in only 7–10% of patients, a risk that does not justify routine urethrectomy. However, the presence of TCC invading the prostatic stroma does predict recurrence. These patients *should* undergo prophylactic urethrectomy. All other patients should be followed with serial urethral wash cytologies.

39. Is transurethral resection alone ever curative for invasive TCC?

Only rarely. Patients with small, first-time tumors with only superficial muscle invasion (stage T2) that are completely re-resected after initial resection may be candidates for this. Survival rates equal to those for radical cystectomy have been reported using this approach.

40. What is the role for partial cystectomy for invasive TCC?

Partial cystectomy should be considered in patients with lower grade, unifocal, first-time tumors that are located away from the ureteral orifices and bladder floor and in whom a minimum 2-cm margin of normal tissue can be obtained. Random mucosal biopsies should be obtained at the time of staging evaluation to test for the presence of multifocal dysplasia and/or CIS which, if present, dictate radical rather than partial cystectomy.

41. Is systemic neoadjuvant (precystectomy) or adjuvant (postcystectomy) chemotherapy useful in the treatment of invasive TCC?

Neoadjuvant therapy produces responses in about 50% of patients, but most patients have residual disease in the bladder and require cystectomy. Its effect on survival has been assessed in randomized clinical trials. MVAC (methotrexate, vinblastine, Adriamycin [doxorubicin], and cisplatin) has shown a prolonged interval of disease-free survival. Several studies have suggested a modest increase in survival of patients with poor prognostic factors (perivesical fat invasion or positive nodes) following adjuvant chemotherapy.

42. What are the most popular forms of urinary diversion after radical cystectomy?

The ileal or Bricker conduit has the longest track record of any single technique. This is the simplest and least prone to major complications of all diversions, but it is limited by the need for an external urinary appliance. Various forms of continent urinary diversion were popularized in the 1980s and are now considered the gold standard in terms of improved patient lifestyle.

43. Describe the advantages and disadvantages of end and loop ileal conduit stomas.

The main advantage of a loop stoma is the ease of obtaining an everted bud above skin level. Both types produce equivalent functional results and complication rates in properly selected patients. End stomas are more prone to ischemic complications.

44. Name the four most important factors in obtaining good postoperative results from an ileal conduit stoma.

1. Patient education
2. Planned preoperative stomal site selection
3. Creation of an everted stomal bud without mesenteric ischemia
4. Postoperative support from enterostomal therapists

45. Describe the jejunal conduit syndrome.

This syndrome consists of hyponatremia, hypochloremia, hyperkalemia, and acidosis resulting from the increased absorptive capacity of jejunum (versus ileum). It occurs in patients with jejunal conduits and is related to the length of the conduit and/or impaired renal function.

46. What are the most popular forms of continent urinary diversions?

Continent cutaneous diversions include the Indiana and Kock pouches and their variations. These have internal reservoirs with a valve mechanism to prevent continuous efflux of urine. They require the patient to perform clean intermittent catheterization several times daily to empty.

Orthotopic diversions to the urethra have been used in men and women. These pouches may be formed from ileum, colon, or both and are anastomosed to the urethra. This form of urinary diversion most closely approximates normal voiding, although about 10% of patients require intermittent catheterization to empty completely.

47. How should patients with metastatic or locally unresectable tumors be treated?

With platinum-based combination chemotherapy. The most commonly used regimen is MVAC, but CMV (MVAC without the Adriamycin) and CISCA (cisplatin, Adriamycin, and cyclophosphamide) have been used with similar response rates.

48. What are the characteristics of the T helper cell 1 and T helper cell 2 pathways in the immunologic response to intravesical agents such as BCG and interferon-α?

Both pathways are elucidated by these immunostimulatory agents. Cellular immunity is driven by T helper cell 1, is primarily regulated by production of interferon-γ, and creates tumor antigen–specific cytotoxic T lymphocytes. It is essential for anticancer activity. Humoral immunity is driven by T helper cell 2, is primarily regulated by interleukin-10, and inhibits production of the key cellular immunity substrate, interferon-γ. It has been shown that patients who respond to intravesical agents by higher production of T helper cell 1 have a longer disease-free survival.

BIBLIOGRAPHY

1. Bretton PR, Herr HW, et al: Intravesical BCG therapy for in situ transitional cell carcinoma involving the prostatic urethra. J Urol 141:853, 1989.
2. Catalona WJ, Ratliff TL: BCG and superficial bladder cancer: Clinical experience and mechanism of action. Surg Annu 22:363, 1990.
3. Chechile G, Klein EA, Bauer L, et al: Functional equivalence of end and loop ileal conduit stomas. J Urol 147:582, 1992.
4. Droller MJ: Bladder cancer: State-of-the-art care. CA Cancer J Clin 48:269–284, 1998.
5. Hardeman SW, Soloway MS: Urethral recurrence following radical cystectomy. J Urol 144:666, 1990.
6. Herr HW: Conservative management of muscle-infiltrating bladder cancer: Prospective experience. J Urol 138:1162, 1987.
7. Herr HW, Schwalb DM, Zhang ZF, et al. Intravesical bacillus Calmette-Guérin therapy prevents tumor progression and death from superficial bladder cancer: Ten-year follow-up of a prospective randomized trial. J Clin Oncol 13:1404–1408, 1995.

8. Klein EA, Montie JE, Montague DK, Straffon RA: Jejunal conduit urinary diversion. J Urol 135:244, 1986.
9. Klein EA, Rogatko A, Herr HW: Management of local BCG failures in superficial bladder cancer. J Urol 147:601, 1992.
10. Lamm DL, van der Meijden AP, Akaza H, et al: Intravesical chemotherapy and immunotherapy: How do we assess their effectiveness and what are their limitations and uses? Int J Urol 2(suppl 2):23–35, 1995.
11. Lieskovsky G, Skinner DG: Role of lymphadenectomy in the treatment of bladder cancer. Urol Clin North Am 11:709, 1984.
12. Rowland RG, Mitchell ME, Bihrle R, et al: Indiana continent urinary reservoir. J Urol 137:1136, 1987.
13. Skinner DG, Lieskovsky G, Boyd SD: Continent urinary diversion. J Urol 141:1323, 1989.
14. Spruck CH, Ohneseit PF, Gonzalez-Zulueta M, et al: Two molecular pathways to transitional cell carcinoma of the bladder. Cancer Res 54:784, 1994.
15. Sternberg CN, Yagoda A, Scher HI, et al: MVAC for advanced transitional cell carcinoma of the urothelium. J Urol 139:461, 1988.
16. Tsai YC, Nichols PW, Hiti AL, et al: Allelic losses of chromosomes 9, 11, and 17 in human bladder cancer. Cancer Res 50:44, 1990.
17. Wood DP, Montie JE, Pontes JE, et al: Transitional cell carcinoma of the prostate in cystoprostatectomy specimens removed for bladder cancer. J Urol 141:346, 1989.
18. Wood DP, Montie JE, Pontes JE, et al: The role of magnetic resonance imaging in the staging of bladder cancer. J Urol 140:741, 1988.
19. Zabbo A, Montie JE, et al: Management of the urethra in men undergoing radical cystectomy for bladder cancer. J Urol 131:267, 1984.

28. CARCINOMA OF THE PROSTATE

Martin I. Resnick, M.D.

1. List the different types of prostate cancer. Which one is most common?

Several histologic types of prostate cancer have been identified and include adenocarcinoma, transitional cell carcinoma, and sarcoma. Greater than 90% of patients have adenocarcinoma, which has several variations, including neuroendocrine, endometroid, small cell, and mucinous types.

2. What is the prevalence of carcinoma of the prostate in the United States?

Carcinoma of the prostate is the most common malignancy diagnosed in American men. Approximately 30% of men over 50 years of age have histologic evidence of carcinoma of the prostate. The percentage rises as the population ages.

3. What are the estimated incidence and death rate?

The American Cancer Society estimates that 184,500 new cases of carcinoma of the prostate will be diagnosed and 39,200 men will die of the disease in 2001. The incidence of carcinoma of the prostate peaked several years ago, and the death rate has been declining for the past 5 years.

4. Which men typically are at greater risk for developing carcinoma of the prostate?

African-Americans have a higher risk of developing carcinoma of the prostate than whites. Additionally, they have a higher mortality from the disease. The stage of the disease is usually more advanced at time of diagnosis in African-American patients.

Men with one **first-degree relative** with carcinoma of the prostate have a two-fold increased chance of developing the disease, which increases to nine-fold if two first-degree relatives are affected (e.g., father and brother). Familial predilections are predominant in younger men with the disease (e.g., age 50).

5. In which portion of the prostate does cancer typically form?

Approximately 70% of adenocarcinomas originate in the peripheral zone of the prostate, 20% occur in the transition zone, and 10% in the central zone. Cancers in the fibromuscular stroma usually result from invasion by tumors arising in other zones, particularly the transition zone.

6. What symptoms are associated with carcinoma of the prostate?

In the early stages, patients have no symptoms related to the malignancy. Many may have symptoms similar to those of benign prostatic hyperplasia (e.g., nocturia, urinary urgency, weakness of the urinary stream). In patients with advanced disease, particularly bone metastases, skeletal pain may be a presenting symptom.

7. Describe the typical physical findings.

On digital rectal examination, prostate carcinomas are typically palpable as discrete, hard nodules. In patients with localized tumors, these nodules can be 0.5–1.0 cm in size, and with more advanced disease, the entire prostate may be involved. With the increased use of tumor markers (e.g., prostate-specific antigen and prostate biopsy), more men are being diagnosed with carcinoma of the prostate who have no palpable abnormalities.

8. What is prostate-specific antigen (PSA)? How is it used?

Prostate-specific antigen (PSA) is produced by both normal and malignant prostate epithelial cells. PSA is a serine protease of the kallikrein family and is associated with semen. Serum levels of PSA are elevated in many but not all men with cancer of the prostate but also in some men with benign prostatic hyperplasia and with prostatitis. The marker is used in monitoring patients who have been treated for carcinoma of the prostate. Its use in screening and early detection remains controversial. Free and bound levels of PSA can be measured, which is at times helpful in selecting which patients may require a prostate biopsy.

9. How is the diagnosis of carcinoma of the prostate usually established?

Patients with elevations in PSA and/or palpable abnormalities of the prostate are usually evaluated with ultrasonography and ultrasound-directed biopsies. If abnormalities are noted, these specific areas are biopsied, but if not, systematic or sextant biopsies of the prostate are obtained to establish a diagnosis. These biopsies are usually performed transrectally, and cores of tissue are obtained. It is apparent that the greater the number of biopsies obtained, the greater is the likelihood of establishing a diagnosis of malignancy. Increasingly, urologists are taking more and more biopsies, up to 10–12 at a time.

10. What are the different clinical stages of carcinoma of the prostate?

TNM Classification System of Prostate Carcinoma

Primary tumor (T)	
TX	Primary tumor cannot be assessed
T0	No evidence of primary tumor
T1	Clinically inapparent tumor not palpable or visible by imaging
T1a	Tumor incidental histologic finding in ≤5% of tissue resected
T1b	Tumor incidental histologic finding in >5% of tissue resected
T1c	Tumor identified by needle biopsy (e.g., because of elevated PSA)
T2	Palpable tumor confined within prostate
T2a	Tumor involves one lobe
T2b	Tumor involves both lobes
T3	Tumor extends through the prostatic capsule
T3a	Extracapsular extension (unilateral or bilateral)
T3b	Tumor invades seminal vesicle(s)
T4	Tumor is fixed or invades adjacent structures other than seminal vesicles: external sphincter, bladder neck, and/or rectum
Regional lymph node (N)	
NX	Regional lymph nodes cannot be assessed
N0	No regional lymph node metastasis
N1	Metastasis is in regional lymph node or nodes
Distant metastasis (M)	
MX	Distant metastasis cannot be assessed
M0	No distant metastasis
M1	Distant metastasis
M1a	Nonregional lymph nodes
M1b	Bone(s)
M1c	Other site(s)

11. Is a bone scan useful in diagnosis?

A bone scan is a radionuclide study useful in detecting bone metastases. With the introduction of PSA, its use is limited and it is more commonly obtained in patients with significant elevation of PSA (>20 ng/dl), high-grade, large-volume tumors, or the presence of bone pain.

12. What is Gleason's sum or score?

Gleason's sum or score is based on the pattern of cells constituting the carcinoma. Two regions of the prostate are viewed, each being graded 1–5 (well differentiated to poorly differentiated). A total of the patterns comprise a Gleason's sum—i.e., 2–10 with the more predominent pattern cited first (e.g., 3+4). Tumors may be classified as well differentiated (2,3,4), moderately differentiated (5,6,7), or poorly differentiated (8,9,10). It is becoming increasingly recognized that scores of 6 or less are more prognostically favorable than scores of 7 or greater.

13. What is a radical prostatectomy?

Radical prostatectomy is a surgical procedure used for treating patients with carcinoma of the prostate. The procedure involves removing the entire prostate and seminal vesicles, with anastomosis of the urethra to the bladder. The procedure can be performed through a retropubic, perineal, or laparoscopic approach.

14. How is radiation therapy used?

Radiation therapy can be administered by external beam or placement of radioactive seeds (interstitial, brachytherapy) within the prostate. External sources include cobalt, linear accelerated, protons, and neutrons. Interstitial seeds are varied and include radioactive gold, iodine, iridium, and palladium.

15. What is salvage prostatectomy?

Salvage prostatectomy is performed in patients in whom radiation therapy has failed. A radical prostatectomy is performed to accomplish cure in such patients, but complications such as impotence, incontinence, and rectal injury are greater than when the procedure is performed as initial treatment.

16. What is the purpose of endocrine therapy?

The malignant prostatic cell, like the normal hyperplastic cell, requires testosterone for growth. Endocrine therapy is directed at reducing the circulating levels of testosterone available to the prostate and/or interfering with the metabolism of testosterone within the prostate epithelial cells. Atrophy and death of prostatic cells occur and tumor progression is reduced.

17. How do LH/RH analogs function?

Luteinizing hormone-releasing hormone (LH/RH) analogs reduce circulating LH levels and subsequently interfere with the secretion of testosterone by the Leydig cells of the testicle. Castrate levels of testosterone are maintained in patients treated with these agents.

18. What does total androgen blockade do and how is it carried out?

Total androgen blockade attempts not only to interfere with testosterone produced by the testicle with either castration or an LH/RH analog, but also to interfere with the action of other circulating androgens, particularly those produced by the adrenal gland. Antiandrogens (e.g., flutamide) are effective in interfering with the binding of dihydrotestosterone to a specific cytoplastic receptor. Combination therapy is what is referred to as total androgen blockade.

BIBLIOGRAPHY

1. Gillenwater JY, Grayhack WT, Howards SS, Mitchell ME (eds): Adult and Pediatric Urology, 4th ed. Philadelphia, Lippincott Williams & Wilkins, 2002.
2. Raghavan D, Scher HI, Leibel SA, Lang P (eds): Principles and Practices of Genitourinary Oncology. Philadelphia, Lippincott-Raven, 1997.
3. Vogelzang N, Norman J, Scardino PT, et al (eds): A Comprehensive Textbook of Genitourinary Oncology. Baltimore, Williams & Wilkins, 1996.
4. Han M, Snow PB, Brandt JM, Partin AW: Evaluation of artificial neural networks for the prediction of pathologic stage in prostate cancer. Cancer 91:1661–1666, 2001.
5. Zlotta AR, Schulman CC. Can survival be prolonged for patients with hormone-resistant prostate cancer? Lancet 357:326–327, 2001.

29. BENIGN PROSTATIC HYPERPLASIA

Martin I. Resnick, M.D.

1. Describe the anatomic relationship of the prostate to adjacent structures.

Superiorly, the prostate is attached to the bladder neck, and inferiorly it is bound by the urogenital diaphragm. Posteriorly, the prostate is next to the rectum, and its anterior surface lies against the pubis, to which it is attached by the puboprostatic ligaments. The dorsal venous complex lies between the prostate and the pubis, and Denonvilliers' fascia, a reflection of the peritoneum, lies between the prostate and rectum. Laterally, the prostate is bound by the levator muscles.

2. What does the prostate do?

The specific function of the prostate has not been fully clarified, but it provides the bulk of the ejaculate. The secretions of the prostate include nutrients for sperm cells and proteases (e.g., prostate-specific antigen), which function to liquefy the ejaculate. It is likely that many other functions have not been identified.

3. What is the historic structure of the prostate?

The prostate is composed of stromal and epithelial elements. Organized acinar glands compose the epithelial components, which make up a ductal system that drains into the urethra. The fibromuscular stromal component is made up of smooth and skeletal muscle elements that interact with the epithelial structures.

4. What are the anatomical zones of the prostate?

The prostate comprises three zones of glandular tissue—transition zone, peripheral zone, and central zone. The fibromuscular stroma is located anteriorly.

5. How is testosterone metabolized in the prostate?

Free testosterone enters the prostate cell by passive diffusion and is reduced by the enzyme 5α-reductase to dihydrotestosterone. Dihydrotestosterone becomes bound to a specific protein receptor and is translocated into the nucleus where it stimulates the expression of specific RNA synthesis and thus directs cellular activity.

6. Are the zones of the prostate associated with specific diseases?

Benign hyperplasia of the prostate has its origin in the transition zone. The peripheral zone gives rise to most malignancies of the prostate. The central zone tends to be devoid of specific disease processes.

7. What is the prevalence of benign prostatic hyperplasia (BPH)?

Histologic BPH begins to be detected in men in their early 30s. The prevalence of the disease continues to rise and approaches 90% in men 80 years of age. Symptoms secondary to prostatic enlargement and bladder outlet obstruction increase with aging, and significant symptoms are present in approximately one-fourth of men by the seventh decade of life.

8. List the symptoms associated with BPH.

OBSTRUCTIVE SYMPTOMS	IRRITATIVE SYMPTOMS	OTHER SYMPTOMS
Weakness of urinary stream	Urinary urgency	Hematuria
Hesitancy	Frequency	Urinary tract infection
Terminal dribbling	Nocturia	Urinary retention
Intermittency	Incontinence (at times)	Renal failure (in severe
Sensation of incomplete bladder emptying		obstruction)
Straining to urinate (at times)		

9. What is meant by symptom score?

Various symptom scores have been developed that quantitate the subjective symptoms associated with BPH. Specific symptoms (e.g., nocturia, urinary frequency, urinary urgency) are graded and a total score is derived that relates to the severity of the patient's symptoms. Symptoms are characterized as being mild, moderate, or severe based on the symptom score. Treatment decisions and assessment of outcomes are based on symptom scores. The most commonly used symptom score was developed by the American Urological Association and is now referred to as the International Prostate Symptom Score (IPSS).

International Prostate Symptom Score (I-PSS)

	Not at all	Less than 1 time in 5	Less than half the time	About half the time	More than half the time	Almost always	Your score
1. Incomplete emptying Over the past month, how often have you had a sensation of not emptying your bladder completely after you finished urinating?	0	1	2	3	4	5	
2. Frequency Over the past month, how often have you had to urinate again less than two hours after you finishing urinating?	0	1	2	3	4	5	
3. Intermittency Over the past month, how often have you found you stopped and started again several times when you urinated?	0	1	2	3	4	5	
4. Urgency Over the past month, how often have you found it difficult to postpone urination?	0	1	2	3	4	5	
5. Weak Stream Over the past month, how often have you had a weak urinary stream?	0	1	2	3	4	5	
6. Straining Over the past month, how often have you had to push or strain to begin urination?	0	1	2	3	4	5	

	None	1 time	2 times	3 times	4 times	5 times or more	Your score
7. Nocturia Over the past month, how many times did you most typically get up to urinate from the time you went to bed at night until the time you got up in the morning?	0	1	2	3	4	5	
Total I-PSS Score							

Quality of Life Due to Urinary Symptoms	Delighted	Pleased	Mostly satisfied	Mixed About equally satisfied and dissatisfied	Mostly dissatisfied	Unhappy	Terrible
If you were to spend the rest of your life with your urinary condition just the way it is now, how would you feel about that?	0	1	2	3	4	5	6

The International Prostate Symptom Score (I-PSS) is based on the answers to seven questions concerning urinary symptoms. Each question allows the patient to chose one of five answers indicating incresing severity of the particular symptom. The answers are assigned points from 0 to 5. The toal score can therefore range from 0 to 35 (asymptomatic to very symptomatic). Furthermore, the International Consensus Committee (ICC) recommends the use of only a single question to assess the qality of life. The answers to this question range from "delighted" to "terrible" or 0 to 6. Although this single question may or may not capture the global impact BPH symptoms or quality of life. It may serve as a valuable starting point for a doctor-patient conversation.

The ICC strongly recommends that all physicians who counsel patients suffering from symptoms of prostatism utilize these measures not only during the inital interview but also during and after treatment in order to monitor treatment response.

The ICC under the patronage of the World Health Organization (WHO) has agreed to use the symptom index for benign prostatic hyperplasia (BPH), which has been developed by the American Urological Association (AUA) Measurement Committee, as the official worldwide symptoms assessment tool for patients suffering from prostatism.

10. What are the potential consequences of untreated BPH?

In addition to the significant symptoms that develop, BPH can result in the development of bladder calculi and associated symptoms, urinary retention, hydronephrosis, and in severe cases, chronic renal failure. Several of these conditions respond to treatment (e.g., urinary retention and bladder stones), but others may be permanent (renal failure) and may not respond to removal of the obstructing prostate.

11. When should patients with BPH be treated?

Increasingly, it appears that the severity of symptoms is directing the need for treatment, i.e., the "bother factor." Patients with mild symptoms can be observed. However, those with moderate to severe symptoms require some form of therapy. Other indications for treatment relate to the complications associated with BPH, such as chronic urinary tract infection, bladder calculi, urinary retention, hydroureteronephrosis, and renal failure.

12. What diagnostic studies are useful in evaluating BPH?

In addition to a symptom score, specific studies such as measurement of serum creatinine, urinalysis, residual urine, and urinary pressure-flow studies are helpful in establishing the diagnosis of BPH and in assessing its severity.

13. What is finasteride? How does it work?

Finasteride is a 5-α reductase inhibitor that is used in the treatment of patients with symptomatic BPH. Interfering with the conversion of testosterone to dihydrotestosterone, finasteride typically results in shrinkage of the prostate gland by approximately 25% over 3 months. Symptomatic improvement follows, although patients must be maintained on the medication for at least 1 year. Generally glands $\geq$40 gm respond better to finasteride.

14. Why are alpha-blocking agents effective in treating patients with BPH?

α-Receptors are located in the trigone of the bladder and fibromuscular stroma of the prostate. The fibromuscular stroma is composed in part of smooth muscle, and these, in addition to those located in the bladder neck, relax under α-blockade. Studies have demonstrated that prostates with a greater density of smooth muscle have a greater response to α-blockade.

15. What is a simple prostatectomy?

A simple prostatectomy is performed in patients with symptomatic BPH and involves removing the hyperplastic tissue located within the transition zone. A simple prostatectomy can be performed by transurethral resection or an open procedure, via either a suprapubic or retropubic approach.

16. List the potential complications of transurethral resection of the prostate.

Intraoperative Complications	Postoperative Complications
Hemorrhage	Ureteral stricture
Hyponatremia (due to abosorption	Bladder neck contracture
of irrigating fluid)	Incontinence
	Retrograde ejaculation
	Impotence

17. What is a transurethral incision of the prostate?

Transurethral incision of the prostate involves incising the prostatic urethra in an attempt to reduce urethral resistance and relieve voiding symptoms. The procedure is most efficacious in patients with small prostates and is associated with less morbidity than transurethral prostatic resection.

18. Are other forms of therapy available for treating patients with BPH?

New forms of therapy are being developed, including balloon dilation of the prostatic urethra and use of prostatic stents. Other forms of therapy include microwave thermotherapy, lasers, high-temperature radio frequency transurethral ablation of prostatic tissue, high-intensity focused ultrasound, and use of hot water circulated through the prostatic urethrae.

BIBLIOGRAPHY

1. Gillenwater JY, Grayhack WT, Howards SS, Mitchell ME (eds): Adult and Pediatric Urology, 4th ed. Philadelphia, Lippincott Williams & Wilkins, 2002.
2. Eckhardt MD, van Venrooij GE, Boone TA. Symptoms and quality of life versus age, prostate volume and urodynamic parameters in 565 strictly selected men with lower urinary tract symptoms suggestive of benign prostatic hyperplasia. Urology 57:695–700, 2001.
3. Meigs JR, Mohr B, Barry MJ, et al. Risk factors for clinical benign prostatic hyperplasia in a community-based population of healthy aging men. J Clin Epidemiol 54:935–944, 2001.
4. Schulman CC, Lock TM, Buzelin JM, et al. Long-term use of tamsulosin in benign prostatic hyperplasia. J Urol 166:1358–1361, 2001.
5. Floratos DI, Kiemeny LA, Rossi C, et al. Long-term follow up of randomized transurethral microwave thermotherapy versus transurethral prostatic resection study. J Urol 165:1533–1538, 2001.
6. Helke C, Manseck A, Hakenberg OW, et al. Is transurethral vaporesection of the prostate better than standard transurethral resection. Eur Urol 39:551–557, 2001.

30. SQUAMOUS CELL CARCINOMA OF THE PENIS

Kurt H. Dinchman, M.D.

1. What is the most common form of carcinoma of the penis?
Squamous cell carcinoma.

2. What is carcinoma in situ of the penis?
Carcinoma in situ of the penis, also referred to as erythroplasia of Queyrat or Bowen's disease, may precede and progress to invasive squamous cell carcinoma of the penis.

3. How is circumcision related to the incidence of penile carcinoma?
Squamous cell carcinoma of the penis is rare among men who were circumcised at infancy. Development of squamous cell carcinoma of the penis in uncircumcised men is attributed to chronic irritative effects of smegma and chronic bacterial infection that may be related to smegma in men with poor hygiene.

4. Has the human papillomavirus (HPV) been implicated in penile cancer?
Recent studies have shown that men with HPV and genital herpetic infections have a higher incidence of penile carcinoma.

5. What is the most common presenting manifestation of squamous cell carcinoma?
Squamous cell carcinoma usually presents as a persistent sore or ulcer of the glans and/or the foreskin. The sores are usually painless; for this reason, patients may delay seeking treatment.

6. What are the most common premalignant lesions of the penis?
• Leukoplakia
• Erythroplasia of Queyrat
• Balanitis xerotica obliterans
• Buschke-Löwenstein tumor

7. How is carcinoma of the penis staged?
Accurate assessment of stage is important in determining the type of therapy that the patient requires. Initial diagnosis should be made by an excisional biopsy, which allows accurate assessment of the depth of invasion. The status of inguinal lymph nodes should be assessed by careful physical examination. CT scan of the abdomen and pelvis is also required to assess the status of the pelvic and abdominal lymph nodes.

8. What is the most commonly used staging system for carcinoma of the penis?
The most commonly used staging system is the Jackson staging system. Stage 1 refers to tumors confined to the glans and prepuce; stage 2, to tumors extending into the shaft of the penis; stage 3, to tumors with inguinal metastases that are amenable to surgery; and stage 4, to inoperable inguinal metastases or distant metastases.

9. How is the primary lesion treated in squamous cell carcinoma of the penis?
Removal of the cancer by partial or total penectomy is standard therapy. Partial penectomy requires a 2-cm margin of normal cancer-free penile shaft for effective removal of tumor. For extensive lesions approaching the penoscrotal junction, total penectomy should be performed with both excision of corpora and creation of a perineal urethrostomy. Small lesions involving the fore-

skin may be managed with circumcision alone; however, diligent postoperative follow-up is required because of the high rate of recurrence.

10. What is the most important factor in the prognosis of penile carcinoma?
The most important factor is the presence of inguinal metastases.

11. What is the current recommendation for treatment of Jackson stages 1 and 2 without inguinal lymphadenopathy?
The current recommendation is local excision of the lesion with a wide tumor-free margin and examination of inguinal lymph nodes every 3–4 months for approximately 24 months.

12. What is the current recommendation for treatment of Jackson stages 1 and 2 with invasion of corporal bodies and/or tunica albuginea?
The current recommendation is to perform a superficial lymph node dissection, followed by total lymphadenectomy if the superficial lymph nodes are positive, with either partial or total penectomy.

13. What is the current recommendation for treatment of Jackson stage 3 carcinoma of the penis?
In patients with lymphadenopathy, a 6-week course of antibiotic therapy should be initiated because of the inflammatory inguinal lymphadenopathy frequently associated with ulcerated and/or infected penile lesions. After therapy is completed, the lymphatic tissue should be re-evaluated. Bilateral lymphadenopathy requires bilateral inguinal lymph node dissection, whereas unilateral lymphadenopathy requires a superficial and deep node dissection of the ipsilateral inguinal nodes.

14. What treatment is currently recommended for Jackson stage 4 penile carcinoma?
The usual treatment for such patients is palliative radiotherapy and/or chemotherapy (most commonly a single-agent application of bleomycin, methotrexate, or cisplatin).

BIBLIOGRAPHY

1. DeVita VT, Hellman SA, Rosenberg SA (eds): Cancer: Principles and Practice of Oncology, 5th ed. Philadelphia, Lippincott-Raven, 1997.
2. Resnick MI, Kursh ED (eds): Current Therapy in Genitourinary Surgery, 2nd ed. St. Louis, B. C. Decker–Mosby, 1992.
3. Seidman EJ, Hanno PM (eds): Current Urologic Therapy. Philadelphia, W. B. Saunders, 1994.
4. Walsh PC, Retik AB, Stamey AT, Vaughan ED, Wein AJ (eds): Campbell's Urology, 8th ed., Philadelphia, W. B. Saunders, 2002.

31. PREMALIGNANT LESIONS OF THE PENIS

Kurt H. Dinchman, M.D.

1. What is the most common malignant lesion of the penis?
Squamous cell carcinoma of the penis.

2. What is the significance of premalignant lesions of the penis?
Approximately 30–40% of patients with squamous cell carcinoma of the penis have a history of a preexisting penile lesion.

3. What precancerous lesions may be found on the penis?
• Cutaneous horns
• Balanitis xerotica obliterans
• Leukoplakia
• Condyloma acuminatum
• Bowenoid papulosis
• Kaposi's sarcoma
• Buschke-Löwenstein tumor

4. Which of the above are related to viral etiology?
Condyloma acuminatum, bowenoid papulosis, and Buschke-Löwenstein tumors are related to infections with the human papillomavirus (HPV), whereas Kaposi's sarcoma is seen in patients infected with the human immunodeficiency virus (HIV).

5. What is a cutaneous horn?
A cutaneous horn is a hyperkeratotic lesion and may be related to preexisting lesions, such as a wart or traumatic injury. Because of their malignant potential, such lesions should be excised, and the area of excision should be watched carefully.

6. What is balanitis xerotica obliterans?
Balantis xerotica obliterans is a patchy white lesion involving the glans and prepuce. Such lesions predispose patients to painful erosions and fissures, along with obstructive symptoms due to meatal stenosis. Treatment consists of a biopsy followed by local application of steroids to the lesions. Meatotomy may be needed to alleviate outlet obstruction. Close observation is required to look for changes of malignant transformation.

7. What is leukoplakia of the penis?
Leukoplakia is a hyperkeratotic lesion of the prepuce or glans that is associated with chronic irritation. Although the malignant potential of such lesions is low, circumcision for lesions involving the prepuce or removing the source of irritation on the glans is the therapeutic regimen of choice, along with close observation.

8. What is condyloma acuminatum?
Also called venereal or genital warts, condyloma acuminatum is a common form of sexually transmitted disease caused by a family of related viruses grouped under the name human papillomaviruses (HPV). Recent reports from the Centers for Disease Control show new cases at approximately 1 million per year. HPV is also considered the main etiologic agent in cervical cancer and dysplasia.

9. How is condyloma acuminatum detected?

Most cases of condyloma acuminatum are detected by the patient as clusterlike lesions on a narrow stalk or sessile base. Frequently patients are evaluated after HPV is discovered on a cervical smear of a female partner on a routine Papanicoloau test. In addition to appearing on the foreskin, glans, and shaft, such lesions may be found on the wall of the scrotum, perineum, and anus. Careful inspections of the distal urethra are warranted to rule out urethral condyloma.

10. How is condyloma acuminatum treated?

Treatment depends on the extent of the disease. Isolated lesions on the shaft may be treated with podophyllin or trichloroacetic acid solution. Surgical excision and electrocautery are also acceptable methods for isolated lesions. More extensive disease may be treated with laser ablation. Nd:YAG and CO_2 lasers have been used successfully with good control of lesions and satisfactory cosmetic results. Intraurethral and meatal condyloma have been treated successfully with 5-fluorouracil cream.

11. Define Buschke-Löwenstein tumor.

Buschke-Löwenstein tumor, also known as giant condyloma, is similar to condyloma acuminatum in appearance but may cause invasive erosion into surrounding tissue. Surgical excision is the treatment of choice.

12. Define bowenoid papulosis.

Bowenoid papulosis is a papulelike lesion of genitalia with pathologic features similar to carcinoma in situ; a connection to HPV has been made in multiple studies. All modalities outlined for the treatment of condyloma acuminatum may be used. To date, no invasive form of the disease has been documented.

13. Why is recognition of Kaposi's sarcoma important?

Kaposi's sarcoma (KS) consists of dark-colored, bleeding, tender papules of the penile skin. In patients with acquired immunodeficiency syndrome (AIDS), KS may be the initial presenting manifestation. Treatment is palliative, including laser treatment and surgical excision.

14. What is Moh's micrographic surgery (MMS)?

MMS is a surgical technique of removing layers of malignant cutaneous tissue for excision.

15. Is MMS indicated in the treatment of penile cancer?

In patients with small distal lesions, MMS has been shown to have cure rates approaching those of partial penectomy.

BIBLIOGRAPHY

1. Gillenwater JY, Grayhack JT, Howards SS, Duckett JW (eds): Adult and Pediatric Urology, 3rd ed. St. Louis, Mosby, 1996.
2. Resnick MI, Elder JS: Office urology. Urol Clin North Am 15(4):1988.
3. Resnick MI, Kursh ED (eds): Current Therapy in Genitourinary Surgery, 2nd ed. St. Louis, B. C. Decker–Mosby, 1992.
4. Walsh PC, Retik AB, Stamey AT, Vaughan ED, Wein AJ (eds): Campbell's Urology, 8th ed. Philadelphia, W. B. Saunders, 2002.

32. URETHRAL CANCER

J. Stephen Jones, M.D.

1. Compare male and female urethral cancer histology.

Most urethral cancers in both sexes are squamous cell carcinoma. Less common is transitional cell cancer, which may coexist with bladder cancer, especially in women. Male transitional cell cancer (15%) is usually found in the prostatic urethra. Adenocarcinoma accounts for 10–15% of cases in women and is associated with a worse prognosis. Adenocarcinoma is uncommon in males, except when prostatic adenocarcinoma extends into the urethra.

2. What are the etiologic factors associated with urethral cancer development?

The only known association is with chronic irritation. This usually involves urethral stricture disease in men and urethral diverticulae in women.

3. How does urethral cancer present?

Females: Hematuria or urethral bleeding is the most common symptom. Irritative or obstructive voiding symptoms are often suggestive of advanced disease. Pain and a palpable indurated mass are the most suggestive clinical findings.

Males: Men present with similar signs and symptoms; in addition, a persistent urethral stricture or urethrocutaneous fistula may also signify the disease. Because most of these symptoms are nonspecific, a delay in diagnosis of several months is common.

4. What is the differential diagnosis of urethral cancer?

Female	Male
Urethral caruncle	Stricture
Bartholin's gland cyst	Perineal abcess
Urethral diverticulum	Urethrocutaneous fistula
Condyloma	Condyloma
Periurethral abcess	Prostatic or penile cancer

5. What are the methods for diagnosis of urethral cancer?

The diagnosis may be suspected by the presenting symptoms and signs described previously, especially the identification of a urethral mass. Cystoscopy usually reveals the lesion, which is best biopsied under anesthesia. This may be done cystoscopically or by needle biopsy. Bimanual physical examination is done at that setting to evaluate any extension or fixation. Voided cytologies usually reveal malignant cellularity.

Retrograde urethrography in men shows a filling defect, but this may be confused for benign urethral stricture. Other radiographs are used primarily to assess extension or metastasis. This includes abdominopelvic MRI or CT, chest radiographs, and bone scan. As with most malignancies, the most common sites of metastases are lymphatics, liver, lung, and bone.

6. How is urethral cancer staged?

The staging system is summarized in the following table.

International Union Against Cancer TNM Staging System for Urethral Cancer

STAGE	DEFINITION
Primary tumor (T)	
Tx	Primary tumor cannot be assessed
T0	No evidence of primary tumor

(continued)

International Union Against Cancer TNM Staging System for Urethral Cancer
(Continued)

STAGE	DEFINITION
Tis	Carcinoma in situ
Ta	Noninvasive papillary, polypoid, or verrucous carcinoma
T1	Tumor invades subepithelial connective tissue
T2	Tumor invades periurethral musculature (corpus spongiosum or prostate)
T3	Tumor invades anterior vagina or bladder neck (corpus cavernosum or beyond prostate or bladder neck)
T4	Tumor invades other adjacent structures
Regional lymph (N)	
Nx	Regional lymph nodes cannot be assessed
N0	No regional lymph node metastasis
N1	Metastasis in a single superficial inguinal lymph node, 2 cm or less in greatest dimension
N2	Metastasis to a single lymph node, >2 cm but <5 cm in greatest dimension, or multiple nodes involved, none >5 cm
N3	Metastasis to a lymph node >5 cm in greatest dimension
Distant metastasis (M)	
Mx	Presence of distant metastasis cannot be assessed
M0	No distant metastasis
M1	Distant metastasis

7. What is the treatment for female urethral cancer?

Low-grade, low-stage cancers may be resected, fulgurated, or treated with laser ablation. However, most urethral cancers are of higher grade and require anterior exenteration with wide excision of the adjacent vaginal wall. Occasionally, resection of the symphysis pubis is required to remove all locally advanced disease. Adjuvant radiotherapy may increase the cure rate. Interstitial radiotherapy, alone or in combination with resection, has shown benefit in women.

8. What is the treatment of male urethral cancer?

Low-grade, low-stage cancers may be treated with resection, fulguration, or laser ablation. Distal cancers of higher grade are best managed by partial penectomy. More proximal high-grade or locally invasive cancers are best managed by aggressive surgical removal of the penis, pubis, prostate, and bladder. Inguinal adenopathy usually represents cancer (unlike penile cancer, in which adenopathy often results from inflammatory changes); therefore, ileoinguinal lymphadenectomy is indicated if enlarged groin nodes are present. Proximal urethral cancers metastasize to the pelvic lymph nodes.

9. How is male urethral cancer managed after cystectomy?

Up to 7% of patients in some series developed urethral cancer during the 5 years following cystectomy for transitional cell carcinoma. For this reason, most patients with a retained urethra should undergo serial surveillance with urethral washing for cytology and possibly urethroscopy. If a urethral cancer occurs after cystectomy, secondary urethrectomy should be performed unless the lesion is clearly superficial and amenable to total endoscopic removal or ablation. Secondary urethrectomy is difficult to perform owing to the scarring at the proximal urethra and the proximity of the small bowel to the obliterated end.

10. What is the prognosis for urethral cancer?

Anterior lesions present at a lower stage and have a better prognosis. Partial or total penectomy offers the opportunity for wide surgical margins. Five-year survival for anterior cancers is 50%, compared with 10–15% for posterior urethral cancer.

REFERENCE

Herr HW: Surgery of penile and urethral carcinoma. In Walsh PC, Retik AB, Vaughan ED (eds): Campbell's Urology, 7th ed. Philadelphia, W.B. Saunders, 1998, pp 3401–3408.

33. TESTICULAR TUMORS IN ADULTS

Eric A. Klein, M.D.

1. What is the most common type of tumor affecting the testis?

More than 90% of testis cancers are germ-cell tumors derived from the germinal epithelium of the mature testis (see table below). The tumors occur in both pure and mixed forms, slightly more commonly on the right, and are bilateral in 1–2% of patients. Approximately 5% of testis cancers are gonadal stromal tumors, derived from cells that support the generation and maturation of sperm. About 1% of testis tumors are metastatic from another site.

Histologic Classification of Testicular Neoplasms

Germ-cell tumors	Other tumors
Seminoma	Epidermoid cyst
Embryonal carcinoma	Adenomatoid tumor
Choriocarcinoma	Adrenal rest
Yolk sac tumor	Adenocarcinoma of the rete testis
Teratoma	Carcinoid
Mixed tumors	
Gonadal stromal tumors	
Leydig-cell tumors	
Sertoli-cell tumors	
Gonadoblastoma	
Mixed tumors	

2. What non–germ-cell cancers affect the testis?

Primary tumors of the other cellular elements of the testis include tumors of specialized stroma such as Leydig-cell tumors. Sertoli-cell tumors, and mixed forms; other stromal tumors include gonadoblastoma, adenocarcinoma of the rete testis, carcinoid, and mesenchymal tumors (see previous table). Secondary tumors include leukemia, lymphoma, and metastases from solid tumors of other sites.

3. Name the histologic subtypes of germ-cell tumors.

Seminoma, embryonal carcinoma, teratoma, choriocarcinoma, and yolk sac tumor.

4. What is the most common histology found in germ-cell tumors?

The most common histologically pure form is seminoma, but mixed tumors occur more frequently than pure ones.

5. What is the most common solid tumor in men between the ages of 15 and 40 years?

Germ-cell tumors of the testis.

6. What are risk factors for germ-cell tumors?

Age, race, and cryptorchidism (with a 3- to 14-fold increased risk) are the only known risk factors. Although testis cancer can occur at any age, the three peaks of incidence are: between ages 20–40, in men >60 years, and in children from birth to age 10. Caucasians are four times more likely to develop testis cancer than African-Americans. Approximately 10% of all testis tumors occur in undescended testes. A cryptorchid testis has a 3–5% chance of developing cancer, with the risk proportional to the degree of maldescent. Intraabdominal testes and dysgenetic testes associated with a chromosomal syndrome (intersex) have the highest risk of malignancy.

7. Does family history increase the risk of testis cancer?

Testis cancer has been reported in fathers and sons, twins, and in two or more male siblings. However, except for the known forms of intersex, a defined familial inheritance pattern has not been established.

8. How does age influence the histology of testis tumors?

The histology of the primary tumor is closely correlated with age. Seminoma and mixed germ-cell tumors are most common in postpubertal men up to age 40 years; yolk sac tumors and pure teratoma predominate in infants, and men >50 years of age are most commonly affected by spermatocytic seminoma, lymphoma, or other secondary tumors.

9. Does testicular trauma cause testis cancer?

Although cancer is often diagnosed after an episode of testicular trauma, no evidence suggests trauma as an etiologic agent. It is more likely that the traumatic episode brings an underlying tumor to attention.

10. What are the most frequent sites of metastasis by nonseminomatous germ-cell tumors?

The retroperitoneal lymph nodes are the most frequent site of metastasis, followed in order by lung, liver, brain, bone, and kidney.

11. What are the primary lymphatic drainage areas of the testes?

Testicular lymphatics exit via the mediastinum testis and coalesce into larger channels in the spermatic cord. These channels travel through the inguinal canal, into the retroperitoneum following the testicular artery, and fan out medially over the great vessels. Primary drainage of the right testis occurs in the interaortocaval area at the level of the L2 vertebral body. The left testis drains to the paraaortic area lateral to the aorta and medial to the ureter.

12. How do germ-cell tumors metastasize to the inguinal nodes?

The scrotal skin and underlying layers are drained by the inguinal and perianal lymph nodes; tumors that invade the scrotum therefore may drain to inguinal nodes. Prior inguinal or scrotal surgery (such as orchidopexy) also may put the inguinal nodes at risk. Massive retroperitoneal adenopathy may lead to retrograde lymphatic deposits in the inguinal region as well.

13. What is the most common presenting complaint in patients with testis tumors?

The most common presenting complaint is painless unilateral swelling or nodule, usually as an incidental finding by the patient or his sexual partner. Scrotal or lower abdominal pain occurs in about one-third of patients. In 10% the presenting symptoms are due to systemic metastasis and may include a neck mass due to supracalavicular nodal disease, cough or dyspnea due to lung metastases, gastrointestinal symptoms or back pain due to retroperitoneal metastases, bone pain, central nervous system symptoms, or gynecomastia.

14. How common is a delay in diagnosis of testis tumors?

Delayed diagnosis is common. Ample evidence suggests that a delay in diagnosis leads to more advanced clinical stage, higher morbidity, and excessive mortality. Both patients and physicians may be the source of delay. Reasons for patient delay include misunderstanding the significance of testicular symptoms, attribution of symptoms to minor testicular trauma, transience of symptoms, and fear of cancer. Reasons for physician delay include attribution of symptoms to a benign condition, such as infection, epididymitis, or hydrocele, and neglect of a testicular examination.

15. Outline the clinical evaluation of a patient with a testis tumor.

Physical examination should include palpation of the testis with particular attention to possible involvement of the spermatic cord, scrotum, or skin by the primary tumor. Examination of the abdomen, chest, and cervical regions may disclose obvious metastases. A scrotal ultrasound may confirm the presence of an intratesticular mass. Serum tumor markers including alpha fetoprotein (AFP), the beta subunit of human chorionic gonadotrophin (βHCG), and lactic acid dehydrogenase (LDH) should be measured. A chest x-ray and CT scan of the chest, abdomen, and pelvis are performed routinely.

16. What is the *sine qua non* for the diagnosis of a germ-cell tumor?
Inguinal orchiectomy with pathologic examination of the testis.

17. How are germ-cell tumors staged?
According to the *1998 American Joint Commission on Cancer Staging Manual,* germ-cell tumors are staged by assessing four parameters: (1) the extent of the primary tumor (T category); (2) the presence or absence of regional lymph nodes (N category); (3) the presence or absence of distant metastases (M category); and (4) the level of serum tumor markers (S category) (see following tables).

Primary Tumor

T STAGE	TUMOR EXTENT	VASCULAR/LYMPHATIC INVASION
Tx	Cannot be assessed	—
T0	No evidence of primary tumor (histologic scar)	—
Tis	Intratubular germ-cell neoplasia (carcinoma in situ)	—
T1	Limited to testis and epididymis, may involve tunica albuginea	Absent
T2	Limited to testis and epididymis, may involve tunica vaginalis	Present
T3	Invades spermatic cord	Present or absent
T4	Invades scrotum	Present or absent

Regional Lymph Nodes

N STAGE	SIZE	NUMBER
Nx	Cannot be assessed	—
N0	None	None
N1	<2 cm	<5
N2	2–5 cm or histologic extranodal extension	>5
N3	≥ 5 cm	Any

Distant Metastasis

M STAGE	SITE
Mx	Cannot be assessed
M0	None
M1a	Nonregional nodes or pulmonary
M1b	All other

Serum Tumor Markers

S STAGE	LDH	HCG (MIU/ML)	AFP (NG/ML)
S0	NL	NL	NL
S1	<1.5 × NL	<5,000	<1,000
S2	1.5–10 × NL	5,000–50,000	1,000–10,000
S3	>10 × NL	>50,000	>10,000

AFP = alpha fetoprotein, HCG = human chorionic gonadotropin, LDH = lactic acid dehydrogenase, NL = normal.

18. What serum tumor markers are important in germ-cell tumors?
AFP, HCG, LDH, and placental alkaline phosphatase (PLAP) are useful for diagnosis, staging, monitoring response to therapy, predicting prognosis, and monitoring for tumor recurrence.

19. What is AFP, and which histologic types secrete it?

AFP is a 70-kD single-peptide chain glycoprotein present in the developing fetus but in only minute amounts in adults. Serum AFP elevations (above 10 ng/dl) are detectable in 50–70% of patients with germ-cell tumors, including embryonal carcinoma, yolk sac tumor, and mixed tumors containing these elements.

20. What is HCG, and which histologic types secrete it?

HCG is a 38-kD glycoprotein composed of alpha and beta subunits. The alpha subunit is homologous to the alpha peptides of several other hormones, including luteinizing hormone (LH), thyroid-stimulating hormone (TSH), and follicle-stimulating hormone (FSH). The beta subunit is antigenically distinct and is the clinically relevant marker for germ-cell cancer. Elevated βHCG levels (above 5 mIU/ml) are found in 40–60% of patients with testis cancer, including choriocarcinoma, embryonal carcinoma, and some cases of pure seminoma.

21. What other diseases may cause elevations in serum AFP and βHCG?

Hepatocellular, pancreatic, gastric, and lung cancers and benign liver conditions, including hepatitis and cirrhosis, may cause elevations in serum AFP levels. Multiple myeloma and hepatocellular, pancreatic, gastric, lung, and bladder tumors may cause elevated serum βHCG.

22. What are the serum half-lives of AFP and βHCG?

The half-life of AFP is 5–7 days; of βHCG, 24–36 hours.

23. What is the significance of elevated levels of LDH and PLAP?

Elevations in serum LDH usually indicate advanced or bulky metastatic disease. PLAP, a fetal isoenzyme of alkaline phosphatase, is secreted by some seminomas.

24. What cytogenetic abnormalities are characteristic of germ-cell tumors?

A duplication of the short arm of chromosome 12, known as isochromosome 12p or i(12p).

25. Does an elevated serum βHCG after orchiectomy always indicate the presence of residual tumor?

No. Some assays for βHCG cross-react with LH and may lead to a false-positive interpretation. The typical scenario is in patients who are clinically free of disease but who have physiologically elevated concentrations of LH after unilateral orchiectomy and slightly elevated βHCG levels. This cross-reactivity can be distinguished from a true elevation of βHCG by repeating the assay 48 hours after the intramuscular injection of 200 mg testosterone, which suppresses the secretion of LH. Any elevations in βHCG attributable to cross-reactivity should return to normal after testosterone injection.

26. What is the significance of an elevated serum βHCG in a patient with a histologically pure seminoma?

It suggests the presence of syncytiotrophoblasts that secrete HCG, but these tumors behave identically to non–HCG-secreting pure seminomas and are treated as such. The syncytiotrophoblastic elements may not be apparent by light microscopy, but can usually be demonstrated by immunohistochemistry.

27. What is the significance of an elevated serum AFP in a patient with a germ-cell tumor?

Elevated serum AFP always implies the presence of nonseminomatous elements, and such tumors should be treated as mixed or nonseminomatous tumors.

28. Do normal serum markers after inguinal orchiectomy preclude the presence of residual active cancer?

No. Small-volume metastases may produce insufficient amounts of these substances to be detectable in the blood, and even massive amounts of teratoma are usually marker-negative.

29. What pathologic factors in the primary tumor are associated with a high risk of metastases?
- Advanced local stage (T2, T3, or T4)
- Presence of lymphatic or vascular invasion
- Percentage of embryonal carcinoma

30. Name the histologic variants of pure seminoma.

There are three histologic variants of pure seminoma: classic, anaplastic, and spermatocytic. Classic seminoma accounts for 85% of seminomas, the anaplastic variant for 5–10%, and the spermatocytic variant for the remainder of cases.

31. What are the histologic and clinical characteristics of anaplastic and spermatocytic seminoma?

Anaplastic seminoma is characterized by increased mitotic activity, more local invasion, and a higher likelihood of metastatic disease at presentation. However, at each stage anaplastic seminomas have cure rates similar to classic seminoma. Spermatocytic seminoma is characterized by cells resembling maturing spermatogonia. Spermatocytic tumors are biologically indolent and have a uniformly good prognosis.

32. What is meant by a nonseminomatous tumor?

These tumors are composed histologically of embryonal carcinoma, teratoma, choriocarcinoma, and yolk sac elements alone or in combination. Tumors with both seminomatous and nonseminomatous elements behave and are treated as nonseminomatous tumors. Tumors with more than one element of any type are called "mixed" nonseminomatous germ-cell tumors.

33. Define teratoma. Distinguish between its mature and immature forms.

Teratoma is a tumor that contains elements derived from more than one germ-cell layer (mesoderm, ectoderm, and endoderm). Mature teratoma contains benign-appearing differentiated structures such as glands, cartilage, bone, muscle, or neural tissue. Immature teratoma consists of undifferentiated tissue from the three layers. Occasionally, malignant changes are seen in otherwise mature tissue, leading to teratoma with malignant differentiation.

34. What is the treatment for clinical stage $T_{1-2}N_0M_0$ pure seminoma?

Inguinal orchiectomy and radiation therapy to the retroperitoneal and ipsilateral iliac lymph nodes, which yields a 95% 5-year NED (no evidence of disease) survival rate. Recently, surveillance for low-stage seminomas has been advocated by some as a way of avoiding the cost and toxicity of radiotherapy. However, the toxicity of radiotherapy in this setting is usually minor and self-limited, and surveillance requires more intensive follow-up and the potential for a much greater burden of therapy if relapse occurs.

35. Describe treatment for low-volume clinical stage $T_{1-2}N_{1-2}M_0$ (retroperitoneal lymph nodes of <5 cm) seminoma?

Inguinal orchiectomy and radiation therapy to the retroperitoneal and ipsilateral iliac lymph nodes, which yield 90% 5-year NED survival.

36. What is the treatment for advanced ($T_{any}N_3M_{0-1}$) seminoma?

Inguinal orchiectomy followed by platinum-based combination chemotherapy. More than 90% of patients will have a complete response to this therapy and most will remain disease-free at 5 years.

37. Describe the management of a residual mass in the retroperitoneum after chemotherapy for seminoma.

Treatment is controversial. Treatment approaches have included retroperitoneal lymphadenectomy, radiation therapy, and observation. Surgery in this setting is difficult owing to severe fibrosis, and a clean retroperitoneal dissection is usually not attainable. Most residual masses less than 3 cm do not contain viable tumor and probably do not require surgical excision.

38. What is the treatment for a clinical stage $T_{1-2}N_0M_0$ nonseminomatous tumor?

Inguinal orchiectomy with a careful pathologic analysis to determine the presence of adverse factors that increase the likelihood of retroperitoneal metastases (see question 29). In patients with no adverse histologic factors, either surveillance or nerve-sparing retroperitoneal lymphadenectomy (RPLND) may be offered. In patients with one or more adverse histologic factors, RPLND should be performed. In Europe and some U.S. centers, primary chemotherapy has also been used in this setting. However, no randomized trials have compared primary chemotherapy with surveillance or RPLND, and its use remains controversial.

39. What are the advantages and disadvantages of surveillance vs. RPLND for clinical stage $T_{1-2}N_0M_0$ nonseminomatous tumors?

The main advantage of surveillance is the avoidance of a major surgical procedure in the 70% of patients who are cured by orchiectomy alone. The disadvantage of surveillance is the more intensive follow-up regimen required and the uncertainty about cure. The main advantage of RPLND is complete pathologic staging in all patients, early identification of the 30% who have occult retroperitoneal metastases, and the identification of a small subset who require adjuvant chemotherapy. In the past, the main disadvantage of RPLND was loss of seminal emission, but nerve-sparing techniques result in preservation of emission and ejaculation in virtually 100% of patients with Stage I disease.

40. Describe nerve-sparing RPLND.

The key element in nerve-sparing RPLND is the prospective identification and preservation of postganglionic sympathetic nerves that arise from the lumbar sympathetic chains and form an anastomosing network (the hypogastric plexus) anterior to the abdominal aorta and surrounding the origin of the inferior mesenteric artery. Nerves from the hypogastric plexus travel anteriorly along the aorta, across the aortic bifurcation, and descend into the pelvis to innervate the bladder neck and enter the seminal vesicles, vas deferens, prostate, and external urinary sphincter, and subserve emission and ejaculation. Older techniques of RPLND routinely disrupted these nerves and often resulted in failure of seminal emission, leading to dry ejaculation.

41. Describe the treatment for a clinical stage $T_{1-2}N_0M_0$ nonseminomatous tumor found to have metastatic cancer at the time of RPLND.

Treatment depends on the number, size, and histology of the involved nodes. For patients with N1 disease (see table following question 17), the risk of relapse is about 25–30%, and most patients are observed. For N2 or greater disease, the risk of relapse is 50%, and 2 cycles of adjuvant chemotherapy are recommended. If the nodes contain mature teratoma only, observation is usually recommended regardless of the number of size of nodes involved.

42. Describe treatment for small-volume (<5 cm retroperitoneal mass) clinical stage $T_{1-2}N_{1-2}M_0$ nonseminomatous tumors.

Treatment depends upon the level of postorchiectomy tumor markers. If the markers are normal, RPLND is performed; if metastatic disease is confirmed, patients are generally treated with adjuvant chemotherapy, although observation may be advised if the volume of metastases is small or only mature teratoma is found. Tumors with elevated postorchiectomy serum markers are treated with systemic chemotherapy followed by surgical resection of any residual metastases.

43. What is the treatment of advanced ($T_{any}N_3M_{0-1}$) nonseminomatous germ-cell tumors?

The recommended treatment is systemic platinum-based multiagent chemotherapy, followed by surgical excision of residual pulmonary or retroperitoneal masses. If the initial diagnosis is made by lymph node or retroperitoneal biopsy, the ipsilateral testis should also be removed. A recent international consensus has classified advanced stages of germ-cell tumors into prognostic groups based on their likelihood of cure and agreed-on recommended chemotherapy regimens for each risk group (see the following tables).

Good Prognosis Group

CRITERION	NSGCT	SEMINOMA
PRIMARY SITE	TESTIS/RP	ANY
METASTASES	NO NPVM	NO NPVM
AFP	<1000	NL
HCG	<5000	ANY
LDH	<1.5 × ULN	ANY

NL = normal, NPVM = nonpulmonary visceral metastasis, NSGCT = nonseminomatous germ-cell tumor, RP = retroperitoneum, ULN = upper limits of normal

Intermediate Prognosis Group

CRITERION	NSGCT	SEMINOMA
PRIMARY SITE	TESTIS/RP	ANY
METASTASIS	NO NPVM	NPVM
AFP	1000–10,000	NL
HCG	5000–50,000	ANY
LDH	>1.5 to 10 × ULN	ANY

NSGCT = nonseminomatous germ-cell tumor, NPVM = nonpulmonary visceral metastasis, RP = retroperitoneum, ULN = upper limits of normal

Poor Prognosis Group*

CRITERION	NSGCT
PRIMARY SITE	MEDIASTINUM
METASTASIS	NPVM
AFP	>10,000
HCG	> 50,000
LDH	>10 × ULN

NPVM = nonpulmonary visceral metastasis, NSGCT = nonseminomatous germ-cell tumor, ULN = upper limits of normal
*Note there are no poor prognosis seminomas.

Prognosis Based on Risk Group (5-Year Survival)

GROUP	RELAPSE-FREE SURVIVAL (%)	OVERALL SURVIVAL (%)
GOOD	89	92
INTERMEDIATE	75	80
POOR	41	48

Recommended Treatment by Risk Group

RISK GROUP	THERAPY
GOOD	EP × 4 or BEP × 3
INTERMEDIATE	BEP × 4
POOR	VIP or EIP × 4

B = bleomycin
E = etoposide (VP16)
P = cis-Platinum
V = vinblastine
I = ifosfamide

44. Describe the clinical presentation of gonadal stromal tumors.

Gonadal stromal tumors usually present similar to germ-cell tumors, with a painless mass or swelling. Except for Leydig-cell tumors, which may present with feminization or other endocrinologic manifestations, these tumors are not usually suspected before orchiectomy.

45. Do gonadal stromal tumors produce clinically useful tumor markers?

These tumors do not secrete AFP or HCG, but some (especially Leydig-cell tumors) do produce estrogens and estrogen metabolites, which may be useful for monitoring for tumor recurrence.

46. How are gonadal stromal tumors treated?

About 90% of these tumors are benign and are cured by inguinal orchiectomy. RPLND may be considered if the histologic appearance suggests malignancy.

47. What other mesenchymal tumors may occur in the testis?

The most common mesenchymal tumors are fibromas, angiomas, leiomyomas, and neurofibromas, although any other stromal element may give rise to a tumor. These are important chiefly to be distinguished from germ-cell tumors.

48. Describe epidermoid cysts and their treatment.

Epidermoid cysts are round, sharply circumcised lesions composed of fibrous tissue and keratinized squamous epithelium. They are uniformly benign and treated by inguinal orchiectomy, although some have advocated partial excision, especially in children. This lesion may be suspected on testicular ultrasound because of its well-defined edge and associated calcification.

49. Name the most common secondary tumor of the testis.

Lymphoma, which typically causes diffuse enlargement of the involved testis and may be the initial presenting sign of disease.

50. What are the most common metastatic tumors to the testis?

Adenocarcinomas of the prostate, lung, gastrointestinal tract, and kidney and melanoma.

BIBLIOGRAPHY

 1. Donohue JP, Zachary JM, Maynard BR: Distribution of nodal metastases in nonseminomatous testis cancer. J Urol 128:315, 1981.
 2. Donohue JP, Foster RS, Rowland RG, et al: Nerve-sparing retroperitoneal lymphadenectomy with preservation of ejaculation. J Urol 144:287, 1990.
 3. Fleming ID, Cooper JS, Henson DE, et al (eds): AJCC Cancer Staging Handbook, 5th ed. Philadelphia, Lippincott-Raven, 1998.
 4. International Germ Cell Consensus Classification: A prognostic factor-based staging system for metastatic germ cell cancers. International Germ Cell Cancer Collaborative Group. J Clin Oncol 15:594, 1997.
 5. Jewett MA, Kong YS, Goldberg SD, et al: Retroperitoneal lymphadenectomy for testis tumor with nerve sparing for ejaculation. J Urol 139:1220, 1987.
 6. Klein EA, Kay R (eds): Testis cancer in adults and children. Urol Clin North Am 20(1):1993.
 7. Klein EA: Tumor markers in testis cancer. Urol Clin North Am 20:67, 1993.
 8. Lange PH, Neurin P, Fraley EE: Fertility issues following therapy for testicular cancer. Semin Urol 2:264, 1984.
 9. Lowe BA: Surveillance vs nerve sparing RPLND in stage I nonseminomatous germ cell tumors. Urol Clin North Am 20:75, 1993.
10. McLeod DG, Weiss RB, Stablein DM, et al: Staging relationships and outcome in early stage testicular cancer: A report from the testicular cancer intergroup study. J Urol 145:1178, 1990.
11. Marshall FF, Elder J: Cryptorchidism and Related Anomalies. New York, Praeger, 1982.
12. Motzer RJ, Bosl GJ: Role of adjuvant chemotherapy in patients with stage II nonseminomatous germ-cell tumors. Urol Clin North Am 20:11, 1993.

13. Recker F, Tscholl R: Monitoring of emission as direct intraoperative control for nerve sparing retroperitoneal lymphadenectomy. J Urol 150:1360, 1993.
14. Sheinfeld J, Bajorin D: Management of the postchemotherapy residual mass. Urol Clin North Am 20:133, 1993.
15. Vugrin D, Whitmore WF, Golbey RB: VAB-6 combination chemotherapy without maintenance in treatment of disseminated cancer of the testis. Cancer 51:211, 1983.
16. Wishnow KW, et al: Prompt orchiectomy reduces morbidity and mortality from testis cancer. Br J Urol 65:629, 1990.

34. TESTICULAR TUMORS IN CHILDREN

Robert Kay, M.D.

1. What is the most common type of testicular tumor in children?

Yolk sac tumor. It represents 60%–63% of all testicular tumors in children.

2. Is a yolk sac tumor the same as embryonal cell tumor in an adult?

No. Yolk sac tumors differ histologically and biologically from embryonal cell tumors, and the treatment is different.

3. How do children with a testicular tumor usually present?

Most children with testicular tumors present with an asymptomatic mass. It may be misdiagnosed as a hydrocele, delaying diagnosis for up to 6 months.

4. What are the best diagnostic tests for a testicular tumor?

Ultrasound may be definitive with testicular tumors. If a child has a scrotal mass in which the testis cannot be felt or if the diagnosis is unclear, an ultrasound should be obtained. It can clearly delineate the testis and determine if there is an intratesticular mass.

Serum alpha-fetoprotein levels should also be analyzed. Alpha-fetoprotein is a protein that occurs in the fetus but disappears after birth. It is also produced by yolk sac tumors. Although elevated levels may be seen in a newborn and in the first six months of life, it is an excellent tumor marker that can be used both preoperatively and postoperatively to follow the tumor.

5. What tests should be ordered after a diagnosis of yolk sac tumor is made?

Assuming the alpha-fetoprotein was ordered preoperatively or immediately postoperatively, one should obtain a chest x-ray and an ultrasound or computed tomographic (CT) scan of the retroperitoneum to assess for retroperitoneal metastasis. This will allow the physician to stage the patient clinically.

6. What is the half-life of alpha-fetoprotein? How long before elevated levels return to normal?

The half-life of alpha-fetoprotein is 5 days. Thus, five half-lives or approximately 25–30 days should elapse before normal values are seen.

7. What are the survival statistics for children with yolk sac tumors?

Greater than 90% of children with yolk sac tumors will survive.

8. Besides yolk sac tumors, are other testicular tumors malignant?

Most other testicular tumors are benign. The second most common tumor in children, the teratoma, is always benign in infants and children. Although most gonadal stromal tumors are benign, the very rare case of a malignant gonadal stromal tumor has occurred.

9. Does radiation therapy have a role in the treatment of prepubertal testicular tumors?

No. Surgery is curative in almost all cases, and only in the unusual metastatic yolk sac tumor is chemotherapy needed. Chemotherapy is effective, so radiotherapy does not play a role except in the palliative care of the child or in metastatic disease that is resistant to chemotherapy.

10. Can tumors be seen in the newborn?

Almost all types of testicular tumors may be seen in the newborn. However, juvenile granulosa cell tumor and yolk sac tumor are the most common tumors in the neonatal period. The tumors present as a hard mass and must not be misdiagnosed as in utero torsion of the testis.

11. What other testicular tumors occur in children?

Classification of Prepubertal Testicular Tumors

Germ cell tumors
  Yolk sac
  Teratoma
  Mixed germ cell
  Seminoma
Gonadal stromal tumors
  Leydig cell
  Sertoli cell
  Juvenile granulosa cell
  Mixed
Gonadoblastoma
Tumors of supporting tissues
  Fibroma
  Leiomyoma
  Hemangioma
Lymphomas and leukemias
Tumor-like lesions
  Epidermoid cysts
  Hyperplastic nodule secondary to congenital adrenal hyperplasia
Secondary tumors
Tumors of the adenexa

12. Which testicular tumor leads to precocious puberty in children?
Leydig cell tumor.

13. Is a retroperitoneal node dissection routinely indicated in yolk sac tumor?
No. The tumor metastasizes via both the hematogenous and lymphogenous system. A retroperitoneal node dissection should be done only if there is radiologic evidence of metastatic disease.

14. What is occult testicular leukemia?
Occult testicular leukemia refers to children with acute lymphogenous leukemia in remission but in whom routine biopsy of testis reveals disease confined to the testis. This occurs in 11% of patients with acute lymphogenous leukemia.

15. Why would leukemia present in the testis but not be detected anywhere else?
Although there are different theories, most believe there is a blood testis barrier. This allows the testis to be a protected haven from chemotherapy; thus, isolated cells are not destroyed by the systemic treatment.

16. Which prepubertal tumor of the testis is seen in genetic disorders such as Peutz-Jeghers syndrome?
Sertoli cell tumor.

17. What is the most likely diagnosis in a child who has congenital adrenal hyperplasia (CAH) and presents with a bilateral testicular mass?
The most likely diagnosis is hyperplastic nodules (testicular tumor of CAH).

18. Is teratoma in children identical to teratoma in adults?

No. Teratoma in children is always benign. In contrast, teratoma in adults may undergo malignant changes and subsequent metastasis. Teratoma in children may be enucleated because of its universal benign behavior.

BIBLIOGRAPHY

1. Berg NB, Schenkman NS, Skoog SJ, Davis CJ: Testicular masses associated with congenital hyperplasia: MRI findings. Urology 47:252–253, 1996.
2. Connolly JA, Gearhart JB: Management of yolk sac tumors in children. Urol Clin North Am 20:7–14, 1993.
3. Grady R, Ross JH, Kay R: Epidemiologic features of teratomas of the testis in a prepubertal population. J Urol 158:1191–1192, 1997.
4. Grady R, Ross JH, Kay R: Patterns of metastatic spread in prepubertal yolk sac tumor of the testis. J Urol 153:1259–1261, 1995.
5. Kay R: Genital tumors in children. In Kelalis PP, King LR, Belman AB (eds): Clinical Pediatric Urology, 3rd ed. Philadelphia, W. B. Saunders Co., 1992, pp 1457–1467.
6. Kay R: Prepubertal Testicular Tumor Registry. Urol Clin North Am 20:1–5, 1993.
7. Kay R, Kaplan GW: Testicular tumors in infants and children. Am Urol Assoc Update Ser 9:114–118, 1992.
8. Lange PH, Vogelzang NJ, Goldman A, et al: Marker half-life analysis as a prognostic tool in testicular cancer. J Urol 128:708, 1982.
9. Levy D, Kay R, Elder J: Neonatal testis tumors: A review of the Prepubertal Testis Tumor Registry. J Urol 151:715, 1994.
10. Rich MA, Keating MA, Levin HS, Kay R: Tumors of adrenogenital syndrome: Aggressive conservative approach. J Urol 160:1838–1848, 1998.

35. LAPAROSCOPIC SURGERY FOR GENITOURINARY TUMORS

Inderbir S. Gill, M.D., M.Ch.

1. What is laparoscopic surgery?

The term *laparoscopy* implies performing endoscopic surgery of the abdominal cavity through keyhole incisions. Carbon dioxide is instilled into the peritoneal cavity to a pressure of 10–15 mm Hg in order to distend the abdomen and provide clear visualization. The real-time laparoscopic pictures are relayed by an attached camera to a television monitor, and surgery is performed while looking at the television monitor. Various specially designed instruments are inserted into the abdomen through individual ports, allowing specific surgical procedures to be performed with great precision.

2. What laparoscopic procedures are being performed in the field of genitourinary oncology?

Urologic laparoscopic surgery is a rapidly evolving subspecialty. Currently, laparoscopic techniques are being used in the treatment of tumors of the adrenal gland, kidney, ureter, prostate, bladder, and testis.

3. What role does laparoscopy have in the treatment of adrenal cancer?

Laparoscopic radical adrenalectomy for solitary adrenal metastasis or small, locally confined adrenal cancers has been reported in a limited number of patients. Although laparoscopic adrenalectomy is replacing open surgical techniques in the treatment of the vast majority of benign surgical adrenal disease, open surgery still remains the preferred treatment for adrenal cancer in most cases. Surgery for localized adrenal cancer involves a radical adrenalectomy, occasionally with en bloc resection and/or lymphadenectomy, which may be best accomplished by the open approach. Thus, larger adrenal tumors with evidence of local invasion of adjacent tissues or presence of a thrombus in the main adrenal vein or inferior vena cava are best treated by open surgery. However, smaller, solitary adrenal metastatic lesions without evidence of local infiltration have been excised laparoscopically. In this regard, meticulous preoperative scanning and imaging by CT and MRI are critical to confirm absence of local periadrenal infiltration of adjacent structures, to visualize fat planes between the adrenal gland and the inferior vena cava/aorta, and to confirm the absence of venous thrombus. Therefore, laparoscopic adrenalectomy for adrenal metastasis or cancer is advanced surgery and should be performed only by the experienced laparoscopist.

4. Has laparoscopy been applied to benign adrenal tumors?

Yes. Laparoscopic adrenalectomy is probably now the preferred technique for the majority of surgical adrenal disease, including pheochromocytoma, aldosteroma, Cushing's disease, Cushing's adenoma, and selected incidentalomas (incidentally detected adrenal tumors). At centers of excellence, the primary adrenal-specific contraindication to laparoscopic adrenalectomy is a large, locally invasive adrenal cancer.

5. What are the current indications for a laparoscopic radical nephrectomy?

Laparoscopic radical nephrectomy for kidney cancer is slowly but surely reaching "established" status. Currently, laparoscopic radical nephrectomy is being performed at an increasing number of centers for selected patients with T_1–$T_2N_0M_0$ kidney tumors. The technique of laparoscopic radical nephrectomy mirrors that of its open surgical counterpart, in that the tumor-bearing kidney, including en bloc adrenal gland covered by Gerota's fascia, is removed while observing established principles of oncologic surgery. The renal artery and vein are laparoscopically controlled before mobilization of the cancerous kidney. Laparoscopic radical nephrectomy can be performed by either the transperitoneal approach or the retroperitoneal approach. Approximately 1000 laparoscopic radical nephrectomies have been reported worldwide. Although short-term results have been excellent, long-term data are currently lacking. In a multi-institutional analysis of 157 laparoscopic radical nephrectomies with a mean follow-up of 19.2 months, 5-year actuarial disease-free patient survival was 91%. No patient had renal fossa or port-site seeding, and 5 patients with T_2 disease developed retroperitoneal/metastatic recurrences. The cancer mortality rate was 0.

6. How is the patient positioned during a laparoscopic radical nephrectomy?

In the 45-degree to 60-degree flank position for the transperitoneal approach, and in the 90-degree flank position for the retroperitoneal approach.

7. Is laparoscopic partial nephrectomy now a viable treatment option?

Laparoscopic partial nephrectomy has been performed in fewer than 200 patients worldwide. The last edition of this book mentioned that, at that writing, laparoscopic partial nephrectomy was not a viable treatment option. Things have obviously progressed a lot since then. The largest experience in over 75 cases comes from the Cleveland Clinic, where reproducible techniques have been developed for transient atraumatic clamping of the renal artery and vein, excision of the tumor in a bloodless field, suture repair of the collecting system (if indicated), and renal parenchymal suture reconstruction. In the initial 50 cases, mean O.R. time was 3 hours, blood loss was 270 cc, warm ischemia time was 23 min, and hospital stay was 2.2 days. Complications occurred in 6 (12%) patients. As such, this author believes that laparoscopic partial nephrectomy has significant potential in the future armamentarium of nephron-sparing surgery. Advances in tissue glue technology and development of laparoscopic techniques of renal hypothermia will further advance the application of laparoscopic partial nephrectomy.

8. Can laparoscopic radical nephroureterectomy be performed for upper tract urothelial transitional cell carcinoma (TCC)?

Yes. In patients with upper tract TCC who are candidates for a radical nephroureterectomy, the laparoscopic approach is an excellent alternative to open surgery. The Gerota's fascia–covered kidney, adrenal gland, and ureter with adjacent bladder cuff can be excised en bloc laparoscopically. Extreme care is taken not to violate Gerota's fascia intraoperatively, and at the end of the procedure, the specimen is extracted *intact* enclosed within an impermeable plastic sac.

9. You are performing a laparoscopic radical nephrectomy in a 70-year-old man with pre-existing cardiac valvular disease. Intraoperatively, the patient suddenly becomes hypotensive and the anesthesiologist auscultates a "mill-wheel" cardiac murmur. What is occurring and how would you manage it?

The appearance of a mill-wheel murmur is a classic sign of gas embolism. Management of gas embolism includes immediate desufflation (removal of carbon dioxide from the abdomen) and placing the patient in a steep left lateral decubitus (right side up) Trendelenburg position to minimize right ventricular outlet obstruction. Often, aspiration of the gas embolus via a central venous catheter may be required. Although typical, a mill-wheel murmur is not the earliest sign of a venous gas embolism. An exponential, rapid decrease in end-tidal CO_2 within the space of a dozen breaths is the earliest sign of a gas embolus, which results from a sudden interruption of pulmonary blood flow by the embolus. Auscultation of a mill-wheel murmur, severe hypotension, and a sudden decline in oxygen saturation appear somewhat later and are more ominous findings. Although a rare occurrence, gas embolism remains one of the most dreaded complications associated with laparoscopy. Since a decrease in end-tidal CO_2 is one of its earliest signs, capnometric monitoring is used routinely during all laparoscopic cases.

10. Are there any special considerations in regards to anesthesia during laparoscopic surgery?

An expert anesthesiologist familiar with the nuances of laparoscopic surgery is a vital member of the laparoscopic surgical team. Laparoscopic cases may be long in duration, with the patient situated often in a flank and/or Trendelenburg position; a cuffed endotracheal tube is mandatory to guard against pulmonary aspiration intraoperatively. Because laparoscopic surgery causes minimal fluid losses as compared to open surgery, intraoperative intravenous (IV) fluid requirements are lesser. Vigorous fluid replacement may cause pulmonary edema in patients with a borderline cardiac status. Controlled ventilation with high minute volumes is necessary to compensate for the pulmonary and diaphragmatic alterations caused by the prolonged pneumoperitoneum and the head-down position. Nitrous oxide may cause bowel distention and its use as an anesthetic agent should be avoided. Furthermore, although not combustible, nitrous oxide can support combustion and must not be used when using electrosurgical instruments.

11. You are performing a laparoscopic radical nephrectomy in a 50-year-old man without preexisting cardiac disease. The operation has been proceeding smoothly for the past 3 hours, with stable vital signs. However, the anesthesiologist notes that over the past 20 minutes, the patient's blood pressure has started dropping, ventilation has become more difficult, and some arrhythmias have developed. You have detected no problems through the laparoscope—what is going on?

Tension pneumoperitoneum is a consequence of persistently elevated intraabdominal CO_2 pressures (of >15–20 mm Hg). When such high intraperitoneal pressures have been present for a long period, inferior vena cava compression occurs, leading to decreased venous return and hypotension. Additionally, pressure on the diaphragm makes ventilation more difficult. Increased amounts of CO_2 get absorbed into the blood stream, resulting in acidosis, hypoxemia, hypercarbia, and arrhythmias with ultimate cardiovascular collapse. Treatment consists of immediate desufflation, correcting the Trendelenburg position, hyperventilation with 100% oxygen, and IV fluids.

12. How has laparoscopy been applied to prostate cancer?

Again, in the previous edition of this book, there was only a dismissive mention of the words "laparoscopic radical prostatectomy"! In the short time since, laparoscopic radical prostatectomy has emerged as the singlemost visible advance in minimally invasive urologic surgery, thanks largely to the French team of Guillonneau and Vallencien. Laparoscopic radical prostatectomy is not an established procedure at this writing, and its merits and demerits compared with open surgery are hotly debated. However, more than 1500 procedures have already been performed worldwide. Data from multiple institutions regarding continence, potency, surgical margins, and quality-of-life questionnaires will be necessary to determine the true place of laparoscopic radical prostatectomy in comparison with the open retropubic and perineal approaches.

13. What are the current indications for laparoscopic PLND for prostate cancer?

Laparoscopic PLND is indicated in patients who have a high likelihood of lymphatic metastatic disease, the identification of which would spare the patient a subsequent open radical prostatectomy or definitive radiotherapy altogether. The availability of prostate-specific antigen (PSA) testing, transrectal ultrasonography, and the Partin nomogram have been a major advance. Current indications for laparoscopic PLND include patients with clinical stage B_2/C disease, Gleason score $\geq$ 7, PSA $\geq$ 10, or an elevated acid phosopatase. With these indications, the node-positive rate approaches 40%. In the early 1990s, laparoscopic PLND was the most commonly performed laparoscopic urologic procedure. However, in recent years, owing to the previously mentioned advances, laparoscopic PLND is now an infrequent procedure, representing less than 5% of the author's total laparoscopic workload.

14. What are the anatomic boundaries of a limited laparoscopic PLND?

At most centers, a limited PLND is preferred over an extended PLND, because 85–90% of lymphatic metastases from prostate cancer involve the obturator-hypogastric nodal chain. Only 15% of patients have "skip-lesions" involving the common iliac/aortic nodes while sparing the obturator-hypogastric nodes. Furthermore, the incidence of complications is significantly higher

(12–25%) during an extended PLND as compared to a limited PLND. The boundaries of a limited laparoscopic PLND include the external iliac vein anterolaterally, the obturator nerve posteriorly, the pelvic side wall laterally, the pubic periosteum distally, and the hypogastric bifurcation proximally.

15. What is the false-negative rate of a laparoscopic PLND?
≤10%.

16. During a laparoscopic PLND the urine in the Foley catheter becomes pink-tinged. What does this indicate?
Hematuria and/or pneumaturia are the initial signs of bladder injury. The bladder should be filled with indigo carmine-stained saline through the Foley catheter and leakage into the peritoneal cavity is assessed laparoscopically. If a cystotomy is identified, it should be repaired either laparoscopically or by converting to open surgery. The most common postoperative complication after laparoscopic PLND is urinary retention. Other infrequent complications include bowel injury, ureteral injury, inferior epigastric artery injury, obturator nerve palsy, and rarely, osteitis pubis.

17. During a laparoscopic PLND, the end-tidal CO_2 reading increases to 50 mm Hg. How should this be managed?
The safest thing to do is to desufflate immediately. The anesthesiologist will proceed to hyperventilate the patient. This is usually a problem in patients with preexisting pulmonary disease. After the end-tidal CO_2 has decreased appropriately, the procedure may be resumed, albeit at a lower pneumoperitoneum pressure.

18. Have laparoscopic techniques been applied to testicular cancer?
Yes. Laparoscopic retroperitoneal lymph node dissection (RPLND) has been performed in patients who are candidates for open RPLND. In addition to patients with stage I nonseminomatous germ cell testicular tumor, laparoscopic RPLND also has been performed in a few centers in patients with postchemotherapy residual retroperitoneal masses.

19. How about bladder cancer?
Laparoscopic radical cystectomy with urinary diversion has been performed in a limited number of patients. Various laparoscopically created urinary diversions include ileal conduit, rectosigmoid pouch, and even orthotopic ileal (Studer) neobladder. However, these techniques are still in their infancy.

20. What are the contraindications for laparoscopic surgery?
General contraindications for laparoscopic surgery include severe cardiopulmonary risk factors, uncorrected coagulopathy, and abdominal sepsis and distention.

21. What are the advantages and disadvantages of laparoscopic surgery?
Minimally invasive surgery decreases the trauma of access while allowing the actual surgical procedure to be performed in a manner comparable to open surgery. Accordingly, significant advantages result, including decreased postoperative morbidity, quicker convalescence, decreased analgesic requirements, and a superior cosmetic result. However, there are certain disadvantages: Typically, the learning curve for laparoscopic surgery is steep, and consequently, the operative times are longer than for a comparable open procedure. Special training is required to become facile at laparoscopic surgery. In terms of cost, laparoscopic surgery is in general somewhat more expensive than open surgery. However, not factored into this equation are the significant although intangible cost advantages of decreased postoperative patient discomfort, a superior sense of patient well-being, a better cosmetic result, and a quicker return to employment.

22. What are some of the misconceptions about laparoscopic surgery?

Because laparoscopy is performed through keyhole incisions, the visualization and exposure are considered to be inferior by some. This is completely untrue. The excellent optics and magnification afforded by the laparoscope provide outstanding visualization, which is actually superior to that obtained during conventional surgery.

23. What are some of the anticipated advances of laparoscopic techniques in the field of genitourinary oncology?

Precise, targeted ablation of solid tumors will be increasingly performed by minimally invasive, and ultimately noninvasive techniques. For example, **laparoscopic cryoablation** is currently being investigated for select patients with small (<4 cm) exophytic renal tumors that would otherwise be amenable to open partial nephrectomy. Cryoablation in this setting is precisely monitored by a combination of laparoscopic visualization and real-time endoscopic ultrasound monitoring. Alternative energy sources with potential laparoscopic application include radio frequency and interstitial laser. As experience and facility in laparoscopic technique increase, a majority of renal tumors can be approached in this way. Currently, large tumor size per se is not an absolute contraindication to the laparoscopic removal of adrenal and renal tumors up to 12 cm in size. Increasing applications for laparoscopic prostate and bladder surgery are anticipated.

BIBLIOGRAPHY

1. Cadeddu JA, Ono Y, Clayman RV, et al: Laparoscopic nephrectomy for renal cell cancer: Evaluation of efficacy and safety: A multi-center experience. Urology 1998;52: 773–777.
2. Heinford T, Sung GT, Gill IS et al: Laparoscopic adrenalectomy for cancer. J Urol 165:2, 2001.
3. McDougall EM, Gill IS, Clayman RV: Laparascopic urology. In Gillenwater JY, Grayhack JT, Howards SS, Duckett JW (eds): Adult and Pediatric Urology, 3rd ed. St. Louis, Mosby, 1996, pp 829–912.
4. Gill IS, Meraney AM, Schweizer DA, et al: Laparoscopic radical nephrectomy in 100 patients: A single center experience from the United States. Cancer 92;1843–1855, 2001.
5. Gill IS, Desai MM, Kaouk JH, et al: Laparoscopic partial nephrectomy for renal tumor: Duplicating open surgical techniques. J Urol (in press) 2002.
6. Gill IS, Sung GT, Hobart MG, et al: Laparoscopic radical nephroureterectomy for upper tract transitional cell carcinoma: The Cleveland Clinic experience. J Urol 164:1513, 2000.
7. Shalhav AL, Dunn MD, Portis AJ, et al: Laparoscopic nephroureterectomy for upper tract transitional cell cancer: The Washington University experience. J Urol 163:1100, 2000.
8. Guillonneau B, Vallancien G: Laparoscopic radical prostatectomy: The Montsouris experience. J Urol 163:418, 2000.
9. Gill IS, Fergany A, Klein E, et al: Laparoscopic radical cystoprostatectomy with ileal conduit performed completely intracorporeally: The initial 2 cases. Urology 56:26–29, 2000.

III. Congenital and Acquired Disease

36. CONGENITAL RENAL CYSTIC DISEASE

Jonathan H. Ross, M.D.

1. Explain the difference between polycystic kidney disease and a multicystic kidney.

The polycystic kidney diseases are congenital cystic diseases of the kidneys in which otherwise normal renal elements become cystically dilated. In contrast, the cysts of a multicystic kidney are not due to dilatation of specific renal elements, but rather, the entire kidney is dysplastic and composed of immature dysplastic stroma and cysts of various sizes.

2. What is the prognosis for an infant with bilateral multicystic kidneys?

Dismal. Multicystic kidneys do not function. As in renal agenesis, this results in anhydramnios and fatal pulmonary hypoplasia.

3. What is the most common cause of an abdominal mass in a newborn?

A multicystic dysplastic kidney. A hydronephrotic kidney, usually due to ureteropelvic junction obstruction, is a close second.

4. How are most multicystic kidneys currently diagnosed?

By prenatal ultrasound. Historically, only palpable multicystic kidneys were detected. Most went undetected and probably regressed. Many adults with an incidentally noted solitary kidney probably had a multicystic kidney originally.

5. What entities may be confused with a multicystic kidney?

Any of the other congenital cystic kidney diseases may be confused with a multicystic kidney, but these are quite rare. The most important distinction is between a multicystic kidney and a severe ureteropelvic junction obstruction.

6. How do you distinguish a multicystic kidney from a ureteropelvic junction obstruction?

The distinction can usually be made by ultrasound. The cysts of a multicystic kidney do not communicate. The cystic dilatation of a hydronephrotic kidney communicates throughout. Therefore, if communications between cysts can be demonstrated, then the kidney is hydronephrotic. If any uncertainty remains, a renal flow scan should be obtained. On a renal scan, multicystic kidneys appear photopenic, whereas even severe ureteropelvic junction obstructions generally demonstrate some function. In rare equivocal cases, an antegrade nephrostogram may be obtained.

7. Are there any other urologic anomalies associated with multicystic dysplastic kidneys?

Yes. Contralateral ureteropelvic junction obstruction and vesicoureteral reflux are the most common.

8. Are there any absolute indications for surgical removal of a multicystic kidney?

Hypertension or massive size.

9. What features distinguish autosomal-recessive polycystic kidney disease (ARPKD) from autosomal-dominant polycystic kidney disease (ADPKD)?

ARPKD Versus ADPKD

	ARPKD	ADPKD
Gross appearance	Massively enlarged but still reniform	Renal contour distorted by cysts of varying sizes
Portion of nephron that is cystically dilated	Collecting ducts and tubules only	All portions of the nephron, including the glomeruli
Lesions in other organs	Proliferation and dilatation of biliary ducts with periportal fibrosis	Hepatic, pancreatic and splenic cysts, and cerebral berry aneurysms
Age of onset	Infancy/childhood	Usually adulthood

10. Which polycystic kidney disease occurs in children?

This is a trick question. ARPKD is typically a disease of infancy and childhood, and ADPKD usually presents in adulthood. However, a few patients with ADPKD become symptomatic in childhood.

11. Do infants and older children with ARPKD generally present with the same problems?

No. All children with ARPKD have renal and hepatic involvement, but the renal involvement tends to be more prominent in infants. In the most severe cases, extensive renal involvement is present and death occurs due to pulmonary hypoplasia. Older children tend to present with complications of hepatic fibrosis, such as bleeding esophageal varices or hepatosplenomegaly due to portal hypertension.

12. What is the outlook for patients with ARPKD?

Not as grim as it used to be. Because of improvements in neonatal intensive care, the 2-year survival rate for those presenting in the neonatal period is roughly 50%. However, nearly all patients develop end-stage renal disease by adulthood (50% by adolescence). Hepatic involvement is variable. Some patients require treatment for portal hypertension, whereas others have subclinical disease detectable only by ultrasound or biopsy. Hepatic failure does not occur.

13. Can ARPKD be detected by prenatal ultrasound?

Yes, in about 50% of cases.

14. How may ADPKD present in childhood?

It presents rarely in infancy with nephromegaly or pulmonary hypoplasia. Older children may develop the same spectrum of problems seen more commonly in adults: Hematuria, urinary tract infection, flank pain, hypertension, proteinuria, palpable kidneys, or intracerebral hemorrhage.

15. Although most affected children with ADPKD are asymptomatic, can they be detected by ultrasound?

Ultrasound can detect 22% of affected individuals in the first decade of life, and 66% during the second decade.

16. Can ADPKD be detected prenatally?

Prenatal ultrasound is abnormal in a minority of affected fetuses. DNA probes have been used for prenatal diagnosis, but this technique is expensive and not readily available.

17. What is the prognosis for ADPKD presenting in childhood?

Approximately one-half of patients with clinical manifestations in infancy die of respiratory failure or sepsis. Cases that become evident later in childhood rarely progress to renal failure before adulthood.

18. How is ADPKD in childhood treated?

The same as in adulthood—aggressive management of complications such as hypertension and urinary tract infection.

19. Can simple renal cysts be diagnosed in childhood?

Yes, but they are rare. Any young child with a renal cyst requires careful evaluation of family members (including renal ultrasonography of both parents) and periodic follow-up to rule out polycystic kidney disease.

20. Describe familial juvenile nephronophthisis (FJN).

FJN is a type of hereditary interstitial nephritis associated with medullary and cortico-medullary cysts. Most cases are inherited as an autosomal recessive trait. The disease usually progresses to renal failure by the second or third decade of life.

CONTROVERSY

21. What is the appropriate management of multicystic dysplastic kidneys detected by prenatal ultrasonography?

The options for managing a multicystic dysplastic kidney are to remove it, follow it, or ignore it. Surgical excision is supported by the reports of hypertension and malignancy (both Wilms tumor and renal cell carcinoma) occurring in patients with multicystic kidneys. However, the number of reported cases is small, and the total number of multicystic kidneys, although unknown, is undoubtedly large. Therefore, the risk for any given patient is probably extremely small and may not justify the surgical risk of excision.

Most pediatric urologists therefore recommend following patients with multicystic kidneys with periodic ultrasound and blood pressure monitoring. Obviously, any patient developing hypertension or a renal mass should undergo nephrectomy. Some surgeons also remove multicystic kidneys that fail to regress. Conversely, once a multicystic kidney has regressed on ultrasound, monitoring is discontinued.

However, this approach is not entirely logical. It bases management on the progression (or regression) of the cystic component of these lesions (the part discernible on ultrasound). Yet, the hypertension and tumors reported undoubtedly arise from the stromal component. Must patients therefore undergo periodic flank ultrasounds for life? Would it be simpler just to remove the multicystic kidney in infancy—an operation which can be done as an outpatient procedure through a relatively small incision? Or, given the anecdotal nature of reports of hypertension and tumors, and the difficulties of ultrasonographic follow-up, perhaps they should just be ignored? After all, that is how nearly all of them were successfully managed before the era of prenatal ultrasound (because we did not know they were there). Perhaps this is a case "Where ignorance is bliss, 'tis folly to be wise." To address such issues, a multicystic kidney registry has been instituted by the Section of Urology of the American Academy of Pediatrics.

BIBLIOGRAPHY

1. Cendron M, Elder JS, Duckett JW: Perinatal urology. In Gillenwater JY, Grayhack JT, Howards SS, Duckett JW (eds): Adult and Pediatric Urology, 3rd ed. St. Louis, Mosby, 1996, pp 2075–2169.
2. Gagnadoux AF, Habib R, Levy M, et al: Cystic renal diseases in children. Adv Nephrol 18:33–58, 1989.
3. Glassberg KI, Stephens FD, Lebowitz RL, et al: Renal dysgenesis and cystic disease of the kidney: A report of the Committee on Terminology, Nomenclature and Classification, Section on Urology, American Academy of Pediatrics. J Urol 138:1085–1092, 1987.
4. Kaplan BS, Kaplan P, Rosenberg HK, et al: Polycystic kidney disease in childhood. J Pediatr 115: 867–880, 1989.
5. Lippert MC: Renal cystic disease. In Gillenwater JY, Grayhack JT, Howards SS, Duckett JW (eds): Adult and Pediatric Urology, 3rd ed. St. Louis, Mosby, 1996, pp 931–971.

6. Perez LM, Naidu SI, Joseph DE: Outcome and cost analysis of operative versus nonoperative management of neonatal multicystic kidneys. J Urol 160:1207–1211, 1998.
7. Ross JH, Elder JS: Renal dysplasia, hypoplasia, multicystic kidney, and polycystic kidney disease in childhood. In Resnick MI, Kursh ED (eds): Current Therapy in Genitourinary Surgery. St. Louis, Mosby, 1992, pp 198–202.
8. Rudnick-Schoneborn S, John U, Deget F, et al: Clinical features of unilateral multicystic renal dysplasia in children. Eur J Pediatr 157:666–672, 1998.
9. Susskind MR, Kim KS, King LR: Hypertension and multicystic kidney. Urology 34:362–366, 1989.
10. Wacksam J, Phipps L: Report of the Multicystic Kidney Registry: Preliminary findings. J Urol 150:1870–1872, 1993.

37. CUSHING'S SYNDROME

David A. Goldfarb, M.D.

1. What is Cushing's syndrome?

Cushing's syndrome is an endocrine disorder characterized by the excessive secretion of glucocorticoids (cortisol).

2. How does it differ from Cushing's disease?

Cushing's disease refers to a type of Cushing's syndrome produced by pituitary adenomas or hyperplasia. It is a subset of patients with Cushing's syndrome.

3. What are the causes of Cushing's syndrome?

ACTH-Dependent	*ACTH-Independent*
Pituitary (70%)	Adrenal adenoma (10%)
Ectopic ACTH (10%)	Adrenal carcinoma (5%)
Excessive corticotropin releasing factor production (2%)	Adrenal hyperplasia (3%)

4. What are the clinical findings?

Patients with Cushing's syndrome have a characteristic appearance with a round face, truncal obesity, and increased scapular fat pad (buffalo hump). Other features include thin skin, easy bruisability, and proximal muscle weakness. Many patients have hypertension, diabetes mellitus, or psychiatric symptoms.

5. How is the diagnosis made?

When the diagnosis is suspected clinically, the following biochemical tests can be performed:

1. **AM and PM cortisol.** Normal serum cortisol is highest in the early morning and lowest in the evening. This normal diurnal variation is lost in Cushing's syndrome, with high levels of cortisol remaining unchanged through the day.

2. **24-Hour urinary cortisol.** This is the best and most widely available test to measure the integrated cortisol secretion over a 24-hour period. It is elevated in Cushing's syndrome.

3. **Overnight dexamethasone suppression test (DST).** Serum cortisol is measured at 8 AM following 1 mg of dexamethasone given at 11 PM the evening before. Failure to suppress AM cortisol is consistent with Cushing's syndrome.

4. **Low-dose DST.** Plasma and 24-hour urinary cortisol are measured at baseline and after 2 days of dexamethasone (0.5 mg every 6 hr). Failure to suppress cortisol secretion is diagnostic for Cushing's syndrome.

6. How can the different pathologies be differentiated biochemically?

Plasma ACTH should be routinely assessed. A **low plasma ACTH** value suggests primary adrenal cortical disease. When this value is elevated, it suggests pituitary disease or ectopic ACTH syndrome.

Suppression of cortisol secretion after **high-dose DST** (2.0 mg every 6 hr for 2 days) suggests pituitary disease, whereas failure to suppress cortisol occurs with primary adrenal disease and ectopic ACTH syndrome. The false-positive and false-negative rates are 20%.

7. How are patient evaluated radiographically?

1. When the plasma ACTH is low, computed tomography (CT) or magnetic resonance imaging (MRI) of the adrenals should be performed. In most cases, a mass will be identified, although in a few cases hyperplasia may be found.

2. When the plasma ACTH is normal or minimally elevated, an MRI of the pituitary should be obtained. The examination is only 70–80% sensitive in identifying an adenoma.

3. When the plasma ACTH is significantly elevated, ectopic ACTH is likely, but a pituitary tumor needs to be evaluated and an MRI of the pituitary should be obtained.

4. When the MRI fails to disclose a pituitary tumor in ACTH-dependent Cushing's syndrome, petrosal venous sinus sampling can be performed. This is a highly sensitive and specific test to differentiate the causes of Cushing's syndrome, but it is invasive.

5. When ectopic ACTH is suspected, a CT of the abdomen and chest should be obtained to identify the responsible tumor.

8. What is the treatment of Cushing's disease?

Pituitary tumors are treated by transsphenoidal pituitary surgery. Eighty percent of cases respond. Radiation therapy can be used for surgical failures.

9. How are benign vs. malignant adrenal tumors differentiated?

Size is the single most important feature. Tumors >6 cm should be considered malignant until proven otherwise. Biochemical profiling is not reliable for differentiating benign from malignant tumors, with the exception that DHEA-S may be subnormal in adenoma patients and greatly elevated in carcinoma patients. Adenoma patients are generally younger than carcinoma patients.

10. How are adrenal tumors treated?

For small tumors, laparoscopic adrenalectomy has emerged as the treatment of choice. In the absence of an experienced laparoscopist, small tumors can be treated by using an extra-peritoneal approach, such as a flank or posterior incision. If the tumor is large and suspicious for cancer, an anterior transperitoneal approach (subcostal incision) or thoracoabdominal approach should be used. Nonetheless, large tumors may be removed laparoscopically by an experienced team provided an adequate clean tissue plane can be dissected around the adrenal.

11. Is any preoperative treatment required?

For adrenal tumors a steroid preparation should be administered. The contralateral adrenal is suppressed, and until it recovers, supplemental steroid will be required. This recovery may take up to 2 years, and up to 25% of patients may never be steroid-free.

12. Who are candidates for medical treatment?

- Patients who are not surgical candidates due to concomitant medical illness
- Patients in whom transsphenoidal surgery and radiation have failed
- Patients with ectopic ACTH and no identifiable tumor

13. What are available adrenolytic agents?

Mitotane (o, p'DDD) (patients may require supplemental steroids), aminoglutethimide (patients may require supplemental steroids), ketoconazole, and metyrapone.

14. When is bilateral adrenalectomy indicated?

- Macronodular adrenal hyperplasia, which is bilateral
- Medical treatment failures in a patient who is otherwise a surgical candidate

BIBLIOGRAPHY

1. Atkinson AB: The treatment of Cushing's syndrome. Clin Endocrinol 34:507–513, 1991.
2. Orth DN: Differential diagnosis of Cushing's syndrome. N Engl J Med 325:957–959, 1991.
3. Sheeler LR: Cushing's syndrome. Urol Clin North Am 16:447–456, 1989.
4. Straffon RA: Cushing's syndrome and Cushing's disease. In Resnick MI, Kursh ED (eds): Current Therapy in Genito-urinary Surgery, 2nd ed. St. Louis, Mosby, 1992, pp 1–3.

5. Trainer PJ, Grossman A: The diagnosis and differential diagnosis of Cushing's syndrome. Clin Endocrinol 34:317–330, 1991.
6. Vaughan ED, Blumenfeld JD: The adrenals. In Walsh PC, Retik AB, Stamey TA, Vaughan ED Jr (eds): Campbell's Urology, 6th ed. Philadelphia, W. B. Saunders, 1992, pp 2360–2412.
7. Daitch JA, Goldfarb DA, Novick AC: Cleveland Clinic experiences with adrenal Cushing's syndrome. J Urol 158:2051–2055, 1997.
8. Findling JW, Raff H: Diagnosis and differential diagnosis of Cushing's syndrome. Endocrinol Metab Clin North Am 30:729–747, 2001.
9. Goldfarb DA: Comtemporary evaluation and management of Cushing's syndrome. World J Urol 17: 22–25, 1999.

38. ADULT POLCYSTIC KIDNEY DISEASE

Charles S. Modlin, Jr., MD

1. What is the incidence and prevalence of adult polycystic kidney disease?
Adult polycystic kidney disease (APKD) is one of the most common systemic hereditary diseases in the United States, affecting more than 500,000 Americans. Over 5 million persons worldwide are at risk for the disease. APKD affects between 1 in 400 and 1 in 1000–1250 live births. Approximately 6000 new cases occur each year in the United States. APKD accounts for 10–12% of all patients on maintenance hemodialysis. In the United Sates, the annual cost of treating APKD is estimated to exceed $1 billion.

2. Explain the genetic aspects of APKD.
APKD is the most prevalent hereditary renal disorder and is a mendelian autosomal dominant transmitted trait, with nearly 100% penetrance if the carrier lives long enough. Because the disease is characterized by variable expressivity and some cases may represent a spontaneous mutation (<10% cases), as many as 50% of affected patients have no family history of renal disease. APKD consists of at least three phenotypically indistinguishable but genetically distinct entities, caused by mutations in three autosomal genes: PKD1 (chromosome 16p13.3) is present in about 85% of patients; PKD2 (chromosome 4q13q23) in 10%; and PKD3 (unknown chromosome) in a few families. Type 1 progresses more rapidly than type 2. Offspring of affected persons have a 50% chance of acquiring the disease, making reproductive counseling important. Both sexes are affected equally.

3. What are the other cystic diseases of the kidney?

Hereditary	Nonhereditary
1. Infantile (autosomal-recessive) polycystic kidney disease	Medullary sponge kidney
	Multicystic kidney disease
2. Juvenile nephronophthisis/ medullary cystic disease complex	Multiocular cystic kidney disease
	Glomerulocystic kidneys
3. Congenital nephrosis	Acquired cystic disease of dialysis
4. von Hippel-Lindau disease	Multiple simple renal cyst
5. Tuberous sclerosis	Lymphoma or multiple renal masses
6. Other multiple malformation syndromes	

4. Does APKD occur only in adults?
No. Although the highest incidence occurs in patients 45–65 years of age and clinical manifestations of the disease are very uncommon in children and generally occur in the fourth and fifth decades, recent experience with prenatal ultrasonography indicates that the disease begins in utero in most patients. Overlap in the clinical presentation, radiologic features, and pathologic findings is evident in glomerulocystic kidney disease (most often found in infants and children) and APKD.

5. Does adult APKD affect organs other than the kidney?
Yes. Although renal cysts and renal failure are the cardinal manifestations of APKD, APKD is a systemic disease with multiple extrarenal manifestations encompassing both cystic involvement of the organs and connective tissue abnormalities, which often produce significant clinical symptoms. Hepatic cysts are the most common extrarenal manifestation of APKD with variable prevalence (10–75%) depending on the age of the patient. Hepatic cystic disease is mot severe in patients with the most severe renal cystic disease and worst renal function. Liver function, liver enzymes, bilirubin, and portal pressures usually remain normal, although hepatic cyst infection, hemorrhage, portal hypertension, cholangiocarcinoma, and bilary obstruction have been described.

Other organs commonly associated with cyst formation in APKD include the pancreas (10%), spleen (<5%), arachnoid, thyroid, lung, pituitary gland, breast, peritoneum, parathyroid, pineal body, epididymis, testes, seminal vesicles, endometrium, and ovaries. Other associated organ system abnormalities include:

1. **Cardiac:** mitral and aortic valvular prolapse, regurgitation, annuloaortic ectasia
2. **Intestinal:** diverticulosis, diverticular disease complications
3. **Neurologic:** intracranial saccular aneurysms, frequency 0–41%, arteriovenous malformations, cerebral complications due to hypertensive cerebral hemorrhage of cerebral ischemia/ infarction (first-line diagnosis procedure is nonenhanced head CT scan followed by contrast CT scan and lumbar puncture reserved for patients with no blood detected on CT). An APKD patient with a positive family history of intracranial aneurysm rupture is 5 times more likely to have a rupture than an APKD patient with a negative family history. Screening all patients is controversial, but is indicated for those with sudden onset headaches with unusual character or severity, photophobia, nausea, vomiting, lethargy, and confusion.
4. **Vascular:** vertebral, thoracic, and abdominal aortic aneurysms have been described.

A relationship between APKD and renal cell carcinoma has not been conclusively established. Despite the large number of extrarenal manifestations of APKD, patients with APKD have better survival rates on dialysis than do general dialysis patients.

6. What is the pathogenesis of the cystic disease and extrarenal manifestations in APKD?

The exact pathogenesis of the pathologic finding of APKD is now known. Theories involve failure of union of the branches of the ureteral bud with the metanephrons, failure of involution by the first generation of nephrons that subsequently detach and dilate, partial obstruction of normal tubules by hyperplastic cells, defective tubular basement membrane, and disordered tubular cell growth.

Recent research in cell biology has shown the three forces involved in cyst formation to be epithelial proliferation, fluid accumulation, and matrix remodeling. During the course of APKD, growth of multiple cysts distorts the kidneys and causes atrophy of adjacent renal parenchyma and tubular obstruction. Cysts may arise from Bowman's capsule, from any nephron segment, or from the collecting duct. Most commonly, the cysts arise from the tip of Henle's loop, Bowman's space, and the proximal convoluted tubule. Epithelial proliferation is believed to result from abnormalities in the regulation of cell growth. Fluid accumulation may result from a combination of tubular obstruction and altered tubular secretion. The basement membrane surrounding the cysts is composed of abnormal protein and is of altered metabolism. The observed extrarenal cardiac and intracranial abnormalities in APKD are compatible with a defect in the composition of the extracellular matrix.

7. What are the renal pathologic findings of APKD?

The main structural change is cyst formation (cortex and medulla), which vary in size and symmetry. The pathologic findings reflect the number and size of the cysts. The increase in renal size precedes renal impairment. The fluid is clear and straw-colored in uncomplicated cysts, to hemorrhage or purulent. True unilateral APKD is probably extremely rare. In true unilateral APKD, the cysts are lined by flattened or cuboidal epithelium, stromal changes are nonspecific (tubular atrophy, vascular and glomerular sclerosis); dystrophic calcification is common.

8. Do all patients with APKD develop renal failure?

No. The severity of renal disease varies considerably among patients. The course of APKD in a particular patient is determined by the extent and severity of both renal and extrarenal manifestations. The development of bilateral renal cysts leads to functional changes of the kidneys. Early functional changes include impaired renal concentrating ability and hypertension (related to increased activity of the renin-angiotensin-aldosterone system). Renal insufficiency develops in approximately 50% of patients with APKD. Churchill calculated that patients with sonographically identifiable APKD have a 2% chance of developing end-stage renal disease (ESRD) by age 40 years, a 23% chance by age 50 years, and a 48% chance by age 73 years. Renal disease seems to follow a more aggressive course in patients with the APKD1 gene. The rate of renal deterioration correlates with the rate of cyst growth. In earlier reports, the mean life expectancy of APKD patients was 4–13 years after clinical presentation, and death was usually attributed to uremia, heart failure, or cerebral hemorrhage. Because of improvements in dialysis, transplantation, and managing complications associated with APKD, the prognosis appears to be improving dramatically.

9. How is APKD diagnosed?

A strong family history may suggest the diagnosis; however, characteristic symptoms and physical findings with radiologic imaging are used to confirm it. The characteristic radiographic findings are bilaterally enlarged kidneys with variably sized innumerable renal cysts. Renal ultrasonography may demonstrate enlarged kidneys, ascites, hepatomegaly, and renal cysts. Early diagnosis is important for genetic counseling and for screening siblings of affected patients for potential kidney transplant donation.

Ultrasonography and CT are sensitive in establishing the diagnosis. Current ultrasound technology can image cysts as small as 5 mm in diameter. Ultrasound is the preferred imaging technique because of its noninvasiveness, low cost, general availability, and lack of ionizing radiation. Negative studies in individuals over age 40 years most likely indicate that the disease will not develop. CT is advantageous when ultrasound is equivocal and also is useful in the diagnosis of renal complications associated with polycystic kidneys (calculi, hemorrhage, cystic and perinephric infection, coexistent tumor, urinary tract obstruction). The exact role or MRI is not established but may have a role in the differentiation of infected and hemorrhagic cysts. Uncomplicated cysts on MRI resemble simple cysts (homogeneous on T1-weighted images, homogeneous and high-intensity on T2), and hemorrhagic cysts are usually hyperintense at all pulse sequences, but this depends on the age of the blood.

Other less commonly used radiologic tests include excretory urography with nephrotomography (sensitive in young children), radionuclide imaging (cysts are photopenic masses), and indium 111-labeled white blood cells or gallium-67 citrate scans to differentiate infected cysts. Angiography and retrograde pyelography are used in selected situations.

It is possible to diagnose APKD before either cysts or symptoms develop. Gene-linkage techniques can be used to test for the presence of the APKD gene-carrier state. Even prenatal diagnosis is possible with the use of DNA obtained from aminocentesis or chorionic-villus sampling. The identification of a gene-carrier state, however, does not predict the clinical course.

10. How many cysts must there be before polycystic kidney disease can be diagnosed?

Most studies consider the presence of at least three bilateral renal cysts in a person with a family history of dominantly expressed renal cystic disease highly suggestive of the disease. This arbitrary number of cysts has been chosen to differentiate patients with simple renal cyst from those with polycystic kidney disease. The prevalence of simple cysts increases with age (0.1% of children); therefore, any cysts in a child with a family history are suggestive, whereas in an adult, the diagnosis is more certain in the presence of numerous cysts or if extrarenal manifestations of the disease are also present.

11. At what age does the absence of renal cysts exclude the diagnosis?

Negative studies in individuals over 40 years most likely indicate that the disease will not develop. Eleven to 24% of gene carriers of ADPKD1 do not have ultrasonographically detectable renal cysts before the age of 30 years.

12. Describe the most common associated physical findings.

Palpable flank mass(es) represent the most common physical findings in patients with APKD and must be differentiated from other causes of flank masses. Hepatomegaly and splenomegaly are often detected as well.

13. List and describe the associated laboratory and clinical findings in patients with APKD.
- Loss of renal concentrating ability (first indicator of renal impairment). Urinalysis may reveal proteinuria (usually <1 gm/day) and microscopic or gross hematuria, pyuria, or bacteriuria
- Polycythemia may develop secondary to increased erythropoietin production
- Azotemia (elevated blood urea nitrogen and serum creatinine) in advanced cases
- Anemia (related to uremia or recurrent cyst hemorrhage)

14. Describe the most common signs, symptoms, and related complications of adult polycystic kidney disease.

The most common signs and symptoms are:

1. **Palpable flank/abdominal masses**

2. **Hypertension:** commonly present on initial exam and antedates renal dysfunction. Normotension at diagnosis may be associated with better patient survival.

3. **Pain:** abdominal and flank pain may require cyst decompression (percutaneous, alcohol sclerosis, laparoscopic, open) or nephrectomy

4. **Hematuria:** (50% of patients) gross or microscopic is presenting symptom in 35% of patients. One must exclude other causes of hematuria in APKD (i.e., infection, stones, tumors). Trauma may precipitate hematuria. Usually resolves spontaneously with bed rest, analgesics, and hydration. Angiography/embolization is necessary in selected cases.

5. **Nephrolithiasis:** (20% of patients) (usually uric acid or calcium oxalate) associated with a metabolic abnormality (distal acidification defect, abnormal ammonium transport, low urine pH, hypocitraturia) and/or obstruction and urinary stasis. Noncontrast CT scan sensitive in diagnosis.

6. **Urinary tract infection:** (50–60% of patients) predominantly in women. Differentiate between parenchymal and cyst infection. Cystic infections are difficult to eradicate. Lipid-soluble antibiotics (i.e., trimethoprim sulfate, chloramphenicol, ciprofloxacin, vancomycin, clindamycin, erythromycin) penetrate the cyst wall more dependably.

7. **End-stage renal disease (ESRD):** ESRD develops in roughly 50% of patients by age 60 years and develops approximately 10 years earlier in African-Americans than Caucasians. Dialysis and/or transplantation prolongs life by an average of 14 years.

15. What is the treatment of APKD?

The main goal of therapy is the preservation of renal function by controlling hypertension and urinary tract infections. Angiotensin-converting enzyme (ACE) inhibitors have proven helpful in controlling hypertension, but hypertension is also volume dependent; combination sodium restriction/diuretic may prove helpful. A low-protein diet also may slow progression of renal insufficiency once renal function begins to deteriorate. Treatment is largely directed at treatment of individual complications. Analgesics usually provide pain relief and hematuria is usually treated conservatively. Consider activity limitations to avoid direct trauma. Pretransplant nephrectomy is performed only in selected cases (recurrent bleeding, infection, pain, massively enlarged kidney[s] precluding allograft placement) because these kidneys often help alleviate the severe anemia of renal failure (erythropoietin production) and contribute to fluid/electrolyte management in dialysis and transplant patients. Nephrolithiasis in APKD patients with early disease and normal renal function is treated with conventional methods (percutaneous, extracorporeal shock-wave lithotripsy) but with lower success rates. Potassium citrate is useful. Dissolution of uric acid stones can be reliably achieved. Many patients ultimately require dialysis or transplantation.

16. Can cyst decompression prevent the progression of renal failure and control hypertension?

It is the rare case (i.e., ureteral obstruction caused by ureteral compression by an enlarged cyst) in which surgical decompression improves upon renal function or control of hypertension.

17. What are the results of dialysis and transplantation in patients with APKD?

Survival of APKD patients with ESRD is as good or even better than other nondiabetics treated with dialysis or renal transplant, particularly at more marked ages. The main causes of death in

APKD patients on renal replacement therapy are cardiac (38%) and cerebrovascular events (12%). It appears that less anemia is one of the factors that provide cardiac protection in the patient with APKD on dialysis compared to other patients with ESRD.

18. If APKD is hereditary, can family members safely donate kidneys?
Yes. Current ultrasound and genetic technology can reliably assess family members for the presence of APKD, especially those older than ages 25–35. Family members interested in living related donations who are without evidence of disease may serve as potential kidney donors.

19. Briefly describe the future goals of research and treatment of APKD.
Future goals of research into APKD revolve around identifying the key processes and contributing factors that promote decline in renal function in APKD. Development of dietary and pharmacologic treatments to prevent or slow the formation and growth of cysts and observed changes in the basement membrane and interstitium would reduce the morbidity and mortality of APKD.

BIBLIOGRAPHY

1. Andreoni KA, Pelletier RP, Elkhammas EA, et al: Increased incidence of gastrointestinal surgical complications in renal transplant recipients with polycystic kidney disease. Transplantation 67:262–266, 1999.
2. Bear JC, McManamon P, Morgan J, et al: Age at clinical onset and at ultrasonographic detection of adult polycystic kidney disease: Data for genetic counseling. Am J Med Genet 18:45–53, 1984.
3. Beebe DK: Autosomal dominant polycystic kidney disease. Am Fam Physician 53:925–931.
4. Bennett WM, Elzinga LW: Clinical management of autosomal dominant polycystic kidney disease. Kidney Int 44(suppl 42):S74–S79, 1993.
5. Bennett WM, Elzinga L, Golpher TA, Barry JA: Reduction of cyst volume for symptomatic management of autosomal dominant polycystic kidney disease. J Urol 137:620–622, 1987.
6. Bennett WM, Elzinga L, Pulliam JP, et al: Cyst fluid antibiotic concentrations in autosomal dominant polycystic kidney disease. Am J Kidney Dis 6:400–404, 1985.
7. Churchill DN, Bear JC, Morgan J, et al: Prognosis of adult onset polycystic kidney disease re-evaluated. Kidney Int 26:190–193, 1984.
8. Dedeoglu IO, Fisher JE, Springate JE: Spectrum of glomerulocystic kidneys: A case report and review of the literature. Pediatr Pathol Lab Med 16:941–994, 1996.
9. Elzinga LW, Barry JM, Bennett WM: Surgical management of painful polycystic kidneys. Am J Kidney Dis 22:532–537, 1993.
10. Fick GM, Gabow PA: Natural history of autosomal dominant polycystic kidney disease. Annu Rev Med 45:23–29, 1994.
11. Gabow PA: Autosomal dominant polycystic kidney disease. N Engl J Med 329:332–342, 1993.
12. Goldman SM, Hartman DS: Autosomal dominant polycystic kidney disease. In Pollack H (ed): Clinical Urography. Philadelphia, W. B. Saunders, 1990, pp 1092–1112.
13. Grantham JJ: Pathogenesis of autosomal dominant polycystic kidney disease: Recent developments. Contrib Nephrol 122:1–9, 1997.
14. Grantham JJ: The etiology, pathogenesis, and treatment of autosomal dominant polycystic kidney disease: Recent advances. Am J Kidney Dis 28:788–803, 1996.
15. Grantham JJ: Ethical issues and genetic counseling. Contrib Nephrol 115:39–43, 1995.
16. Grantham JJ: Polycystic kidney disease: Huge kidneys, huge problems, huge progress. Trans Am Clin Climatol Assoc 108:164–170, 1996.
17. Grantham JJ: Mechanisms of progression in autosomal dominant polycystic kidney disease. Kidney Int 52(suppl 63):S93–S97, 1997.
18. Grunfeld JP, Bennett WM: Clinical aspects of autosomal dominant polycystic kidney disease. Curr Opin Nephrol Hypertens 4:114–121, 1995.
19. Ho-Hsieh H, Novick AC, Steinmuller D, et al: Renal transplantation for end-stage polycystic kidney disease. Urology 30:322–325, 1987.
20. Johnson AM, Gabow PA: Identification of patients with autosomal dominant polycystic kidney disease at highest risk for end-stage renal disease. Am Soc Nephrol 8:1560–1567, 1997.
21. Lieske JC, Toback FG: Autosomal dominant polycystic kidney disease. J Am Soc Nephrol 3:1142–1150, 1993.

22. MacDermot DK, Saggar-Malik AK: Prenatal diagnosis of autosomal dominant polycystic kidney disease (PKD1) presenting in utero and prognosis for very early onset disease. J Med Genet 35:13–16, 1998.
23. Marsick R, Limwongse C, Kodish E: Genetic testing for renal diseases: Medical and ethical considerations. Am J Kidney Dis 32:934–945, 1998.
24. McCarthy S, McMullen M: Autosomal dominant polycystic kidney disease: Pathophysiology and treatment. Am Nephrol Nurses Assoc J 24:45–51, 1997.
25. National Institutes of Health, National Institute of Diabetes, Digestive and Kidney Diseases: Patient survival. In 1996 Annual Data Report. Bethesda, Md, U.S. Renal Data System, 1996, pp E.1–E.94.
26. Parfrey PS, Bear JC, Morgan J, et al. The diagnosis and prognosis of autosomal dominant polycystic kidney disease. N Engl J Med 323:1085–1090, 1990.
27. Perrone RD: Extrarenal manifestations of ADPKD. Kidney Int 51:2022–2036, 1997.
28. Pirson Y, Chauveau D, van Gijn J: Subarachnoid hemorrhage in ADPKD patients: How to recognize and how to manage? Nephrol Dial Transplant 11:1236–1238, 1996.
29. Pirson Y, Christophe JL, Goffin E: Outcome of renal replacement therapy in autosomal dominant polycystic kidney disease. Nephrol Dial Transplant 11(suppl 6):24–28, 1996.
30. Reeders ST, Zerres K, Gal A, et al. Prenatal diagnosis of autosomal dominant polycystic kidney disease with a DNA probe, Lancet 2:6–8, 1986.
31. Ritz E, Zeier M, Geberth S, Waldherr R: Autosomal dominant polycystic kidney disease (ADPKD)— mechanisms of cyst formation and renal failure. Aust N Z J Med 23:35–41, 1993.
32. Ritz E, Zeier M, Schneider P, Jones E: Cardiovascular mortality of patients with polycystic kidney disease on dialysis: Is there a lesson to learn? Nephron 66:125–128, 1994.
33. Sessa A, Ghiggeri GM, Turco AE: Autosomal dominant polycystic kidney disease: Clinical and genetic aspects. J Nephrol 10:295–310, 1997.
34. Torres VE, Wilson DM, Hattery RR: Renal stone disease in autosomal dominant polycystic kidney disease. Am J Kidney Dis 22:513–519, 1993.
35. Wang D, Strandgaard S: The pathogenesis of hypertension in autosomal dominant polycystic kidney disease. J Hypertension 15:925–933, 1997.
36. Zeier M, Jones E, Ritz E: Autosomal dominant polycystic kidney disease—the patient on renal replacement therapy. Nephrol Dial Transplant 11(suppl 6):18–20, 1996.

39. ACQUIRED CYSTIC DISEASE
OF THE KIDNEY

Stuart M. Flechner, M.D.

1. What is acquired renal cystic disease (ARCD)?

ARCD is the term used to describe the development of cystic degeneration of the kidneys in patients without a congenital predisposition to form renal cysts. Usually, 25% or more of the mass of one or both kidneys is involved when the diagnosis is made, predominantly in patients with chronic renal failure. The association of ARCD with renal failure, especially in patients treated with hemodialysis, was first described by Dunnill in 1977. However, reports of cysts in the kidneys of autopsied patients with renal failure date to the 19th century.

2. How many cysts are required to diagnose ARCD?

There is no precise number. However, a generally accepted concept is at least 4–5 individual cysts that encompass about 25% of the renal mass.

3. Where do the cysts form?

Multiple cysts are usually found in both kidneys, predominantly in the renal cortex, although cysts may be found in the medulla or the corticomedullary junction. Because end-stage renal disease (ESRD) kidneys are usually small and contracted, the cysts cause an increased renal mass. The cysts also have been shown to be associated with multiple small renal adenomas and frank renal cell carcinomas. These tumors are often of proximal renal tubular origin.

4. How is ARCD different from other forms of renal cystic disease?

The aging kidney has a propensity to form benign simple cysts, which may develop in either kidney and be single or multiple. However, in ARCD many tens or hundreds of cysts can develop.

Two main types of congenital polycystic renal diseases are found. One is genetically transmitted in an autosomal dominant fashion and the other in an autosomal recessive. Usually, a family history of these forms of cystic kidney disease is present; they are also usually associated with cyst formation in other organs, such as the liver and the gastrointestinal tract. In contrast, ARCD is found in renal failure patients, absent a family history of cystic disease, and is isolated to the kidney. In addition, microdissection studies have shown that ARCD cysts lack the arboral-like proliferation found in cases of congenital cystic disease of the kidney.

5. How often are cysts found in renal failure patients?

This depends on a number of factors that may influence the time that patients undergo evaluation for cystic disease. The prevalence of ARCD in dialysis patients undergoing autopsy is reported to be between 28% and 47%. ARCD is reported to exist in 14–25% of dialysis patients undergoing random radiologic screening studies. It appears that about one-third of patients develop ARCD within the first 3 years of dialysis. However, for those who survive on dialysis for 5–10 years, the number who develop ARCD approaches 80–90%. Interestingly, males appear to have a two-fold increased risk for the development of ARCD. Cyst formation also has been observed in children and adolescents before the initiation of dialysis.

6. Does the type of renal replacement therapy affect the risk for ARCD?

The early reports of ARCD were confined to patients undergoing chronic hemodialysis, and indeed the artificial kidney and/or dialysis tubing were once suggested to be linked to the pathogenesis of cyst formation. However, cysts have been reported in patients with slowly progressive renal insufficiency prior to the initiation of dialysis. Therefore, the length of time an individual suffers from chronic renal insufficiency may be the most important risk factor for ARCD. For this reason, younger patients may be at greatest risk for ARCD during their lifetime.

7. Are some patients more likely to form cysts?

Yes. ARCD develops more commonly in patients with tubulointerstitial diseases. It is less likely to be found in patients with membranoproliferative glomerulonephritis. It is rarely found in type I diabetics with renal failure. Apparently, there is no strong relationship between family history and acquired renal cystic disease.

8. Do the cysts ever go away?

Some evidence suggests that successful renal transplantation, with the return of near-normal renal function, can cause a regression of established ARCD in native kidneys. In addition, new cases of ARCD are uncommon in successfully transplanted patients. However, a few new cases of ARCD have been identified in patients with acceptable renal transplant function, and these may be associated with polycythemia post-transplant.

9. Why do cysts form in end-stage renal disease (ESRD) kidneys?

The pathogenesis is currently not known. Animal research and clinical observations have led to a number of theories:

1. **Occlusive theory.** Obstruction of renal tubules by a combination of interstitial fibrosis, epithelial proliferation, and/or intratubular oxalate crystal leads to cyst formation.

2. **Chemical theory.** Toxic endogenous substances or metabolites accumulated in renal failure, such as polyamines or exogenous substances from dialysis tubing or the artificial kidney, could be responsible.

3. **Ischemic theory.** Experimentally, ischemia and obstruction to a renal segment can induce cyst formation. Both are present in ESRD kidneys.

4. **Growth factor theory.** Currently unidentified polypeptides with renotrophic activity could be locally released and induce cystic degeneration.

5. **Immune theory.** Uremia is known to be immunosuppressive. ESRD kidneys may be susceptible to escape mechanisms, predisposing to cellular proliferation.

6. **Hormonal theory.** The increased incidence of ARCD in males suggests that alterations of sex steroid production and metabolism induced by uremia may predispose to cyst formation. An up-regulation of epidermal growth factor receptors in renal tissue has been shown to result from altered androgen/estrogen ratios in uremic males.

10. Where do cysts come from?

Cysts are generally 1–25 ml in size and contain clear fluid in which oxalate crystals are often found. They have regular cuboidal or columnar epithelium, but papillary hyperplasia and thickened basement membranes are generally observed. Microdissection studies have confirmed that cysts are always in continuity with renal tubules and may represent fusiform tubular dilations or saccular outpouchings. The lumens of over 80% of the proximal and distal tubules are patent. Such data suggest that cyst formation results from dilation and hyperplasia of remaining nephrons rather than obstruction and fibrosis.

11. Do cysts cause any clinical symptoms?

Yes. Depending upon their relative size and position in the kidney, they may result in hematuria, stone formation, infection, hypertension, and pain. Although these symptoms tend to be reported infrequently, they may be significant and require nephrectomy for resolution. The evaluation of hematuria in a patient with ARCD may include CT, renal ultrasound, urine cytology, urine culture, cystoscopy, and retrograde pyelography.

12. Are there any other reasons to worry about cysts in ESRD kidneys?

Several studies have confirmed the association between ARCD and renal tumors. There have been a number of case reports of patients with ARCD who have developed metastatic renal cell carcinomas. Tumors may be found in areas of the kidney where cystic degeneration is prominent, as well as areas without cystic involvement. It is possible that some tumors arise from the hyperplastic multi-layered epithelium, often with papillary projections, found in many cysts. Conversely, about 80% of reported patients on dialysis with renal adenocarcinomas have had ARCD.

Estimated Occurrence of Renal Adenocarcinoma

GROUP	CASES/1000 POPULATION
General population	1.3
Renal insufficiency	1.5
ESRD population	6.0
Kidneys with cysts	22.8
ESRD patients with ARCD	45.5

13. Are all renal tumors found in ARCD patients malignant?

No. A compilation of several pathologic studies reveals the following: about 20–40% of patients with ARCD have small solid renal tumors. This compares with a 10–20% incidence in an age-matched general autopsy poplulation. Only about 1–2% of patients with ARCD will develop a frank renal adenocarcinoma, and about 15% of those with cancer will develop metastases. Similar to that observed with cyst formation in ESRD kidneys, males also exhibit an increased (seven-fold) risk for developing renal adenocarcinoma when ARCD is present. The risk for neoplastic transformation appears to correlate more with the length of time renal failure is present rather than patient age. Therefore, younger patients with ESRD are at greatest risk and require close monitoring.

14. How is a small renal tumor identified as malignant?

This remains a highly controversial issue in urology. Some believe size of the lesion is an accurate discriminator because lesions < 3 cm in diameter rarely if ever metastasize; they are considered to be adenomas. Others believe that renal adenomas are small renal adenocarcinomas and will demonstrate malignant behavior in time. The association of clinical symptoms at the time of presentation also has been suggested as a marker for more rapid growth—e.g., gross hematuria would be most unlikely to result from a small, slow-growing adenoma. Currently, the presence of tissue invasion and/or metastases continues to be the only truly diagnostic feature separating these two entities.

15. What is the best way to determine if an ARCD kidney contains a renal tumor?

The **renal ultrasound** evaluation of the kidneys is uniformly considered the most accurate and efficient way to screen ESRD kidneys for cystic disease. In most cases, cysts can be confidently identified. The CAT scan is more accurate than ultrasound, but it is more costly and delivers contrast and radiation. Magnetic resonance imaging (MRI) using gadolinium has gained popularity as an imaging technique in ESRD patients. It too is a costly test. On very rare occasions, other modalities such as angiography and isotopic renal scans may provide additional information. The altered architecture of the kidney caused by ARCD makes delineation of renal masses more difficult than in otherwise normally functioning kidneys.

16. Because renal adenocarcinoma may develop in ARCD kidneys, how often should a patient be evaluated?

This controversial question involves the true incidence of kidney cancer in ESRD patients, the cost of large-scale screening programs, and the ultimate benefit to patients. Important facts that apply to this consideration are the average life expectancy of new patients beginning dialysis in the United States (under 5 years for patients > 50 years of age), and the infrequent finding of kidney cancer (< 2%) as a cause of death in dialyzed patients.

A reasonable approach would be to perform an ultrasound examination when the diagnosis of ESRD is made and then repeat the study after about 3 years. For example, higher risk groups, such as young males in good health on hemodialysis, should undergo closer scrutiny than elderly females on peritoneal dialysis with cardiac disease.

17. What is the best treatment for a solid renal mass in an ARCD kidney?

If a solid renal mass >3 cm in diameter is found or a smaller mass associated with symptoms is uncovered, the patient should undergo **radical nephrectomy.** This approach should be modified only by coexisting medical conditions that may significantly limit life expectancy or preclude the safe administration of anesthesia and surgery. Smaller asymptomatic masses may either be removed or followed with CT scans. Elective nephrectomy can be done if progression is demonstrated. Newer laparoscopic approaches using minimally invasive surgical techniques are currently gaining wider acceptance.

18. Do both kidneys with ARCD need to be removed if a patient has a solid mass?

No. However, if the presence of a solid renal mass is suspected in the contralateral kidney, often it is easier for the patient to have both kidneys removed at one time. If the contralateral kidney is left in situ, it must be closely screened by ultrasound for the development of solid masses. The availability of laparoscopy has diminished the morbidity of bilateral nephrectomies in ESRD patients. The hand-assisted technique is useful to remove bilateral cystic kidneys

BIBLIOGRAPHY

1. Boileau M, Flechner SM, Foley R, Weinman E: Renal adenocarcinoma and end-stage kidney disease. J Urol 139:603–606, 1987.
2. Concolino G, Lubrano C, Ombres M, et al: Acquired cystic kidney disease: The hormonal hypothesis. Urology 41:170–175, 1993.
3. Dunnill MS, Millard PR, Oliver D: Acquired cystic disease of the kidneys: Hazard of long-term intermittent dialysis. J Clin Pathol 30:868–877, 1997.
4. Ishikawa I, Yasuhito S, Naoto S, et al: Ten-year prospective study on the development of renal cell cancer in dialysis patients. Am J Kidney Dis 26:452–458, 1990.
5. Takebayashi S, Hidai H, Chiba T, Irisawa M, Matsubara S. Renal cell carcinoma in acquired cystic kidney disease: volume growth rate determined by helical computed tomography. Am J Kidney Dis 36:759–766, 2000.
6. Levine E, Slusher S, Grantham J, Wetzel L: Natural history of ARCD in dialysis patients: A prospective CT study. AJR 156:501–506, 1991.
7. Lien Y, Kam I, Shanley P, Schroter G: Metastatic renal cell carcinoma associated with ARCD 15 years after transplantation. Am J Kidney Dis 28:711–715, 1991.
8. Mindell HJ: Imaging studies for screening native kidneys in long-term dialysis patients. Commentary. AJR 153:768–769, 1989.
9. Vandeursen H, Van Damme B, Baert J: Acquired cystic disease of the kidney analyzed by microdissection. J Urol 146:1168–1169, 1991.
10. Querfeld U, Shneble F, Waldherr R, et al: Acquired cystic kidney disease before and after renal transplantation. J Pediatr 121:61–64, 1992.
11. Ravine D, Gibson RN, Donlan J, et al: Ultrasound renal cyst prevalence study: Specificity data for inherited renal cystic disease. Am J Kidney Dis 22:803–807, 1993.
12. Tantravahi J, Steinman TI. Acquired cystic kidney disease. Semin Dialysis 13:330–334, 2000.
13. Nascimento AB, Mitchell DG, Zhang XM, Kamishima T, Parker L, Holland GA: Rapid MR imaging detection of renal cysts: Age-based standards. Radiology 221:628–632, 2001.

40. URETEROPELVIC JUNCTION OBSTRUCTION

Allen D. Seftel, M.D.

1. What is ureteropelvic junction obstruction?

It is a blockage of the ureter at the level of the renal pelvis–proximal ureteral junction.

2. What are the causes?

The causes may be divided into congenital or acquired. **Congenital** ureteropelvic junction obstruction is an entity that is often now found prenatally. Inasmuch as prenatal ultrasonography is routinely performed, it will present as one of the differential diagnoses of prenatal or postnatal hydronephrosis or abdominal mass in the newborn. Acquired ureteropelvic obstruction may be the result of ureteral manipulation, urinary calculi, or retroperitoneal disease. Acquired disease is usually found in the adult.

3. What are the physical findings and symptoms?

In the child, one may be able to appreciate an abdominal mass. In the older child or adult, flank abdominal pain may be present. If significant obstruction to urinary outflow is present, it may be accompanied by nausea and vomiting.

4. How is the diagnosis of ureteropelvic junction obstruction made?

The diagnosis is usually confirmed by a radiologic study. These include renal ultrasonography, intravenous pyelography, retrograde pyelography, or radionuclide renogram.

5. What are the causes of congenital anatomy?

It is believed that it is caused by a disorganization of the renal pelvis–upper ureteral junction during the recanalization process in utero. Disorganization of the smooth muscle leads to a lack of motility or perhaps collagen deposition and a lack of peristalsis, with narrowing at this site.

6. How is this entity treated?

A pyeloplasty is usually performed in the neonate. There are several types of pyeloplasty procedures, the most common being the dismembered pyeloplasty.

7. Are there any other causes of pediatric ureteropelvic junction obstruction?

It may be that vesicoureteral reflux may cause a secondary ureteropelvic junction obstruction. This is most commonly found in children.

8. How does one make a diagnosis of ureteropelvic junction obstruction in children?

Diuretic renal nuclide scanning is usually performed either to make the diagnosis of ureteropelvic junction obstruction or to confirm the diagnosis.

9. Is ureteropelvic junction obstruction more common in male or female children?

It is common in boys more than girls by a 5:2 ratio.

10. In ureteropelvic junction obstruction more common on the right, left, or both (bilateral)?

In children, it is more common on the left than the right, again with a 5:2 ratio. Bilateral obstruction occurs in 15% of cases.

11. How does ureteropelvic junction obstruction usually present in the adult?

Flank pain, flank mass, or a urinary tract infection.

12. How is ureteropelvic junction obstruction diagnosed in the adult?

Diagnosis usually is made by intravenous pyelography, renal ultrasonography, or diuretic renal scanning.

On the pelvis, 4–0 chromic sutures are placed at the margins where excess pelvis will be excised. A small tacking suture is placed in the proximal end of the ureter to minimize handling and traumatic injury. The ureter is then incised for approximately 1–2 cm on the lateral portion of the ureter. (From Novick AC (ed): Stewart's Operative Urology, 2nd ed. Baltimore, Williams & Wilkins, 1989, with permission.)

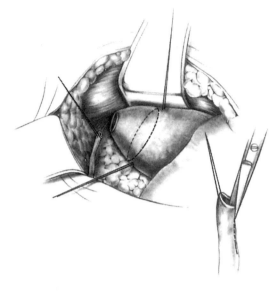

A 4–0 or 5–0 chromic suture is then placed at the apex of the incised ureter to the inferior portion of the pelvis. A pair of forceps is used to spread the internal diameter of the ureter to facilitate the placement of this suture. (From Novick AC (ed): Stewart's Operative Urology, 2nd ed. Baltimore, Williams & Wilkins, 1989, with permission.)

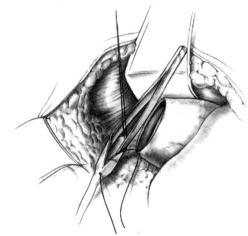

13. What are the causes of this obstruction in an adult?

1. A crossing renal vessel at the ureteropelvic junction
2. Previous passage of a urinary calculus
3. Manipulation of the urinary system with either a ureteroscope or nephroscope
4. A retroperitoneal process impinging on the ureter externally (e.g., inflammation or enlarged lymph nodes)
5. Nonurologic malignancies such as gynecologic cancers or colonic cancers can cause obstruction through either enlarged lymph nodes or actual compression of that area by the tumor burden
6. Abdominal and aortic aneurysm leakage may produce an inflammatory response in the

retroperineal area near the upper uteropelvic junction, causing ureteropelvic junction obstruction as well

7. Infection, either hematogenous or ascending

14. How is the obstruction treated in the adult?

Commonly, a **dismembered pyeloplasty** is performed in the adult. Other types of pyeloplasties also may be performed via minimally invasive therapy, such as **endopyelotomy.** This procedure, performed via percutaneous opening through the skin to the kidney and allowing access to the ureteropelvic junction from above, is being performed more commonly. Another minimally invasive technique gaining widespread acceptance is known as **retrograde endopyelotomy,** which is most commonly performed when the ureteropelvic junction obstruction is short. Balloons, small knives, or even laser may be frequently used to incise the ureteropelvic junction from below. The outcome of these procedures depends on operator experience and the location and size of the stricture, as well as patient selection.

BIBLIOGRAPHY

1. Robson WL, Rogers RC, Leung AK: Renal agenesis, multicystic dysplasia, and uretero-pelvic junction obstruction—a common pathogenesis? Am J Med Genet 53:302, 1994.
2. Shafik A: Ureteric profilometry. A study of the ureteric pressure profile in the normal and pathologic ureter. Scand J Urol Nephrol 32:14–19, 1998.
3. Cvitkovic Kuzmic A, Brkljacic B, Rados M, Galesic K: Doppler visualization of ureteric jets in unilateral hydronephrosis in children and adolescents. Eur J Radiol 2001 39:209–214, 2001.
4. Hibi H, Yamada Y, Mizumoto H, et al: Retrograde ureteroscopic endopyelotomy using the holmium: YAG laser. Int J Urol 9:77–81, 2002.
5. Conlin MJ: Results of selective management of ureteropelvic junction obstruction. J Endourol 16:233–236, 2002.

41. VESICOURETERAL REFLUX

Jeffrey S. Palmer, M.D. and Jack S. Elder, M.D.

1. What is vesicoureteral reflux?
Vesicoureteral reflux refers to the regurgitation of urine from the bladder into the ureter and usually into the kidney.

2. What is low-pressure reflux?
Low-pressure reflux is vesicoureteral reflux that occurs during bladder filling.

3. What is high-pressure reflux?
High-pressure reflux is vesicoureteral reflux that occurs during micturition. Reflux may occur during bladder filling, voiding, or both.

4. Describe the anatomy of the normal ureterovesical junction.
The smooth muscle of the renal calyces, pelvis, and extravesical ureter is composed of helically oriented fibers that allow peristaltic activity. The ureter passes obliquely through the bladder wall for 1 to 2 cm, and the fibers are reoriented into a longitudinal plane, making the ureter incapable of peristalsis in that location.

5. What is the trigone?
The trigone is the triangle formed by the two ureteral orifices and the bladder neck.

6. What is Waldeyer's sheath?
It is the external layer of longitudinal smooth muscle surrounding the ureter. This sheath passes through the bladder wall. As this layer enters the bladder lumen, the fibers diverge to join with the contralateral ureter, forming the deep trigonal layer.

7. How does vesicoureteral reflux occur?
Reflux occurs when the intravesical (intramural) ureteral length is too short. Usually, the ureter is positioned superolateral to the normal position.

8. Discuss the causes of vesicoureteral reflux.
Vesicoureteral reflux has numerous causes. The most common is termed primary reflux and is thought to be a congenital condition. If the ureteral bud is too close to the urogenital sinus on the wolffian (mesonephric) duct, then it may not acquire sufficient mesenchymal tissue around it to have sufficient support to prevent reflux.

Reflux also may occur in association with high-pressure voiding states, including posterior urethral valves, certain cases of neuropathic bladder, and detrusor sphincter dyssynergia. Furthermore, reflux may occur in association with a duplex collecting system, in which the kidney is drained by two ureters and in children with bladder exstrophy. In children with an ectopic ureterocele, the insertion of the lower pole ureter into the bladder may be altered, allowing reflux. In children with an ectopic ureter draining into the bladder neck, reflux into the upper pole ureter may occur. Reflux also may occur following bladder surgery. For example, if one divides the trigone during a bladder operation, the ureteral orifice(s) may retract, allowing reflux to occur.

9. What is the normal ratio of the length of the intramural ureter to the diameter of the ureteral orifice?
Normally, the ratio of the length of the intramural ureter to the diameter of the ureteral orifice is 2.5:1. If this ratio is less, reflux occurs.

10. What is the prevalence of primary vesicoureteral reflux?
The prevalence has been estimated to be as high as 1 in 100.

11. What is the ratio of girls to boys with reflux?
Boys and girls have a similar incidence of reflux. However, because girls are more likely to develop a urinary tract infection, reflux is diagnosed more commonly in girls, and the male:female ratio is approximately 1:6.

12. Who is more likely to have high-grade reflux, boys or girls?
Boys are more likely to have grade IV or V reflux.

13. What is the race distribution of reflux among American girls?
White girls are 10 times more likely to have reflux than black girls. White girls are more likely to have reflux when evaluated for urinary tract infections.

14. Define secondary reflux. Give examples.
Secondary reflux is an anatomic or clinical abnormality in which reflux occurs. Examples include ureterocele, in which reflux may occur from distortion of the base of the bladder from a ureterocele, posterior urethral valves, and neuropathic bladder.

15. What is the significance of vesicoureteral reflux?
Vesicoureteral reflux directly or in association with urinary tract infection may result in renal injury, termed reflux nephropathy.

16. How does a urinary tract infection cause renal injury?
If bacteria from the bladder ascend to the renal pelvis and renal parenchyma, a process that is facilitated by reflux, renal injury may occur by several mechanisms.
1. The bacteria may produce an endotoxin that has a direct effect on the renal tubule.
2. By chemotaxis, there is granulocyte aggregation in the area of the bacteria, resulting in capillary obstruction, which causes focal renal ischemia. During ischemia, the purine pool is consumed owing to anaerobic metabolism. During reperfusion, the remaining hypoxanthine pool is metabolized to xanthine, which, in the presence of xanthine oxidase, is converted to uric acid and superoxide. Superoxide can be converted to peroxide and hydroxyl radicals, both of which may cause cell damage. Experimentally, this ischemic damage has been prevented by treatment with allopurinol, which blocks xanthine oxidase and thus prevents toxic oxygen radical formation during reperfusion.
3. During the inflammatory response, endotoxin causes complement activation, which by chemotaxis leads to phagocytosis. The respiratory burst of phagocytosis results in the release of superoxide with formation of peroxide and hydroxyl radicals. All tissues in the body contain superoxide dismutase, which rapidly degrades superoxide, which naturally occurs in the presence of oxygen. However, urine contains no superoxide dismutase, allowing these radicals to act on the renal tubules unopposed. In addition, lysosomal enzymes are released during phagocytosis, which also may damage renal tubules.

17. How common is primary reflux in children with a urinary tract infection (UTI)?
Approximately 50% of children with a urinary tract infection have reflux. The incidence of reflux in children with urinary tract infections is similar in boys and girls. Primary reflux is less common in African-American children than in Caucasian children.

18. Who should be evaluated for reflux?
Any child with pyelonephritis (i.e., febrile UTI), all boys with a UTI, all girls < 5 years old with a UTI, and girls > 5 years with two or more episodes of cystitis.

19. How is reflux detected?

Reflux is usually detected by performing a voiding cystourethrogram (VCUG). This study is performed by inserting a catheter into the bladder, distending the bladder with contrast material, and observing the bladder and kidneys during bladder filling and voiding. In boys, the study is performed using fluoroscopy, because it is important to assess the urethra for an abnormality (e.g., posterior urethral valves). In girls, the VCUG may be performed either with serial x-rays performed during bladder filling and voiding, or with fluoroscopy.

An alternative method of assessing reflux is to perform the radionuclide cystogram. In this study, a solution containing a radiopharmaceutical is instilled into the bladder and the bladder and kidneys are monitored with a gamma camera during bladder filling and voiding. There is much less radiologic detail with this study, but also much less radiation exposure to the gonads.

20. Describe the grading system for vesicoureteral reflux.

Numerous grading systems have been used over the years. The current system is that adopted by the International Reflux Study in Children and is termed the International System. The five grades are:

Grade I: The contrast material enters the ureter but does not enter the renal pelvis.

Grade II: The contrast material reaches the renal pelvis but does not distend the collecting system.

Grade III: The collecting system is filled and either the ureter or pelvis is distended but the calyceal demarcations are not distorted.

Grade IV: The dilated ureter is slightly tortuous and the calyces are blunted significantly.

Grade V: The entire collecting system is tremendously dilated without a visible papillary impression, and there is significant ureteral tortuosity.

21. What is the typical distribution of grades of vesicoureteral reflux?

Approximately 5–8% have grade I, 35% grade II, 25–35% grade III, 15–25% grade IV, and 5% grade V. Approximately half of children have bilateral reflux.

22. Name the relative advantages and disadvantages of performing a VCUG compared to a radionuclide cystogram in the initial evaluation of a child for reflux.

The International System for grading reflux is based on the VCUG. The grading system has important prognostic features that allow one to predict the likelihood of spontaneous reflux resolution. In addition, the radiographic VCUG allows one to see certain features in the bladder that may predispose to reflux, such as a duplication of the upper urinary tract, paraureteral diverticulum, and ectopic insertion of the ureter. During a VCUG in girls, signs of voiding dysfunction, as well as intrarenal reflux, may be seen. The main disadvantage of the VCUG (radiographic) is the higher radiation exposure. The nuclear cystogram causes only 1–2% of the radiation exposure to the gonads compared to a standard radiographic VCUG. Currently, most obtain a VCUG as the initial study and utilize the radionuclide cystogram for follow-up studies.

23. Can ultrasound be used to detect vesicoureteral reflux?

Only 25% of children with primary reflux have hydronephrosis, which is the most common sonographic finding in children with reflux. Consequently, a VCUG must be done to determine whether a child has reflux.

24. What is intrarenal reflux?

Intrarenal reflux is the reflux of urine into the renal parenchyma during voiding. If intrarenal reflux exists in conjunction with infection, renal inflammation occurs. In general, intrarenal reflux occurs in compound papillae, which are located in the polar regions of the kidney. Most papillae are convex, with slit-like openings of the collecting ducts opening obliquely onto the papilla. In concave or flat papillae, however, collecting ducts open at right angles and allow reflux.

25. When is vesicoureteral reflux most likely to cause renal injury?

Reflux is most likely to cause renal injury during the first year of life, although it may occur at any age in association with urinary infection.

26. Does sterile reflux cause renal injury?

In general, sterile reflux is not thought to cause renal injury. However, if a high-pressure voiding situation exists, as in a boy with posterior urethral valves, a neuropathic bladder, or detrusorsphincter dyssynergia, renal injury may occur in the absence of infection.

27. What is the likelihood of renal scarring in patients with reflux?

Approximately 85% with grade V reflux, 50% of children with grade IV, 30% of those with grade III, 15% of those with grade II, and 5–10% of those with grade I reflux have renal scarring. Thus, renal scarring is more common in those with higher grades of reflux.

28. What is the long-term significance of renal scarring?

The main complications of renal scarring are hypertension, which occurs in approximately 10% of children with renal scarring, and renal insufficiency or end-stage renal disease.

29. What is the association between reflux and hypertension?

One of the most common causes of severe hypertension in children and young adults is reflux nephropathy. The etiology is segmental ischemia and renin-driven hypertension due to arterial damage in the area of renal scarring. Hypertension is related to the grade of reflux, but eliminating the reflux does not reverse the predisposition to hypertension if scarring is present.

30. Of children with reflux, what proportion of their siblings also have reflux?

Approximately 30–35% of siblings have reflux. In most series, 75% of siblings with reflux are asymptomatic, i.e., they have not had urinary tract infections. The incidence of sibling reflux is unrelated to the index patient's reflux grade, sex, or renal scarring.

31. Should all siblings of index patients with reflux undergo a VCUG?

Most recommend that if a sibling is < 2–3 years old, then a radionuclide cystogram should be obtained. In children > 3 years, a renal ultrasound is appropriate, and if an abnormality is discovered, then a VCUG should be performed.

32. What are the signs of reflux on an IVP?

Renal scarring (blunted calyx, thin parenchyma, or global atrophy), hydronephrosis, caliectasis, and vertical striations of the upper ureter.

33. Which imaging studies are commonly used to detect renal scarring? What are the characteristic findings?

A dimercaptosuccinic acid (DMSA) renal scan may show areas of diminished uptake in the cortex. Single photon emission computed tomography (SPECT) increases the sensitivity of DMSA slightly in detecting scarring. On an intravenous pyelogram (IVP), renal scarring is evident as a blunted calyx, renal cortical thinning, or cortical atrophy of a segment of the entire kidney. Ultrasound also may demonstrate global atrophy or atrophy of a part of the kidney, but calyceal morphology usually is indistinct.

34. Which study is most sensitive in detecting renal scarring?

The DMSA renal scan is the most sensitive study. Renal scarring also may be apparent on a MAG-3 or glucoheptonate renal scan, but these studies are not thought to be as sensitive as the DMSA scan. Ultrasound is one of the least sensitive methods of detecting renal scarring.

35. What is the Weigert-Meyer rule?

This rule applies to children with complete duplication of the urinary tract, which results from two ureteral buds leading to the formation of two separate ureters and separate renal pelves within one kidney. The ureter to the upper segment arises from a cephalad position on the mesonephric duct, remains attached to the mesonephric duct longer during embryogenesis, and thus migrates farther, ending inferomedial to the ureter draining the lower segment. Thus, the ureter draining the lower pole is more cephalolateral, and the ureter draining the upper pole is more inferomedial in the bladder, and is prone to becoming ectopic.

36. What is the significance of the Weigert-Meyer law in reflux?
Because the ureter draining the lower pole of the kidney drains in a more lateral position in the bladder, its intramural tunnel is shorter, predisposing to reflux.

37. How common is upper urinary tract duplication?
Approximately 1 of 125 individuals have duplication of the upper urinary tract.

38. In a child with complete duplication of the urinary tract and reflux, into which segment(s) does the reflux occur typically?
Approximately 85% have reflux only into the lower pole, whereas 15% have reflux into both the upper and lower pole systems.

39. Describe the natural history of vesicoureteral reflux (VUR).
With growth and maturation of bladder function, reflux often resolves spontaneously. The likelihood of spontaneous resolution is related directly to reflux grade. Approximately 90% of children with grade I reflux, 75% with grade II, 50% with grade III, 40% with grade IV, and 5% or fewer of those with grade V reflux show spontaneous resolution.

40. How is a patient's age related to the likelihood of spontaneous resolution of reflux?
The younger the child, the greater is the likelihood that reflux will resolve.

41. Are children with upper urinary tract duplication as likely to show spontaneous resolution as those with single systems?
Comparing identical reflux grades, the likelihood of spontaneous reflux resolution in children with complete duplication is slightly less than in those with a single system.

42. What is the likelihood of spontaneous resolution of reflux in a child with bilateral grade III or IV reflux?
Approximately 10% will have spontaneous resolution.

43. What is the mean age at diagnosis of reflux?
The mean age is 2 to 3 years.

44. What is the mean age at spontaneous resolution of reflux?
Approximately 5 to 6 years.

45. At what age is reflux no longer likely to resolve?
In most children with reflux, reflux is unlikely to resolve beyond 10 or 11 years. However, in children with grade II reflux, spontaneous resolution has been shown to occur at 14 to 15 years.

46. How are children with reflux managed medically?
Medical management involves assessment of a child's voiding habits and patterns of infection. In children who are toilet trained, regular frequent voiding is encouraged. In children with bladder instability (urge incontinence), often anticholinergic therapy (e.g., oxybutynin chloride, propantheline bromide) is administered. In addition, constipation should be managed aggressively.

Antimicrobial prophylaxis is administered in an attempt to prevent urinary tract infection. In general, trimethoprim/sulfamethoxazole, trimethoprim, or nitrofurantoin is used, because these drugs have the least effect on the bacterial flora in the stool, which is the source of urinary tract infections. The dosage used for prophylaxis is approximately 1/4 to 1/3 the dosage commonly used to treat a UTI.

The child should have a urinalysis and/or culture performed every 3–4 months. Every 12–18 months, a follow-up cystogram is done to monitor the reflux, usually with a nuclear cystogram. In addition, an upper tract study such as an ultrasound, an IVP, or a DMSA scan is performed to assess renal growth. Children with reflux who are not placed on prophylaxis have a much higher incidence of renal scarring than those receiving prophylaxis.

47. What is a breakthrough UTI?

This term refers to a urinary tract infection that occurs while the patient is receiving prophylaxis.

48. What is the incidence of breakthrough UTI in children with VUR?

Approximately 25–35% with reflux have a breakthrough UTI.

49. Of children with grade I to III reflux managed medically, what is the likelihood of reappearance of reflux after one normal cystogram?

Approximately 20% will show reflux on a follow-up study.

50. Of children with no reflux on one side and contralateral grade I–III reflux, what is the likelihood of reflux on the nonrefluxing side on a follow-up cystogram?

Approximately 20% of those with no reflux on one side will show reflux into that ureter on a subsequent study.

51. What constitutes a failure of medical management?

A child who develops a breakthrough UTI, is allergic to antimicrobial medication, is poorly compliant, or has persistent reflux until the age of 10 or 11 years should be considered unresponsive to medical management.

52. Define bladder instability.

It is uninhibited detrusor (bladder) contractions that persist beyond 2–4 years, the usual age at which toilet training occurs. In a neurologically normal child, typical symptoms include urgency with urge incontinence and frequency.

53. What is the significance of bladder instability in children with reflux?

Bladder instability is common in children with reflux and may worsen their reflux grade. Children with bladder instability are managed with anticholinergic medication (e.g., oxybutynin chloride, propantheline bromide) and regular timed voiding. Children with bladder instability managed with anticholinergic therapy and antimicrobial prophylaxis are more likely to show spontaneous resolution than those who are treated with prophylaxis alone.

54. What are the indications for surgical management of children with reflux?

In general, ureteroneocystostomy is recommended for all children with grade V reflux. In children with lesser grades of reflux, failure of medical management constitutes a strong indication. Thus, breakthrough UTI, noncompliance with medical management, allergies to prophylactic medications, and persistent reflux, particularly in 10-year-old children, are indications. Currently, most pediatric urologists recommend antireflux surgery for primary grade IV reflux because of its low likelihood of spontaneous resolution and the high risk of renal scarring.

55. What are the principles of surgical management for vesicoureteral reflux?

The principles of antireflux surgery include creation of an intramural ureter that is 4–5 times as long as wide. The ureter is placed in the submucosal layer between the mucosa and detrusor (muscle).

56. What types of open surgical techniques are used to correct reflux?

The term for this operation is ureteroneocystostomy. The most common method of correcting reflux consists of opening the bladder, mobilizing the ureter, and advancing it across the trigone (Cohen or transtrigonal repair). Alternatively, the ureter may be reinserted in a higher more medial position in the bladder and brought down to its normal position (Leadbetter-Politano). In extravesical repairs, the ureter is anchored in the bladder base and the bladder muscle is sutured around the ureter (Lich-Gregoir; detrusorrhaphy). Recent advances in laparoscopic equipment have enabled minimally invasive techniques to repair reflux using both intravesical and extravesical techniques. Further studies will be necessary to determine their role in treating reflux in the future.

57. In a child with duplication of the urinary tract and reflux into the lower pole, how is the reflux managed surgically?

In these children, the ureters are in a single sheath near the bladder and share a common blood supply. Even though only the lower pole ureter may reflux, it is necessary to perform a "common sheath" ureteroneocystostomy, in which both ureters are mobilized together and reimplanted as one unit. Alternatively, the refluxing lower pole ureter may be detached from the bladder and anastomosed to the upper pole ureter near the bladder (ureteroureterostomy).

58. What is the success rate of ureteroneocystostomy?

Approximately 95–98% of children undergoing ureteroneocystostomy have a successful surgical result.

59. What are the complications of ureteroneocystostomy?

Obstruction of the ureterovesical junction and reflux each occurs in approximately 1–2% of cases.

60. In children with primary reflux, which patients are most likely to experience a complication?

Children who have untreated voiding dysfunction are most likely to have a surgical complication.

61. What is J-hooking of the ureter?

In children undergoing a Leadbetter-Politano repair, if the ureter is anastomosed to a mobile portion of the bladder, kinking of the ureter may occur where it inserts into the bladder. In most of these patients, when the bladder is empty, there is normal urinary drainage, but with bladder filling, the lower ureter becomes kinked and progressive hydroureteronephrosis occurs. This condition is termed the **high reimplant syndrome.**

62. If the ureter is extremely wide, what modifications of surgical technique are necessary?

If the ureter is wide, a tunnel of satisfactory length may be difficult to achieve. In these patients the ureter must be tailored, i.e., narrowed, to achieve a sufficient width to allow a successful ureteroneocystostomy. This is done in one of two ways. Excisional tapering may be performed, in which the lateral aspect of the ureter is excised to a point 2–3 cm above the level of implantation. Alternatively, the ureter may be plicated, or folded, to narrow its width.

63. Describe the typical cystoscopic appearances of the ureteral orifice in children with reflux.

Normally, the ureteral orifice has a cone shape. Refluxing ureters may have a stadium orifice, a horseshoe orifice, a golf-hole orifice, or a patulous ureteral orifice. These terms refer to progressively abnormal appearances of the ureter in the bladder.

64. What is the endoscopic form of antireflux surgery?

Reflux may be corrected by injecting a substance deep into the ureter to create an intramural tunnel. This procedure has been called the "STING," which stands for subtrigonal injection. In the past, polytef paste was used. This substance consists of pyrolyzed Teflon particles suspended in glycerin. Migration of these Teflon particles to the pelvic lymph nodes, liver, lung, and brain has been demonstrated in laboratory models, and currently few procedures are performed using Teflon. The first FDA-approved substance is a biodegradable, tissue-augmenting material (Deflux®) of non-animal origin.

65. What are the results of the STING?

The results of the STING are inferior to open surgical management. Approximately 70% of patients have reflux resolution with one procedure. With repeat STING procedures, however, the cure rate is as high as 90–95%.

66. What is the likelihood of new renal scarring in children with grade III or IV reflux?

New renal scarring will develop in approximately 20% managed medically.

67. Can reflux be diagnosed prenatally?

Reflux may be detected prenatally by detecting hydronephrosis. However, reflux is not the most common cause of hydronephrosis in the fetus.

68. Of children with prenatally diagnosed reflux, what proportion are boys?

Approximately 80% are boys, because boys have higher grades of reflux than girls.

BIBLIOGRAPHY

1. Arant BS: Vesicoureteric reflux and renal injury: In-depth review. Am J Kidney Dis 17:491–511, 1991.
2. Arant BS: Medical management of mild and moderate vesicoureteral reflux: Follow-up studies of infants and young children. A preliminary report of the Southwest Pediatric Nephrology Study Group. J Urol 148:1683–1687, 1992.
3. Arant BS Jr, Sotelo-Avila C, Bernstein J: Segmental "hypoplasia" of the kidney (Ask-Upmark). J Pediatr 95:931–939, 1979.
4. Bellinger MF, Duckett JW: Vesicoureteral reflux: A comparison of nonsurgical and surgical management. Contrib Nephrol 39:81–93, 1984.
5. Burns DK, Glazier DB, Zaontz MR: Lessons learned about contralateral reflux after unilateral extravesical ureteral advancement in children. J Urol 160:973, 1998.
6. Elder JS: Importance of antenatal diagnosis of vesicoureteral reflux [Commentary]. J Urol 148:1750–1754, 1992.
7. Elder JS, Peters C, Arant BS, et al: Pediatric vesicoureteral reflux guidelines panel summary report on the management of primary vesicoureteral reflux in children. J Urol 157:1846, 1997.
8. Elder JS, Peters C, Arant BS, et al: Report on the Management of Primary Vesicoureteral Reflux in Children. Santa Ana, Calif, American Urological Association, 1997.
9. Elder JS, Snyder HM, Peters C, et al: Variability in management among physicians treating children with vesicoureteral reflux. J Urol 148:714, 1992.
10. Goldraich NP, Goldraich IH: Followup of conservatively treated children with high and low grade vesicoureteral reflux: A prospective study. J Urol 148:1688–1692, 1992.
11. Goldraich NP, Ramos OL, Goldraich IH: Urography versus DMSA scan in children with vesicoureteric reflux. Pediatr Nephrol 3:1–5, 1989.
12. Kobb SA, Wagner TT, Jayenthi VR: Relationship among dysfunctional elimination syndromes, primary vesicoureteral reflux and urinary tract infections in children. J Urol 160:1019, 1998.
13. Koff SA, Lapides J, Piazza DH: Association of urinary tract infection and reflux with uninhibited bladder contractions and voluntary sphincteric obstruction. J Urol 122:373–376, 1979.
14. Koff SA, Murtagh DS: The inhibited bladder in children: Effect of treatment on recurrence of urinary infection and vesicoureteral reflux. J Urol 130:1138, 1983.
15. Noe HN: The long-term results of prospective sibling reflux screening. J Urol 148:1739–1742, 1992.
16. Olbing H, Claesson K, Ebel D, et al: Renal scars and parenchymal thinning in children with vesicoureteral reflux: A 5-year report of the international reflux study in children (European Branch). J Urol 148:1653–1656, 1992.
17. Palmer LS, Franco I, Rotario P, et al: Biofeedback therapy expedites the resolution of reflux in older children. J Urol 168:1699–1703, 2002.
18. Ransley PG, Risdon: Reflux and renal scarring. Br J Radiol Suppl 14:1–34, 1978.

19. Roberts JA: Vesicoureteral reflux and pyelonephritis in the monkey: A review. J Urol 148:1721–1725, 1992.
20. Rushton HG, Massoud M: Dimercaptosuccinic acid renal scintigraphy for the evaluation of pyelonephritis and scarring: A review of experimental and clinical studies. J Urol 148:1726–1732, 1992.
21. Tamminen-Mobius I, Brunier E, Ebel KD, et al: Cessation of vesicoureteral reflux for 5 years in infants and children allocated to medical treatment. J Urol 148:1662–1666, 1992.
22. Weiss R, Duckett J, et al: Results of a randomized clinical trial of medical versus surgical management of infants and children with grades III and IV primary vesicoureteral reflux (United States). J Urol 148: 1667–1673, 1992.

42. URETEROCELE

Robert Kay, M.D.

1. What is a ureterocele?
A ureterocele is the cystic dilatation of the distal end of the ureter in the intravesical segment.

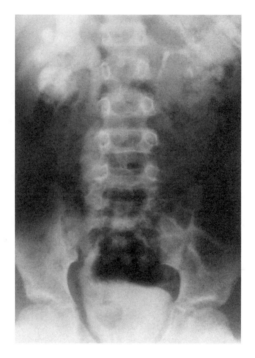

Intravenous pyelogram demonstrating a simple orthotopic ureterocele.

2. In what settings does a ureterocele occur?
Although ureteroceles may occur in single systems (orthotopic ureteroceles), they are most commonly seen in duplicated ureters (ectopic ureteroceles) and come from the ureter draining the upper segment.

3. Why do ureteroceles occur?
There are three current theories to explain the development of ureteroceles:
- Ureteral meatal obstruction
- Inadequate muscularization of the distal ureter
- Excessive dilatation of the distal ureter during development

4. Do ureteroceles occur equally in both sexes?
No. Single-system ureteroceles occur mostly in boys and rarely are seen in girls. Conversely, ectopic ureteroceles, as seen in duplicated systems, occur more frequently in girls than boys.

5. How do ureteroceles present?

Ureteroceles are most commonly diagnosed today by in-utero ultrasound. During fetal ultrasound, a diagnosis of hydronephrosis is made, which is corrected to ureterocele during evaluation in the postpartum period.

Ureteroceles also may be seen during physical examination. An ectopic ureterocele may prolapse through the urethra and present as an intralabial mass, or it may extend underneath the urethra and present between the labia as a cystic mass. Before the advent of ultrasound, urinary tract infection was the most common presentation, and many children still present with this complaint.

6. What is the best way to diagnose a ureterocele?

1. **Ultrasonography** is the best initial step to diagnose a ureterocele. The ultrasound will be ordered as follow-up to the in-utero diagnosis or as evaluation of a urinary tract infection. The technique can evaluate the upper tract and define hydronephrosis. It also may see the cystic mass at the end of the distal ureter and into the bladder.

2. The suspicion of ureterocele on ultrasound may be confirmed by a **voiding cystourethrography.**

3. Finally, a **renal scan** is needed to assess the function of the upper tracts.

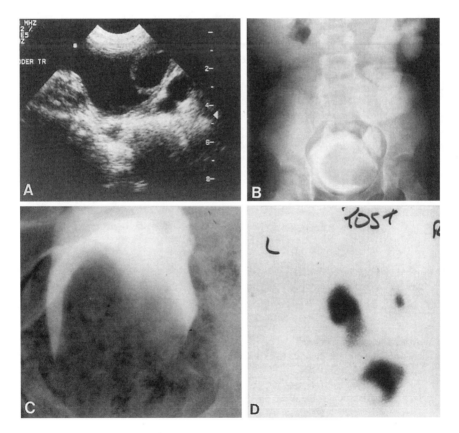

A. Ultrasound demonstrating large ureterocele in bladder. **B.** Intravenous pyelogram revealing large ureterocele in bladder with function of lower pole and dilated ureter. **C.** Cystogram demonstrating large ureterocele. **D.** Renal scan demonstrating hydronephrotic lower pole with nonfunctioning upper pole draining into ectopic ureterocele in bladder.

7. What is the preferred treatment for a single-system (orthotopic) ureterocele?

Although there is a risk of a vesicoureteric reflux, the initial step in treatment is a simple, endoscopic incision of the ureterocele. If reflux occurs and the kidney is salvageable, surgical reimplantation may be performed.

8. List the possible management modalities for ectopic ureteroceles.

1. Endoscopic incision of the ureterocele with possible late bladder reconstruction
2. Upper pole nephrectomy with partial–possible) ureterectomy
3. Upper pole pyelo-pyelostomy for functioning kidneys
4. Upper pole nephrectomy with total ureterectomy and repair of the bladder, including lower pole ureteral reimplantation.
5. Primary excision and bladder reconstruction.

9. What is the functional status of the upper pole associated with an ectopic ureterocele?

The upper pole associated with a ureterocele usually has poor or no function. In many cases, the segment might be dysplastic. In some select cases, however, there is functioning tissue that should be salvaged.

10. Does reflux occur in ureteroceles?

Reflux can occur in up to 50% of ipsilateral ureters that are associated with ureteroceles. This may be due to poor musculature backing and distortion of the bladder wall from the ectopic ureter. It also may be seen in the contralateral ureter, probably due to distortion of the trigone.

11. Can the reflux disappear spontaneously?

Mild reflux in the ipsilateral ureter and contralateral ureter may spontaneously resolve. Significant degrees of reflux, however, do not usually resolve and require surgical reimplantation.

12. Can ureteroceles be bilateral?

Yes. Bilateral ureteroceles may be seen in up to 10% of all cases of ectopic ureteroceles.

13. What is a cecoureterocele?

A cecoureterocele is an ectopic ureterocele that extends suburethrally into the proximal or even distal urethra.

BIBLIOGRAPHY

1. Abrahamsson K, Hansson E, Sillen U, et al: Bladder dysfunction: An integral part of the ectopic uretero-cele complex. J Urol 160:1468–1470, 1998.
2. Balchick RJ, Nasrallah PF: Cecoureterocele. J Urol 137:100, 1987.
3. Blyth B, Passerini-Glazel G, Camuffo C, et al: Endoscopic incision of ureteroceles: Intravesical versus ectopic. J Urol 149:556, 1993.
4. Caldamone AA, Snyder HM, Duckett JW: Ureteroceles in children: Follow-up of management with upper tract approach. J Urol 131:1130, 1984.
5. Churchill BM, Sheldon CA, McLorie GA: The ectopic ureterocele: A proposed practical classification based on renal unit jeopardy. J Pediatr Surg 27:497, 1992.
6. Coplen DE, Duckett JW: The modern approach to ureteroceles. J Urol 153:166–171, 1995.
7. Decter RM, Roth DR, Gonzales ET: Individualized treatment of ureterocele. J Urol 142:535, 1989
8. DeJong TP, Dik P, Klijn AJ, et al: .Ectopic ureterocele: Results of open surgical therapy of 40 patients. J Urol 164:2040–2044, 2000.
9. Gonzales ET: Anomalies of the renal pelvis and ureter. In Kelalis PP, King LR, Belman AB (eds): Clinical Pediatric Urology, 3rd ed. Philadelphia, W.B. Saunders, 1992.
10. Husmann DA, Strand WR, Ewalt DH, Krtamer SA: Is endoscopic decompression of the neonatal extravesical upper pole ureterocele necessary for prevention of urinary tract infection or bladder neck obstruction? J Urol 167:1440–1442, 2002.
11. King LR, Koglowski JM, Schacht MJ: Ureteroceles in children: A simplified and successful approach to management. JAMA 249:1461, 1983.

12. Pfister C, Ravasse P, Barret E, et al: The value of endoscopic treatment for ureteroceles during the neonatal period. J Urol 159:1006–1009, 1998.

13. Retik AB: Ectopic ureter and ureterocele. In Walsh PC, Retik AB, Vaughan ED Jr, Wein AJ (eds): Campbell's Urology, 7th ed. Philadelphia, W. B. Saunders, 1998.

14. Rich MA, Keating MA, Snyder HM, Duckett JW: Low transurethral incision of single system intravesical ureteroceles in children. J Urol 144:120, 1990.

15. Stephens FD: Congenital Malformations of the Urinary Tract. New York, Praeger, 1983, pp 320–322, 329.

16. Tank ES: Experience with endoscopic incision and open unroofing of ureteroceles. J Urol 136:241, 1986.

43. STRESS URINARY INCONTINENCE

Sandip P. Vasavada, M.D.

1. What is urinary incontinence?

Urinary incontinence is not a single disorder. Rather, it is a symptom of some underlying disorder. It is defined as the involuntary loss of urine and is a major clinical problem and a significant cause of disability and dependency.

2. Is urinary incontinence a consequence of aging?

While normal aging is not a cause of urinary incontinence, age-related changes in lower urinary tract function do predispose older individuals to urinary incontinence. These include anatomic or physiologic insults to the lower urinary tract and systemic disturbances common in the older population.

3. What are the types of urinary incontinence?

These may be defined by function or symptoms.

Types of Incontinence

FUNCTIONAL	SYMPTOMATIC
Detrusor overactivity	Total
Detrusor underactivity	Urge
Outlet incompetence	Stress
Outlet obstruction	Overflow
	Transient
	Functional

The essential organs involved relate to the lower urinary tract and consist of the bladder and urethra, and one can distinguish urinary incontinence that is caused by problems at the level of the bladder as compared to urinary incontinence caused by problems at the level of the urethra. More commonly, the symptomatic definition is used. The six symptomatic types are as follows:

1. **Total incontinence.** Urinary loss that is not associated with any particular event.
2. **Urge incontinence.** The inability to delay voiding after perceiving that the bladder is full—i.e., the bladder contracts without its owner's permission.
3. **Stress urinary incontinence.** Urine loss due to increases in intraabdominal pressure (Valsalva maneuver).
4. **Overflow incontinence.** Urinary loss due to obstruction or a poorly contracting bladder that allows for a continuous drip of urine.
5. **Transient urinary incontinence.** Acute urinary loss that is precipitated by a nonurinary tract factor, such as change in medication.
6. **Functional incontinence.** Incontinence occurs despite a normal-functioning lower urinary tract, but the patient has a cognitive disorder.

4. Explain the problem causing stress incontinence.

Stress incontinence is a poor term since *stress* is usually associated with such abnormalities as coronary artery disease and peptic ulcer disease. Here, *stress* is meant as the effect of increased abdominal pressure on the lower urinary tract that occurs during times of coughing, laughing, bending, lifting, and defecating.

Normally, the bladder and functional portion of the urethra are located above the pelvic floor so that both are within the true pelvis as intraabdominal organs. At rest, the urethral pressure is higher than the bladder pressure, preventing urinary leakage. When a Valsalva maneuver increases abdominal pressure, this pressure is transmitted equally onto the bladder and urethra, because both organs are confined within the true pelvis. In stress incontinence, incompetence of the urinary outlet consists of the bladder neck and proximal functional urethra. The weakening of supportive muscular tissue of the pelvic floor also may allow the urethra to move out of the true pelvis during a Valsalva maneuver, which results in unequal transmission of the intraabdominal pressure onto the bladder only and not the urethra. This results in the bladder pressure rising significantly above urethral pressure for that moment and urinary loss.

5. What can cause pelvic floor weakness?
- Anatomic: congenital or traumatic (pelvic floor fracture, pelvic surgery, labor)
- Hormonal
- Neurologic: congenital or traumatic

6. Is the underlying problem in stress incontinence what is meant by urethral incompetence?
Yes! Stress urinary incontinence involves the poor function of the outlet of sphincteric mechanisms. There are, however, degrees of **urethral incompetence,** which are determined by urodynamic investigations of abdominal or Valsalva leak point pressure determination. Patients with lower leak point pressures have worse symptoms and patients with higher leak point pressures do not leak as easily. This is made clear when one realizes that the normal urethra will not leak at any abdominal pressure no matter how hard someone strains. Leakage with a Valsalva maneuver (i.e., cough, sneeze, bending) implies that there is a deficit in urethral function and that leakage can take place with or without hypermobility of the vesicourethral junction. It was formerly believed that two (2) types of stress urinary incontinence existed, one involving the hypermobility of a normally functioning urethral sphincteric mechanism and a second, more severe form of intrinsic sphincteric dysfunction (ISD) due to the above-mentioned urethral sphincteric incompetence. It is now recognized that many women have vesicourethral hypermobility without incontinence, although hypermobility is not the cause of the urinary loss. The only cause of urinary stress incontinence is ISD, which may or may not be associated with hypermobility.

7. What causes urethral incompetence?
It is caused by damage to the sympathetic neural input to the bladder neck and proximal urethra. This area is innervated by the hypogastric nerve, which branches from the thoracolumbar sympathetic outflow tract. Trauma, such as fracture of the pelvis or pelvic surgery, may damage these nerves. Congenital problems such as myelodysplasia (spina bifida) also result in a decrease in innervation to this area of the lower urinary tract, resulting in a nonfunctioning sphincteric mechanism.

8. In that case, are there two types of stress incontinence?
Yes! One type of ISD is associated with hypermobility of the vesicourethral junction and one type has no associated hypermobility, meaning that the bladder outlet is well supported but simply not functioning properly. This concept has changed the outlook on treatment and has helped to explain the failure of bladder neck suspension surgery in the past, leading to the recommendation that women with stress urinary incontinence be treated with either sling surgery or injectable therapy after noninvasive pelvic floor therapy (e.g., Kegel exercises, biofeedback, and electrical magnetic stimulation) has failed to attain the desired response.

9. How does one evaluate a patient complaining of urinary incontinence?

Evaluation of Incontinence

History
    Medical
    Obstetric
Urinary diary
Physical examination
    Observe urinary loss
    Stress test
    Q-tip test
    Bonney/Marshall test
    Vaginal speculum exam
Urinalysis
Urodynamic testing
Cystourethroscopy

10. What is the point of the history?

Because the history is not helpful in arriving at a precise diagnosis, its primary value is to direct further investigative efforts to define the cause of the patient's urinary incontinence. During the history, one attempts to define the type of urinary incontinence while recognizing that significant overlap in many of the "types" of urinary incontinence may occur. In general, pathology in five major areas causes lower urinary tract symptoms:

1. Urinary tract pathology
2. Extrinsic local anatomic changes
3. Neurologic disorders
4. Psychiatric disorders
5. Local effects of systemic disease and/or its treatment

Therefore, specific questions will suggest a category for the patient's problem, placing it into one of the above general areas rather than trying to focus on a specific diagnosis.

11. How is the incontinence documented?

The patient should keep a diary of intake of fluid and output of urine, recording the time and volume of each voiding and incontinent episode. Also, during the physical examination, the physician must be able to reproduce the urinary incontinence and observe it, which may include examination of the patient while he or she is in the standing position.

12. Are there special aspects of the physical examination in female patients?

The proximity of the lower urinary tract to the female reproductive tract makes simultaneous assessment of both a necessity in the proper evaluation of female incontinence problems. For example, estrogen deprivation not only manifests itself with atrophic changes in the vulva and vagina, but also produces a variety of lower urinary tract symptoms due to atrophic urethritis. In addition, both a vesicovaginal fistula or urethral diverticulum may produce incontinence, and a thorough examination may help to detect this particular defect. Prolapse of the bladder, rectum, uterus, or vagina itself also may be affecting voiding function.

13. Explain the specific tests used during the physical examination of a female patient.

1. **Q-tip test.** This helps determine the amount of urethral hypermobility on straining. With the patient in the lithotomy position, the physician inserts a lubricated Q-tip into the urethra to the level of the urethrovesical junction and then measures the angle between the Q-tip and horizontal when the patient strains maximally. Normally, the angle is 10–15° above horizontal at rest with minimal changes on straining. In the patient with genuine stress urinary incontinence, this angle usually increases by >20°, suggesting that the descent of the urethra and bladder neck is due to weakness of the anatomic support.

2. **Stress test.** The patient with a full bladder stands with one leg up on a stool, and while the physician closely observes the urethral meatus, the patient bears down or coughs. If a short spurt of urine escapes simultaneously with the cough, this suggests genuine urinary incontinence. A slight delay in the leakage after the cough suggests an unstable bladder, as contractions in the bladder may have been provoked by the Valsalva maneuver.

3. **Bonney test.** The physician places two fingers in the vagina to elevate the neck of the bladder up toward the pubic bone, taking care not to compress the urethra. Unfortunately, this is extremely difficult to do without compressing the urethra. In a patient who has demonstrated a positive stress test, the Bonney test usually stops the urinary loss by elevating and compressing the urethra.

4. **Marshall test.** In this variation of the Bonney test, the vagina is anesthetized locally to allow a section of the vagina to be grasped with a clamp and elevated in a fashion that does not compress the urethra. Neither the Bonney nor Marshall test is diagnostic, as occlusion of the urethra prevents leakage regardless of the pathophysiology of the urinary incontinence. Therefore, these tests are of limited value.

5. **Speculum evaluation.** A full pelvic examination often reveals evidence for pelvic relaxation with herniation of the bladder (cystocele) or rectum (rectocele) into the vagina. Of course, other disease such as pelvic mass also may be found.

14. Are any laboratory tests necessary?

A urinalysis should be performed. Evidence of hematuria requires further evaluation with urinary cytology, intravenous urography, and cystourethroscopy. Any and all urinary tract infections should be treated appropriately.

15. What is the purpose of urodynamic testing?

Urodynamic studies are the most important set of examinations because they evaluate the motor function of the three specific muscle groups that make up the lower urinary tract: the bladder, smooth muscle of the urethra, and external striated muscle sphincter. When urodynamic testing is combined with contrast placed into the urinary tract, the lower urinary tract may be visualized, and an anatomic and physiologic evaluation can be performed simultaneously; this is called **videourodynamics.** Although this is not necessary for every patient, in patients with confusing symptoms, it helps elucidate the actual dysfunction that is occurring.

Urodynamic tests are done with small catheters that measure the pressure within the bladder and urethra. It is important to do these studies while the patient is in an upright position, especially if the patient denies having any leakage while lying down. The most important of these tests is the cystometrogram, which evaluates the stability of the bladder while it is filling with urine. Unstable bladder contractions are usually interpreted by the patient as the urge to void and, if the pressure is high enough, can result in urge incontinence. The presence of unstable bladder contractions in a patient who has stress incontinence may alter the recommended therapy.

16. When is urodynamic testing indicated?

- Failed previous incontinence surgery
- Previous radical pelvic surgery
- Symptoms of mixed incontinence
- No objective evidence of urinary leakage
- Abnormal neurologic examination
- History of neurologic disorder

17. When is cystoscopy indicated?

1. In patients shown to have an unstable bladder by either history or cystometrogram, it is important to exclude bladder pathology, which could cause the symptoms. Bladder tumors, bladder stones, urinary infections, and even carcinoma-in-situ may result in unstable bladder contractions.

2. If a patient has stress incontinence or another form of incontinence requiring surgical repair, then preoperative cystourethroscopy can prevent errors in patient management. Coexisting disease, if detected before the scheduled incontinence surgery, then can be appropriately handled at the same time. For example, patients who have mixed incontinence may be cured by removal of permanent suture material which has perforated the bladder from previous pelvic surgery.

3. The presence of hematuria, gross or microscopic, demands that cystoscopy be performed.

18. How do you identify patients with a nonfunctioning urethra?

In these patients, urodynamic evaluation is mandatory to evaluate the sphincteric function. Specific tests designed to do this include the **urethral closure profile.** Pressure in the urethra below 20 cm H_2O indicates a poorly functioning urethra (the normal urethral closure pressure is >40 cm H_2O). Leak point pressures can be determined during cystometrography. If the bladder pressure resulting in urinary leakage is <100 cm H_2O, this indicates severe urethral dysfunction.

19. Once the diagnosis of genuine stress incontinence is made, what medical treatments are available?

The only medical treatment that has been helpful is the use of estrogen in postmenopausal women who have demonstrated estrogen deprivation. No other medications have been effective because this is an anatomic disorder.

Treatment of Stress Incontinence

HYPERMOBILITY	URETHRAL INCOMPETENCE
Medical	Slings
Estrogen	Artificial urinary sphincter
Behavioral	Injectables
Pelvic floor exercise	
Bladder drill	
Timed voidings	
Biofeedback	
Surgery	
Abdominal	
Vaginal	

20. Are any other nonsurgical methods helpful?

Most definitely. Noninvasive methods may be helpful in controlling patient symptoms if they are not too severe. These include Kegel pelvic muscle exercises, behavior modification and retraining, and biofeedback. In addition, pelvic floor electrical stimulation with a vaginal probe is effective in approximately 50% of patients with mild stress urinary incontinence, and early results with noninvasive magnetic stimulation to the pelvic floor have been impressive. This stimulation acts directly on the pudendal nerve to cause contraction of the levator muscles and periurethral skeletal muscle and appears to strengthen the sphincter and pelvic floor muscles without actually correcting the underlying anatomic defect.

21. What role does surgery play in the management of stress urinary incontinence?

Some have suggested that the term *stress incontinence* be replaced by the phrase *surgically curable urinary incontinence.* Surgery clearly has been successful in managing patients with genuine stress urinary incontinence, curing about 75% of patients and improving continence in 85%, no matter which technique of surgical repair is used.

A multitude of surgical repairs have been developed in attempts to reduce the amount of surgical trauma and hospitalization time and to return patients to work quicker. However, none of the procedures works 100% of the time, and these new procedures are also attempts to improve surgical success. No one method can be recommended over another, because success relates to the surgeon's experience with a particular procedure and patient selection for that procedure. Some procedures are done via an abdominal surgical approach and others through the vagina.

22. What are the most commonly used materials in vaginal sling surgery?
While traditionally, autologous fascia (rectus or fascia lata) is commonly used, there exists a fair amount of interest in alternative sling materials in order to decrease morbidity and save operative time. These materials include cadaveric tissues (dermis, fascia, dura), bovine tissues, porcine dermis, intestinal submucosa, and a host of synthetic materials, including Prolene mesh and Gortex mesh.

23. What are the major risks of vaginal sling surgery?
Bleeding, infection, bladder/ureteric injury, erosion of graft materials into the urethra or vagina, de novo urge incontinence, recurrent stress incontinence, neurologic injury, and pain.

24. What about patients with intrinsic sphincteric deficiency with urethral incompetence?
Here, standard urethral resuspension procedures will not be effective if the continence mechanism is defective. Rather, compression and coaptation of the urethral mucosa are necessary. The three approaches to this are:
1. **Pubovaginal sling.** An autologous, heterologous, or synthetic material is used as a broad base of support under the urethra and then brought up through the abdominal wall and anchored to either the abdomen or pelvic bones in order to provide compression of the urethra.
2. **Artificial urinary sphincter.** A small cuff is placed around the neck of the bladder, and a hydraulic pump mechanism is placed inside the labia of the patient. When she has the urge to void, she merely pushes the pump once or twice, and this drives the fluid out of the cuff and opens up the neck of the bladder to allow unobstructed voiding.
3. **Injectable treatment.** The use of bovine collagen or silicon-coated carbon beads injected under local anesthesia into the submucosa of the urethra at the level of the bladder neck is extremely effective in controlling urethral incompetence.

25. What is the TVT technique?
The TVT (tension-free vaginal tape) is a technique that uses synthetic Prolene mesh to support the midurethra and to aid patient continence. It was first developed and popularized in Europe and has been used extensively now across the world. Data show between 81% and 92% success rates in intermediate-term follow-up.

BIBLIOGRAPHY

1. Appell RA: Injectables for urethral incontinence. World J Urol 8:208–211, 1990.
2. Appell RA: Primary slings for everyone with genuine stress incontinence? The argument for . . . Int Urogynecol J 9:249–251, 1998.
3. Appell RA: Techniques and results in the implantation of the artificial urinary sphincter in type III stress urinary incontinence by a vaginal approach. Neurourol Urodyn 7:613–619, 1988.
4. Blaivas JG, Fisher DM: Combined radiographic and urodynamic monitoring: Advances in technique. J Urol 125:541–544, 1981.
5. Burgio KL: Behavioral training for stress and urge incontinence in the community. Gerontology 38(suppl 2): 27–34, 1990.
6. Cardozo L: Role of estrogens in the treatment of female urinary incontinence. J Am Geriatr Soc 38: 326–328, 1990.
7. Henalla SM, Kirwan P, Castleden CM, et al: The effect of pelvic floor exercise in the treatment of genuine stress urinary incontinence in women at two hospitals. Br J Obstet Gynaecol 95:602–606, 1988.
8. Kelley MJ, Leach GE: Long term results of bladder neck suspension procedures. Probl Urol 5:94–105, 1991.
9. McGuire EJ: Bladder instability and stress incontinence. Neurourol Urodyn 7:563–567, 1988.
10. McIntosh LJ, Richardson DA: Thirty-minute evaluation of incontinence in the older woman. Geriatrics 49:35–44, 1994.

11. Staskin DR: Sling surgery for the treatment of female stress incontinence. Probl Urol 5:106–122, 1991.
12. Staskin DR, Zimmern PE, Hadley HR, et al: The pathophysiology of stress incontinence. Urol Clin North Am 12:271–278, 1985.
13. Wall LL, Norton PA, DeLancey JOL: Practical Urogynecology. Baltimore, Williams & Wilkins, 1993.
14. Vasavada SP, Comiter CV, Raz S: Vaginal slings in the treatment of stress urinary incontinence. Atlas Urol Clin North Am 8:71–87, 2000.
15. Vasavada SP, Comiter CV, Rovner ES, Raz S: How to prevent complications in vaginal surgery. J Bras Urol 25:152–160, 1999.
16. Rackley et al: Tension free vaginal tape and percutaneous vaginal tape sling procedures. In Cespedes RD, Vasavada SP (eds): Tech Urol 90–100, 2001.

44. VESICOVAGINAL FISTULA

Raymond R. Rackley, MD

1. What is a vesicovaginal fistula (VVF?)

A **vesicovaginal fistula** is an abnormal passage between the bladder and the vagina. The proximity of the lower urinary tract and female reproductive organs renders this anatomic relationship susceptible to numerous iatrogenic and noniatrogenic causes that give rise to the formation of an abnormal communication between the bladder and vagina. Although obstetric trauma is the leading cause of VVF in underdeveloped countries, iatrogenic causes of vesicovaginal fistulas in developed countries are mostly surgical trauma from open pelvic or transvaginal surgery and radiation-induced injury. The increasing use of minimally invasive laparoscopic procedures is gradually resulting in a higher proportion of the total number of lower urinary tract injuries that may give rise to secondary fistula formation.

Etiologies of Vesicovaginal Fistula
  I. Congenital
 II. Acquired
    A. Iatrogenic
      1. Postoperative
        a. Hysterectomy
        b. Incontinence procedures
        c. Anterior colporrhaphy
        d. Pelvic laparoscopy
        e. Gynecologic biopsies
        f. Subtrigonal phenol injection therapy
      2. Radiation injury
    B. Noniatrogenic
      1. Advanced pelvic carcinoma
      2. Obstructed labor
      3. Infectious (tuberculosis)
      4. Foreign body (bladder or vaginal)

2. What are the presenting signs and symptoms of a VVF?

The classic presentation of a patient with a VVF is constant urinary leakage following a pelvic operation. The leakage occurs during the day and night, and in the case of a small fistula with minimal vaginal discharge, it may be associated with a normal voiding pattern. Patients who develop a postoperative urogenital fistula may present very early in their convalescence period with excessive abdominal pain and distention secondary to urinary extravasation, excessive wound or vaginal drainage, hematuria, and even irritative voiding patterns. Some patients experience a painless, watery discharge of varying amounts from the vagina occurring 7 to 14 days after pelvic surgery. A common mistake is to attribute this to serosanguineous drainage, lymphatic fluid, or excessive vaginal discharge, but conformational studies help to establish the correct diagnosis in a timely fashion. Radiation-related fistulas may develop several months or even years after therapy. A radiation-related fistula should be considered a potential complication of recurrent cancer until a biopsy of the edge of the fistula has ruled out this possibility.

3. How is the diagnosis of VVF made?

A complete history is fundamental to the initial diagnostic steps in evaluating a patient for a VVF. The patient's past medical history may provide important clues to the risk factors that lead to the development of VVF and how such risk factors may influence the therapeutic approach selected for repair. Potential risk factors for fistula or recurrent fistula formation are as follows:

1. Prior uterine surgery (cesarean section), radiation therapy, or bladder operation
2. Pelvic endometriosis, previous cervical conization, or extensive vaginal fulguration
3. Hypoestrogenic status or steroid use
4. Sexual practices or use of vaginal pessaries
5. History of urinary tract infections or pelvic malignancies
6. Congenital lower urinary tract or reproductive system malformations
7. History of neurogenic bladder or voiding dysfunction

A complete physical examination is essential for the assessment of all patients undergoing evaluation for a VVF. Special emphasis should be placed on abdominal, genital, pelvic, and neurologic evaluations in an attempt to identify any concomitant pathology that may influence the therapeutic option selected for repair of the lower urinary tract. Identification of previous incisional sites of both the abdominal and vaginal wall is made. Prior or potential reconstructive tissue flap rotations of the abdomen, perineum, or leg, and physical exposure limitations of abdominal or vaginal approaches are assessed.

The pelvic examination and diagnostic steps used to confirm the presence of a VVF are accomplished in three organized steps: (1) confirmation that the water discharge from the vagina is in fact urine; (2) ensuring the urine discharge from the vagina is not due to incontinence via the urethra but in fact results from an abnormal communication between the lower urinary tract and the vagina; and (3) determining the exact location of fistula formation between the lower urinary tract and the vagina.

Confirmation that a continuous watery vaginal discharge is urine may be accomplished by collecting a sample for laboratory measurement of creatinine. The creatinine content of urine is several factors higher than that of serum, lymphatic fluid, fallopian tube discharge, or excessive vaginal exudate. Physical examination with the aid of a speculum usually will identify the inappropriate source of urinary leakage into the vagina. Water-soluble dyes mixed with sterile saline may be instilled into the bladder via a urethral catheter for visualization of inappropriate leakage into the vagina.

4. What special studies should be considered in the evaluation of a VVF?

Cystoscopy, vaginoscopy, and upper tract evaluation should be performed in all patients with a lower urinary tract fistula. Cystoscopic evaluation assesses the following: (1) the relationship between the ureteral orifices and the fistula tract; (2) the size and number of the fistula tract(s); (3) the functional or maximum bladder capacity; and (4) any concomitant bladder pathology such as foreign bodies (suture) or tumors. At the time of cystoscopy, retrograde pyelograms may be performed to evaluate the presence of ureteral involvement with the urogenital injury. Vaginoscopy is an excellent aid to the manual pelvic examination in assessing vaginal wall inflammation and induration. Not only may the quality of vascularity and pliability of the tissue be assessed, but the quantity of vaginal wall in relation to rotational flaps and previous incisions is noted in order to plan tension-free closures and preserve sexual function. A biopsy of the fistula site is essential in the evaluation of the patient with a history of pelvic malignancies.

5. What conservative management options should be considered?

Urinary incontinence from fistula formation represents a major problem for the patient awaiting resolution of continual wetness, undesirable odors, vaginal and bladder infections, and discomfort. In addition to the potential therapeutic benefit of using an indwelling bladder catheter after early detection of a small, uncomplicated VVF, the prolonged use of a bladder catheter to alleviate or dramatically reduce urinary leakage may be warranted for hygienic and psychosocial reasons in a patient awaiting formal surgical repair.

Estrogen replacement therapy should be strongly considered as an adjuvant treatment in the healing of the vagina for postmenopausal or surgically induced menopausal women. Hyperbaric oxygen therapy also has been advocated as an adjuvant treatment to improve healing of VVFs due to radiation-induced ischemic inflammation. The use of adjuvant corticosteroids has been advocated, but concern over the diminished healing capacity associated with steroids and the excellent results obtained without their use in contemporary reports obviate this form of therapy.

For the treatment of small VVFs uncomplicated by ischemia, irradiation, malignancy, and in-flammation, conservative measures at prolonged bladder drainage, fibrinogen occlusion, or addi-tional adjuvant attempts of de-epithelialization of the fistula using silver nitrate, electrocautery, or curettage by metal screws have been proposed. Before epithelialization of the tract has occurred, uninterrupted bladder drainage alone with antibiotic use to maintain a sterile urine may result in successful closure in 10% of patients with an early detected, small, uncomplicated fistula follow-ing hysterectomy.

6. What are the perioperative considerations for a surgical repair?

Surgical principles: Both vaginal and abdominal approaches offer an excellent opportunity for successful outcome of VVF repairs if general surgical tenets are observed. Irrespective of the approach, a successful outcome depends upon the tension-free approximation of tissue that is free of inflammation and well vascularized.

Timing: When conservative measures fail, formal surgical repair is necessary and requires consideration of many individual patient variables and specific reconstructive principles in order to achieve a successful outcome. When VVFs are the result of obstetric injury, the traditional 3–6 months of a delayed approach for repair is warranted in view of the associated ischemic and in-flammatory responses associated with such fistulas. Because of radiation-induced obliterative en-darteritis that reduces tissue vascularity, a waiting period of 12 months is recommended before sur-gical repair of a fistula that develops after radiation therapy is attempted. For uncomplicated VVFs that are generally caused by iatrogenic injury, reports of early (2–3 weeks after time of injury) re-pairs based on the endoscopic resolution of inflammation have shown similar success to the out-comes of empirically delayed (3–6 months after time of injury) repairs. A complicated VVF should be considered for delayed repair in order to maximize the preoperative condition of the patient, as well as tissue construction. Pursuing early repairs of uncomplicated VVFs offers the opportunity to lessen the psychological and medicolegal impact associated with the social inconvenience and morbidity of managing the unexpected nature of a urinary tract fistula. Generally, most fistulas can and should be surgically repaired as soon as they are identified and confirmed.

Surgical approach: The majority of fistulae are amenable to repair via a minimally invasive transvaginal approach, which allows a quicker recovery, less morbidity, and better patient accep-tance over the traditional use of a formal laparotomy and transvesical repair. The reported rates of success (82–100%) for transvaginal repairs are comparable to those for the transabdominal ap-proach. Therefore, the merits of a minimally invasive procedure combined with the versatility for pelvic floor reconstruction and success of reported outcomes makes the transvaginal approach the procedure of choice for most VVF repairs.

An abdominal approach is generally reserved for a minority of women with complicated (mul-tiple) or complex (involvement of more than two organs) fistula repairs; the need to address other pelvic pathology, such as the need for ureteral reimplantation, bladder augmentation, and abdom-inal bladder neck stabilization procedures; or improved surgical access to a high retracted fistula or multiple fistulas in the setting of a narrowed vagina or poor transvaginal exposure due to mus-culoskeletal conditions that preclude proper patient positioning. Although either extraperitoneal or intraperitoneal abdominal approaches may be performed, most surgeons prefer the exposure and versatility of the intraperitoneal approach.

Excision of fistulous tract: Excision of the fistulous tract has been generally recommended in order to assure apposition of fresh tissue at the edges of the defect repair. Disadvantages of per-forming this maneuver on a routine basis include removal of tissue that will aid in the strength of the repair and creating a larger defect that may potentially involve the ureter and complicate a straightforward repair. Furthermore, additional tissue dissection may result in bleeding and its at-tendant destruction of normal tissue, which might be incorporated into the repair. No apparent ad-verse effects on the success of the repair have been seen in cases in which the fistulous tract was not excised.

Interposition of tissue: The interposition of well-vascularized tissue flaps for achieving a re-liable closure is generally reserved for fistulas associated with radiation, obstetric injury, or previously failed surgical repairs. When using the transvaginal approach, the most popular tissue chosen is a pedicled labial fat pad (Martius fat pad flap), which is tunneled to the site of fistula repair. Other choices of interposition tissue flaps with this approach include the medial fibers of the levator ani, the gracilis muscle, a gracilis myocutaneous flap, a peritoneal flap, and gluteal skin flaps. In cases using an abdominal approach, mobilization of the greater omentum may provide the most versatile tissue for constructing an interposition flap. Other choices include the appendix epiploica taken from the sigmoid colon, a rectus abdominis myofascial flap, and the reported use of lyophilized dura mater.

Postoperative care: The choice of postoperative bladder drainage varies according to the type of fistula repaired. For uncomplicated fistula repairs, most surgeons prefer to use some combination of urethral and suprapubic tube drainage to ensure continuous bladder drainage. For complex fistula repairs in which ureteral catheters facilitate the reconstructive repair, these catheters also may be used for temporary urinary diversion in the postoperative period to ensure additional bladder drainage.

Anticholinergics are given to decrease the bladder spasms. Short-term systemic estrogen replacement therapy in postmenopausal or hypoestrogenic patients promotes vaginal wall healing. All forms of vaginal manipulation, such as the use of tampons, vaginal douches, and sexual intercourse, are to be avoided for 2–3 months.

Adjuvant procedures for stress incontinence: The most common cause of incontinence following the repair of a VVF is persistent stress incontinence. In patients without sphincteric compromise, a synchronous colposuspension may be performed via the transabdominal approach for the fistula repair. An organic suburethral sling procedure with or without an interposition flap is a useful technique at the time of a transvaginal approach for a fistula associated with stress incontinence, especially if the fistula repair involves the bladder neck and proximal urethra.

Postoperative complications: Proper intraoperative and postoperative care will avoid many of the early preventable complications (vaginal bleeding and infections, bladder spasms, interpositional flap bleeding or ischemia, and urinary tract infections) specific to VVF repairs. Delayed complications such as dyspareunia due to vaginal stenosis or foreshortening, unrecognized ureteral injury, and recurrent fistula formation may require formal reconstructive procedures.

Urinary diversion: Complex fistula formation due to radiation injury or recurrent pelvic malignancies often may require some form of palliative urinary diversion. Depending on the complexity of associated findings, such as ureteral obstruction or the extent of radiation damage, the choice of urinary diversion has an important physiologic, psychological, and financial impact on the care of the patient. Recent techniques such as the use of ureteral stents and percutaneous nephrostomy tubes have simplified the surgical procedure of urinary bypass. A wide array of formal reconstructive procedures exist for urinary diversion, and the merits of each should be considered for the management of a VVF that is beyond any therapeutic possibility.

BIBLIOGRAPHY

1. Goodwin W, Scardino P: Vesicovaginal and ureterovaginal fistulas: A summary of 25 years of experience. J Urol 123:370–374, 1980.
2. Zimmern PE, Hadley HR, Staskin DR, Raz S: Genitourinary fistulae: Vaginal approach for repair of vesicovaginal fistulae. Urol Clin North Am J 12:361–367, 1985.
3. Wang Y, Hadley HR: The use of rotated vascularized pedicle flaps for complex transvaginal procedures. J Urol 149:509–592, 1993.
4. Rackley RR, Appell RA: Vesicovaginal fistula: Current approach. AUA Update Series 17:162–167, 1998.

45. EXSTROPHY OF THE BLADDER

Jonathan H. Ross, M.D.

1. Define bladder exstrophy.
Bladder exstrophy is a congenital anomaly in which the bladder is exposed and everted on the lower abdominal wall.

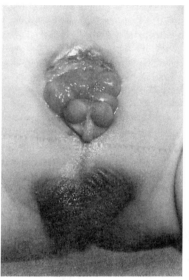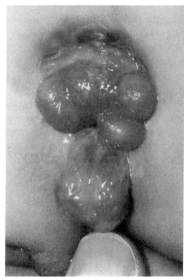

A newborn with bladder exstrophy.

2. Is it common?
No. It occurs in approximately 1 in 35,000 live births. It is three to four times more common in boys than in girls.

3. What causes it?
It is probably caused by a failure of the cloacal membrane to retract. The cloacal membrane covers the mid-lower abdomen in the first weeks of gestation. In the fourth week of gestation, the membrane retracts caudally, allowing the medial migration of the mesoderm on the lateral borders of the membrane to produce the abdominal wall and roll the bladder into a spherical structure. If the membrane persists inappropriately, then this portion of the abdominal wall fails to develop, and when the cloacal membrane ruptures, the bladder is left exposed and everted.

4. What are the usual associated anomalies?
Vesicoureteral reflux is present in most patients. Inguinal hernias are common, particularly in boys. Epispadias (both male and female) and a widely separated pubic symphysis are always present.

5. Are upper urinary tract changes common at birth in patients with bladder exstrophy?
No. But anomalies such as horseshoe kidney and dysplasia have been described. Therefore, newborns should undergo a renal ultrasound.

6. What problems does the exposed bladder mucosa present?

Actually, very few. The main concern is protecting the mucosa from injury and preventing mucosal edema, which will make bladder closure more difficult. To that end, the mucosa is covered with a piece of Silastic or plastic wrap, and care is taken to prevent irritation from diapers and the umbilical cord clamp.

7. List the three operations that most boys with bladder exstrophy undergo.

1. **Primary bladder closure** is usually accomplished in the first days of life. The bladder is closed, but no attempt is made to tighten the bladder neck. Thus, the infants are totally incontinent following the procedure. Iliac osteotomies are performed in most patients at the same time so that the pubic rami can be brought together in the midline, allowing for a more secure bladder closure.

2. **Epispadias repair** is usually performed at 6–18 months of age. It is hoped that the added passive resistance created contributes to increasing bladder size, which facilitates the third operation.

3. **Bladder neck reconstruction.** Bilateral ureteral reimplantation is performed simultaneously to correct vesicoureteral reflux and to move the ureteral orifices away from the caudal portion of the bladder, which is tubularized in reconstructing the bladder neck.

Some centers have recently adopted an approach of total surgical reconstruction at birth, which involves extensive mobilization of the entire bladder, bladder neck, and urethra as an intact unit. The entire lower urinary tract is then tubularized and the bladder and bladder neck are dropped deep into the pelvis to their normal anatomic location. In this way, the bladder closure and epispadias are corrected immediately. Early results suggest that some of these patients will be continent without any further surgery.

8. How successful is the traditional staged approach?

Approximately 70% of patients gain an acceptable level of continence (a dry interval of at least 3.5–4 hr).

9. If patients remain incontinent, what other procedures are available?

The most common reason for failure is a persistently small bladder, which can be corrected with a **bladder augmentation**. Indeed, if the bladder is < 70–80 ml at the time of bladder neck reconstruction, a preemptive augmentation is considered. If persistent incontinence is due to low outflow resistance, then **collagen injection**, a **bladder neck revision**, or placement of an **artificial sphincter** may be undertaken. An ultimate solution, which a minority of patients require, is a **continent urinary diversion**.

10. Name two obstetric/gynecologic complications that occur in women with a history of bladder exstrophy.

Uterine prolapse and fetal malpresentation.

11. What happens if newborns with exstrophy are not operated on?

Actually, they may live long and healthy lives, but intervention is always undertaken. The continuous incontinence is intolerable, and they are at risk for adenocarcinoma in the chronically exposed bladder mucosa. Irritation of mucosa at the ureteral orifices also may lead to hydroureteronephrosis.

12. What is cloacal exstrophy?

Cloacal exstrophy is a rare, complex disorder occurring in 1 in 200,000 live births. It results from premature rupture of the cloacal membrane before separation of the cloaca into an anterior and a posterior portion. This results in two halves of an exstrophied bladder separated by an exstrophied ileocecal segment.

BIBLIOGRAPHY

1. Adams MD, Retik AB: Exstrophy of the bladder. In Resnick MI, Kursh ED (eds): Current Therapy in Genitourinary Surgery. St. Louis, Mosby, 1992, pp 272–275.
2. Canning DA, Koo HP, Duckett JW: Anomalies of the bladder and cloaca. In Gillenwater JY, Grayhack JT, Howards SS, Duckett JW (eds): Adult and Pediatric Urology, 3rd ed. St. Louis, Mosby, 1996, pp 2445–2488.
3. Connor JP, Lattimer JK, Hensle TW, Burbige KA: Primary closure of bladder exstrophy: Long-term functional results in 137 patients. J Pediatr Surg 23:1102–1106, 1988.
4. Gearhart, JP, Canning DA, Peppas DS, Jeffs RD: Techniques to create continence in the failed bladder exstrophy closure patient. J Urol 150:441–443, 1993.
5. Gearhart JP, Jeffs RD: Augmentation cystoplasty in the failed exstrophy reconstruction. J Urol 139:790–793, 1988.
6. Gearhart JP, Jeffs RD: Bladder exstrophy: Increase in capacity following epispadias repair. J Urol 142:525–526, 1989.
7. Gearhart JP, Jeffs RD: State-of-the-art reconstructive surgery for bladder exstrophy at the Johns Hopkins Hospital. Am J Dis Child 143:1475–1478, 1989.
8. Gearhart JP, Mathews R, Taylor S, Jeffs RD: Combined bladder closure and epispadias repair in the reconstruction of bladder exstrophy. J Urol 160:1182–1185, 1998.
9. Lepor H, Jeffs RD: Primary bladder closure and bladder neck reconstruction in classical bladder exstrophy. J Urol 130:1142–1145, 1983.

46. ACQUIRED URETHRAL STRICTURE

Kenneth W. Angermeier, M.D.

1. What is a urethral stricture?

Aurethral stricture is a scar that results from tissue injury. As the scar heals, circumferential contraction may result in narrowing of the urethral lumen.

2. Describe the anatomic divisions of the urethra.

1. **Glanular urethra**—the portion surrounded by the erectile tissue of the glans penis.

2. **Pendulous or penile urethra**—the segment extending from the corona of the glans penis to the distal fusion of the ischiocavernosus muscles.

3. **Bulbous urethra**—the portion covered by the fusion of the ischiocavernosus muscles, extending proximally to the level of the perineal membrane.

4. **Membranous urethra**—the section of the urethra surrounded by the striated urethral sphincter. Embryologically, the membranous urethra extends from the perineal membrane to the verumontanum.

5. **Prostatic urethra**—the portion proximal to the verumontanum and surrounded by the prostate gland.

The prostatic and membranous portions of the urethra are often termed the *posterior urethra*, whereas the combined bulbous, pendulous, and glanular portions are often termed the *anterior urethra*.

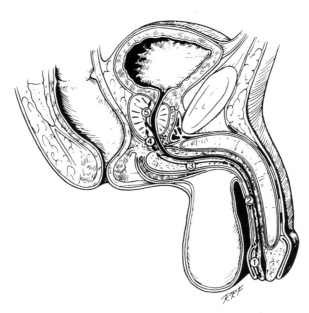

Sagittal section of the penis and perineum demonstrates the divisions of the urethra as enumerated in the text. (From Devine CJ Jr, Angermeier KW: Anatomy of the penis and male perineum. Part 1. American Urological Association Update Series. Vol. 13, Lesson 2, 1994, with permission).

3. Where is the corpus spongiosum in relation to the urethra?

The corpus spongiosum, which consists of erectile tissue, lies in the ventral groove between the two corpora cavernosa. It completely surrounds the anterior urethra throughout its course. The corpus spongiosum expands distally to form a broad cap of tissue, called the glans penis, that encompasses the glanular urethra and proximally to form the bulb of the penis. Within the bulb, the urethra lies closer to the dorsal than the ventral aspect of the corpus spongiosum and exits the dorsal surface of the bulb before its attachment to the perineal body.

4. What are the most common causes of urethral stricture?

In the past, inflammatory urethritis, such as that caused by gonococcal infection, was the leading cause of urethral stricture disease. With the development of modern antibiotic therapy, this is no longer the case. Currently, urethral strictures result most commonly from urethral trauma or instrumentation.

5. How do patients with urethral stricture usually present?

As the urethral lumen gradually narrows, the onset of obstructive voiding symptoms is often insidious. Symptoms may include decreased urinary stream, prolonged voiding time, and hesitancy and/or straining to void. Some patients present with prostatitis or epididymitis, which may be recurrent.

6. What is spongiofibrosis?

Spongiofibrosis is fibrosis or scarring within the corpus spongiosum adjacent to a urethral stricture. It is important to assess the depth of spongiofibrosis, which helps to delineate the severity of stricture disease and affects the success of subsequent treatment modalities.

7. Describe the evaluation of a patient suspected of having urethral stricture.

A retrograde urethrogram is performed, using contrast suitable for intravenous administration. If enough contrast has entered the bladder, the patient is asked to void, and a voiding urethrogram is also obtained. These studies provide information about the location, length, and caliber of stricture disease. Urethroscopy confirms the findings on urethrography and visually assesses the urethral mucosa and associated scarring. Palpation of the urethra also may reveal evidence of spongiofibrosis or periurethral scarring. With experience, one can estimate reliably the depth of spongiofibrosis on the basis of the above information.

8. What is the role of ultrasound in the evaluation of urethral stricture?

Several reports describe the use of ultrasound in the evaluation of patients with urethral stricture, suggesting improved assessment of the depth of spongiofibrosis. In clinical practice, however, it has been the author's impression that the evaluation described in question 7 is sufficient in the majority of cases.

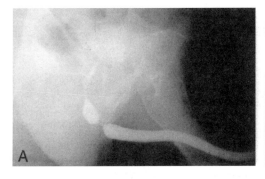

Retrograde urethrogram demonstrating a short, narrow stricture of the mid to proximal bulbous urethra following a straddle injury.

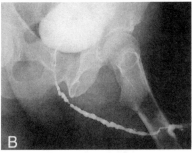

Panurethral stricture disease.

9. Describe the "reconstructive ladder" approach to the treatment of urethral strictures.

The reconstructive ladder approach is based on the concept of beginning with the simplest procedure available and progressing to more complex procedures as initial efforts fail. Management of urethral stricture is initiated with urethral dilation, followed by internal urethrotomy and then by open urethral reconstruction, as necessary. With progress in modern techniques of tissue transfer, this protocol has become outdated. More recently, an anatomic approach has been adopted, which matches a particular treatment modality to the individual patient on the basis of anatomy of the stricture and likelihood of success.

10. How is urethral dilation performed?

In general, urethral dilation should be performed by gradually dilating a stricture over a period of several weeks, increasing the caliber of the dilation by 2–4 French until a maximum of 24–26 French is reached. This approach minimizes further urethral trauma due to dilation. In the past, gradual dilation was accomplished by blind passage of a thin filiform catheter through the area of stricture to serve as a guide, with subsequent dilation by the passage of progressively larger "follower" catheters that attach to the filiform. A more recent technique involves manipulation of a soft wire through the stricture under direct vision with a flexible cystoscope, with subsequent passage of a balloon-dilating catheter over the wire. The balloon is then inflated to dilate the urethra. The radial forces exerted by the balloon catheter may lead to less urethral trauma than the shearing forces generated by filiforms and followers.

11. Can urethral dilation be curative?

Urethral dilation is primarily a management modality in patients with urethral stricture. The interval between dilations often may be progressively increased, eventually to every 6–12 months in optimal circumstances. Discontinuing the dilations almost certainly results in recurrence of the stricture. Infrequently, a patient with minimal stricture in the form of a urethral mucosal scar and minimal to no spongiofibrosis may be cured by dilation alone. Dilation is used primarily as a form of management in patients who are not candidates for more aggressive surgical intervention.

12. Where are the incisions made during endoscopic direct-vision internal urethrotomy (DVIU)?

Traditionally, a cold-knife urethrotome has been used to incise longitudinally through the urethral stricture at the 12-o'clock position. For the procedure to be successful, the incision must be made completely through the spongiofibrosis into the underlying healthy corpus spongiosum. Because of the anatomic position of the urethra, little corpus spongiosum is located dorsally within the bulbous portion. For this reason, some authors advocate incisions at the 10- and 2-o'clock (± 6 o'clock) positions for DVIU within the bulbous urethra.

13. Which patients are good candidates for DVIU?

DVIU may be curative in patients with urethral stricture that involves minimal spongiofibrosis. The best results are seen when the following criteria are met: (1) stricture length ≥ 1 cm, (2) location within the bulbous urethra, and (3) no previous urethrotomy. If the initial attempt is unsuccessful and the stricture recurs, the patient should be re-evaluated both radiographically and endoscopically. If the overall situation is somewhat improved, a second DVIU is reasonable. If the stricture is unchanged or worsened, open urethral reconstruction should be considered.

14. What are the indications for open urethral reconstruction?

In patients who are medically fit for surgery, open urethral reconstruction should be considered for stricture disease associated with moderate-to-severe spongiofibrosis or when more conservative measures have failed. The presence of a fistula or other complicating factors also may necessitate this approach. The length of stricture may vary from 1–2 cm to involvement of nearly the entire anterior urethra (panurethral).

15. What is the optimal form of open urethral reconstruction?

Excision of the stricture with a spatulated primary urethral anastomosis is the optimal reconstruction procedure. Unfortunately, this procedure can be applied only to bulbous urethral strictures of < 3 cm because of limitations in mobilizing the corpus spongiosum to allow a tension-free anastomosis.

16. What is the difference between a "graft" and a "flap"?

Grafts are excised from a donor site and transferred to a host bed from which the graft must revascularize. Skin flaps are transferred to a host site with their underlying tissue and blood supply intact.

17. What is substitution urethroplasty?

Substitution urethroplasty is the basis for many urethral reconstructive procedures. A urethrotomy incision is made into the urethral lumen, and is extended through the entire extent of stricture until normal urethra is identified at both ends. The resulting urethrotomy defect must then be filled using a graft or flap. At times, a segment of severe urethral scar is excised with the remaining "strip" of urethra anastomosed along either the dorsal or ventral aspect, and is followed by substitution inlay.

18. What is the most common graft currently used for urethal reconstruction?

A buccal mucosa graft harvested from the inner cheek.

19. In what situations are grafts most effective in urethral reconstruction?

Grafts provide optimal results when used for bulbous urethral strictures with mild to moderate spongiofibrosis. In this location, an excellent host bed can be obtained by closing the corpus spongiosum over the graft. Alternatively, the graft can be tacked to the corpora cavernosa to close a dorsal urethrotomy defect with similar success. If this is not possible, the bulbospongiosus muscle can be tacked to the graft during closure to provide graft-muscle apposition and allow successful graft take.

20. When may a flap be preferred over a graft during urethral reconstruction?

In general, flaps tend to provide better results for strictures involving the penile urethra and when severe or full-thickness spongiofibrosis is present. Genital skin flaps may be used distally in combination with a proximal graft for long strictures. Alternatively, they can be used alone and configured to reconstruct anterior urethral strictures in virtually any location.

21. What are the most common flaps used in urethral reconstruction?

Genital skin islands mobilized on a dartos fascia pedicle have been found to be a reliable way to fill a urethrotomy defect. Locations of usable penile skin islands include: (1) ventral longitudinal, (2) distal ventral transverse, (3) distal dorsal transverse, and (4) distal circumferential. If penile skin is unavailable, a potential alternative is a scrotal island flap, as some men have an area of truly hairless skin near the inferior midline of the scrotum. Scrotal island flaps are mobilized on a lateral dartos fascia pedicle and are limited to use in the bulbous urethra.

22. What is the surgical approach to the bulbous urethra?

Surgery in this region is accomplished through a perineal incision with the patient in the exaggerated lithotomy position.

23. Are staged procedures ever necessary for urethral reconstruction?

Yes. Although most urethral reconstructive procedures can be performed in one stage, a staged approach is necessary in certain cases, including urethral stricture with severe spongiofibrosis associated with fistula or abscess formation or lack of sufficient well-vascularized local skin for one-stage flap reconstruction.

24. Describe the management of a membranous urethral stricture after transurethral resection of the prostate (TURP).

Development of a membranous urethral stricture after TURP is not uncommon. In this difficult situation, the bladder neck has been resected, and the patient therefore relies solely on the distal urethral sphincter mechanism for continence. DVIU or open reconstruction in this instance carries a high risk of postoperative urinary incontinence, because the striated urethral sphincter encompasses the membranous urethra and may be compromised. Therefore, urethral dilation is the preferred form of management.

BIBLIOGRAPHY

1. Angermeier KW, Devine CJ Jr: Anatomy of the penis and male perineum. Part 2. American Urological Association Update Series. Vol. 13, Lesson 3, 1994.
2. Angermeier KW, Jordan GH, Schlossberg SM: Complex urethral reconstruction. Urol Clin North Am 21:567, 1994.
3. Barbagli G, Palminteri E, Rizzo M: Dorsal onlay graft urethroplasty using penile skin or buccal mucosa in adult bulbourethral strictures. J Urol 160:1307, 1998.
4. Devine CJ Jr, Angermeier KW: Anatomy of the penis and male perineum. Part 1. American Urological Association Update Series. Vol. 13, Lesson 2, 1994.
5. Jordan GH, Schlossberg SM, Devine CJ Jr: Surgery of the penis and urethra. In Walsh PC, Retik AB, Vaughan ED Jr, Wein AJ (eds): Campbell's Urology, 7th ed. Philadelphia, W. B. Saunders, 1998, pp 3341–3369.
6. Jordan GH: Management of anterior urethral stricture disease. Prob Urol 1:199–225, 1987.
7. Jordan GH: Treatment of urethral stricture disease. In Stein BS (ed): Practice of Urology. New York, Norton Medical Books, 1993, pp 1–38.
8. McAnnich JW: Reconstruction of extensive urethral strictures: Circular fasciocutaneous penile flap. J Urol 149:488, 1993.
9. McAninch JW, Laing FC, Jeffrey RB. Sonourethrography in the evaluation of urethral strictures: A preliminary report. J Urol 139:294, 1988.
10. Orandi A: One-stage urethroplasty: Four year followup. J Urol 107:977, 1972.
11. Pansodoro V, Emiliozzi P: Internal urethrotomy in the management of anterior urethral strictures: Long-term follow-up. J Urol 156:73, 1996.
12. Quartey JKM: One-stage penile/preputial cutaneous island flap urethroplasty for urethral stricture: A preliminary report. J Urol 129:284, 1983.
13. Webster GD, Koefoot RB, Sihelnik SA: Urethroplasty management in 200 cases of urethral stricture: A rationale for procedure selection. J Urol 134:892, 1985.
14. Wessells H, McAnnich JW: Use of free grafts in urethral stricture reconstruction. J Urol 155:1912, 1996.

47. POSTERIOR AND ANTERIOR URETHRAL VALVES

Jeffrey S. Palmer, M.D. and Jack S. Elder, M.D.

1. Name the four segments of the male urethra.

1. **Prostatic urethra:** from the bladder neck to the proximal margin of the urogenital diaphragm

2. **Membranous urethra:** traverses the urogenital diaphragm (external or striated sphincter)

3. **Bulbous urethra:** the portion from the distal membranous urethra to the penoscrotal junction

4. **Penile urethra:** the segment traversing the length of the penile shaft, including the glans penis

2. What is the posterior urethra?

The posterior urethra consists of the prostatic urethra and membranous urethra.

3. What is the anterior urethra?

The anterior urethra consists of the bulbous urethra and penile urethra.

4. Define verumontanum.

The verumontanum, located on the dorsal aspect of the prostatic urethra, is a small mound of tissue into which drain the two ejaculatory ducts and the prostatic utricle. It is an important landmark during cystoscopy, as it is just proximal to the external sphincter.

5. What are posterior urethral valves?

Posterior urethral valves are abnormal congenital mucosal folds in the prostatic urethra that look like a thin membrane that impairs bladder drainage.

6. Do girls get posterior urethral valves?

No.

7. What is the incidence of posterior urethral valves?

Approximately 1 in 8000 males.

8. How are posterior urethral valves diagnosed?

Avoiding cystourethrogram (VCUG) must be performed. This involves catheterizing the bladder with a pediatric feeding tube or Foley catheter, infusing contrast material into the bladder under gravity, and observing the bladder fill and empty using fluoroscopic monitoring. The posterior urethra is examined very carefully throughout the procedure. More recently, there have been a few reports of perineal ultrasound diagnosis of posterior urethral valves by demonstrating a dilated prostatic urethra in conjunction with bladder wall hypertrophy.

9. What are the radiographic signs of posterior urethral valves?

A VCUG shows a distended prostatic urethra, the valve leaflets, detrusor (bladder) hypertrophy, possibly with cellules and/or diverticula, bladder neck hypertrophy, and a narrow stream in the penile urethra. In addition, there may be incomplete emptying of the bladder.

10. What other studies should be performed?

Usually, a renal ultrasound shows bilateral hydronephrosis. Another upper tract study such as a renal scan (MAG-3, DTPA, or DMSA) should be performed to ascertain how well the kidneys are functioning.

11. Discuss the three types of congenital posterior urethral valve (PUV).

Hugh Young described three distinct types of congenital PUV. A type I urethral valve is an obstructing membrane that extends distally from each side of the verumontanum toward the membranous urethra where they fuse anteriorly. This type accounts for 90–95% of all cases. Type II valves were described as folds extending cephalad from the verumontanum to the bladder neck. Recently, it has become apparent that type II valves do not exist. A type III valve represents a diaphragm or ring-like membrane with a central aperture just distal to the verumontanum.

There is evidence that types I and III valves represent the same condition. Antegrade cystography (injecting contrast material into the bladder through a small catheter rather than through the urethra) in babies with suspected posterior urethral valves demonstrated the classic radiologic features. Subsequently, during cystoscopy, all of the patients seemed to have a type III valve, but after the cystoscope was inserted, the appearance of the valve changed to a classic type I appearance. Therefore, urethral catheterization seems to disrupt the urethral valve in the vast majority of patients. The subsequent appearance is that of a type I posterior urethral valve.

12. What proportion of boys with urethral valves have vesicoureteral reflux?

Approximately 50% have reflux (half are unilateral and half are bilateral).

13. What are the long-term consequences of posterior urethral valves?

Posterior urethral valves are the most common obstructive cause of end-stage renal disease, and approximately one-third of surviving males develop renal insufficiency or chronic renal failure.

14. How do infants with posterior urethral valves present?

Often the condition is discovered prenatally with the findings of bilateral hydronephrosis and a distended bladder. In a newborn, a palpable abdominal mass (distended bladder, hydronephrotic kidney), ascites, or respiratory distress from pulmonary hypoplasia may be present. Many children with valves present with a febrile urinary tract infection. These infants may have urosepsis, dehydration, uremia, and electrolyte abnormalities. At times, a pneumothorax occurs in these newborns. Often the bladder feels like a small walnut in the suprapubic area. Usually, the urinary stream is poor. Older boys whose obstruction is less severe may have daytime incontinence as the only symptom.

15. In a boy who is found to have posterior urethral valves, what is the appropriate initial management?

Initially, the bladder should be drained with a urethral catheter, ideally a 5 French or 8 French (F) pediatric feeding tube. A Foley balloon catheter should not be used, because it may not drain satisfactorily owing to the balloon's tendency to occlude the ureteral orifices or cause bladder spasm, which can result in secondary distal ureteral obstruction. Broad-spectrum antibiotics are given intravenously to minimize the chance of nosocomial bacterial urinary tract infection. The serum creatinine is measured, and electrolyte abnormalities, including acidosis and hyperkalemia, need to be managed before surgical treatment of the lesion is undertaken. The kidneys should be assessed at minimum with a renal ultrasound.

16. What is the treatment of posterior urethral valves?

The simplest treatment is transurethral valve ablation. If the urethra is sufficient in size, then a small pediatric resectoscope may be used for valve ablation under direct vision. The procedure is performed by incising the valves at the 5- and 7-o'clock positions. Some resect the valves at the 12-o'clock position also. If the urethra is too small to accommodate the pediatric resectoscope, an alternative is to visualize the valves with an 8F cystoscope and ablate the posterior urethral valves under direct vision with a Bugbee electrode passed adjacent to the cystoscope.

If the urethra is too small to accommodate the small cystoscope and Bugbee electrode, then a small insulated crochet hook ("Whitaker hook") may be used. The technique is to pass the hook into the urethra and engage the valve leaflets at the 5- and 7-o'clock positions. The entire instrument, except for the crotch of the hook, is insulated, protecting the urethra from thermal injury. This procedure can be performed while the neonate is awake in the fluoroscopy suite or under anesthesia. This technique is applicable primarily in babies born prematurely or who are small for gestational age, in whom the larger resectoscope is too big for the urethra. Other techniques for valve ablation include a valve rupture using a small Fogarty catheter. In addition, antegrade valve ablation may be performed through a suprapubic cystostomy tract or through a cutaneous vesicostomy.

If the serum creatinine remains significantly elevated despite catheter drainage, then temporary cutaneous vesicostomy is recommended. In this procedure, the dome of the bladder is brought to a point midway between the umbilicus and the pubic symphysis to allow continuous urinary drainage. An alternative is bilateral cutaneous pyelostomies, in which the renal pelvis is exteriorized. This technique provides excellent upper tract drainage. An advantage to this approach is that it allows the surgeon to biopsy the kidneys.

17. What is the role of fetal surgery in the treatment of posterior urethral valves?

Fetal intervention carries a high risk to the fetus with a mortality rate of 43%. Long-term studies indicate that intervention may not be a predictor of possible urinary diversion, nor may it change the prognosis of renal function.

18. Describe the most common complications of valve ablation.

The most common complication of valve ablation through a cystoscope is urethral stricture, which results if the resectoscope or cystoscope is too large for the urethra. Another complication is incomplete valve resection. One may think that injury to the external urinary sphincter also is common, but actually it is quite rare.

19. What are favorable prognostic factors following treatment for posterior urethral valves?

Favorable prognostic factors include the serum creatinine falling below 1.0 mg/dl one month following treatment, absence of vesicoureteral reflux on the VCUG, preservation of the corticomedullary junction of the kidneys by ultrasonography, or evidence of a radiographic "pop-off valve."

20. What is a "pop-off valve"? What are the three types that can occur in boys with urethral valves?

The term *pop-off valve* refers to a mechanism in which the high intravesical or intrapelvic pressure is dissipated, allowing for normal development of one or both kidneys. Examples include (1) urinary ascites, in which urine leaks from the fornices of the kidneys or from a bladder rupture; (2) "VURD" syndrome, in which massive unilateral reflux into a nonfunctioning kidney occurs; and (3) the presence of a large bladder diverticulum, causing aberrant micturition into the diverticulum and taking pressure off the developing kidneys.

21. How is urinary ascites treated?

In patients with urinary ascites secondary to posterior urethral valves, the leakage may be coming from one or both kidneys. At times, however, it may be secondary to a ruptured bladder. In most cases, a temporary cutaneous vesicostomy is necessary to allow decompression. In some neonates, paracentesis (removal of the ascitic fluid) must be done, and occasionally, renal exploration and high urinary diversion must be performed.

22. What proportion of patients with posterior urethral valves have a protective radiographic feature (pop-off valve)?

Approximately 20%.

23. What is VURD syndrome?

Approximately 15% of patients have this condition, in which there is massive reflux into a dysplastic nonfunctioning kidney. VURD stands for vesicoureteral reflux associated with renal dysplasia. The term applies only to children with posterior urethral valves.

24. List the adverse prognostic factors in children with posterior urethral valves.
- Presentation under 1 year of age
- Failure of the serum creatinine to be below 1.0 mg/dl 1 month following initial therapy
- Bilateral vesicoureteral reflux
- Diurnal incontinence beyond 5 years of age
- Prenatal diagnosis in the second trimester

25. What is the overall prognosis for boys with urethral valves?

Approximately 35% have poor renal function; 10% die of renal failure, 20% have end-stage renal disease; and 5% have chronic renal failure that probably will require dialysis.

26. In a neonate with severe posterior urethral valves, what is the likely cause of death?

Pulmonary hypoplasia. Lung development is dependent on a normal volume of amniotic fluid. In the first trimester, amniotic fluid is a transudate from the placenta. During the second and third trimesters, however, the amniotic fluid comes from urine voided by the fetus. In the presence of severe obstructive uropathy, urine output is significantly reduced and pulmonary development is significantly impaired, resulting in pulmonary hypoplasia, i.e., underdeveloped lungs.

27. Does prenatal decompression of the urinary tract improve survival in a fetus with posterior urethral valves?

To date, there have only been a few reports of survival following in utero bladder decompression for posterior urethral valves. Usually, the procedure is performed by inserting a small shunt between the bladder and amniotic space, bypassing the urethral obstruction. The procedure is performed by the perinatologist (obstetrician) using ultrasound monitoring. A few centers have performed cutaneous vesicostomy in utero.

One of the main problems with inserting a vesicoamniotic shunt is making the correct diagnosis of obstructive uropathy in utero, because prune belly syndrome and high-grade vesicoureteral reflux have an appearance similar to that of urethral valves on prenatal ultrasonography. The technique is indicated primarily to prevent pulmonary hypoplasia. If normal amniotic fluid is present, then the baby is not at significant risk for respiratory complications. Consequently, therapy is directed primarily at those with oligohydramnios. If oligohydramnios is detected around 20 weeks' gestation, nearly always irreversible renal dysplasia has occurred, so that even if a technically successful vesicoamniotic shunt is inserted, renal development usually is not improved.

28. What is the "full-valve bladder" syndrome?

In boys born with posterior urethral valves, bladder development is abnormal because of the severe congenital bladder outlet obstruction. In addition, often a urinary concentrating defect results in high urine output. Possible defects in bladder function include (1) reduced bladder compliance: As the bladder fills with urine, the intravesical pressure increases quickly, and this elevated pressure is transmitted to the kidneys, resulting in continued deterioration in renal function; (2) uninhibited bladder contractions, often associated with a nonrelaxing external sphincter (detrusor-sphincter dyssynergia); (3) persistent secondary bladder neck hypertrophy, causing impaired bladder drainage; and (4) myogenic failure with absent bladder contractions. The full-valve bladder syndrome refers to the persistent filling of the bladder secondary to one of these factors, resulting in transmission of elevated intravesical pressures to the kidneys and thereby causing reduction in renal function.

29. At what intravesical pressure is there impaired upper urinary tract drainage?
35 cm of water pressure.

30. What is the treatment for patients with the full-valve bladder syndrome?
Treatment often includes double-voiding, clean intermittent catheterization to allow more effective emptying of the bladder, and anticholinergic medication.

31. In boys with posterior urethral valves, does ureterovesical junction occur?
Some boys with posterior urethral valves develop secondary ureterovesical obstruction, in which there is impaired ureteral drainage into the bladder during bladder filling because the intravesical pressure is higher than in the ureter, but when the bladder is empty, there is normal drainage of urine.

32. When is bladder augmentation recommended in children with posterior urethral valves?
Augmentation cystoplasty may be necessary if there is a noncompliant bladder, severe detrusor-sphincter dyssynergia, or uninhibited bladder contractions that do not respond to medical therapy.

33. What is the source of tissue for augmentation cystoplasty in boys with valves?
Stomach tissue often is recommended for augmentation cystoplasty in boys with posterior urethral valves because it can reduce the acidosis that results from the valve condition, allowing excretion of the hydrogen ion into the urine. The potential complications can be formidable, however. Another option is ureterocystoplasty, in which a dilated ureter associated with a nonfunctioning kidney is used to enlarge the bladder rather than simply performing a total ureterectomy. Finally, the ileum or large bowel may be used.

34. In boys with posterior urethral valves undergoing renal transplantation, what is the prognosis compared to that of a child with glomerulonephritis?
The graft survival rates are identical, but in a few series, the serum creatinine level at 5 years was significantly higher in the group with posterior ureteral valves, probably because of the associated noncompliant or unstable bladder.

35. What is an anterior urethral valve?
An anterior urethral valve is not a true valve. Rather, it is a wide-mouth anterior urethral diverticulum, with the distal lip of the diverticulum filling during voiding, compressing the distal urethra.

36. Where are anterior urethral valves located?
All occur in the bulbous or pendulous urethra.

37. What are the physical findings of an anterior urethral valve?
A cystic mass on the ventral aspect of the penoscrotal junction increases in size during voiding. Prolonged urinary strain often is noted. Compression of the cystic mass may result in urinary dribbling.

38. How is the diagnosis of anterior urethral valves made?
The diagnosis is based on physical findings and voiding cystourethrogram. These patients also should undergo a renal ultrasound and serum creatinine. If there is renal insufficiency, a renal scan should be obtained.

39. How are anterior urethral valves treated?
The treatment is based on the size of the diverticulum and renal function. If the diverticulum is small, the cusp may be ablated by transurethral resection. However, in some neonates with this

condition, open surgical resection of the diverticulum and valve cusp is necessary. A small Silastic urethral stent should be left in the bladder postoperatively for 10–14 days.

If renal function is significantly impaired, temporary catheter drainage of the bladder may be necessary to stabilize the infant and correct electrolyte abnormalities. If the serum creatinine fails to decrease to a satisfactory level, resection of the diverticulum and perinatal urethrostomy will provide reliable drainage. Alternatively, cutaneous vesicostomy should be considered.

BIBLIOGRAPHY

1. Cuckow PM, Dinneen MD, Risdon RA, et al: Long-term renal function in the posterior urethral valves, unilateral reflux and renal dysplasia syndrome. J Urol 158:1004, 1997.
2. Denes ED, Barthold JS, Gonzalez R: Early prognostic value of serum creatinine levels in children with posterior urethral valves. J Urol 157:1441, 1997.
3. Diamond DA, Ransley PG: Fogarty balloon catheter ablation of neonatal posterior urethral valves. J Urol 137:1209, 1987.
4. Cendron M, Duckett JW: Perinatal urology. In Gillenwater JY, Grayhack JT, Howards SS, Duckett JW (eds): Adult and Pediatric Urology, 3rd ed. St. Louis, Mosby, 1996, pp 2095–2169.
5. Duel BP, Mogbo K, Barthold JS, et al: Prognostic value of initial renal ultrasound in patients with posterior urethral valves. J Urol 160:1198, 1998.
6. Elder JS, Duckett JW, Snyder HM: Intervention for fetal obstructive uropathy: Has it been effective? Lancet 2:1007, 1987.
7. Firlit CG, King LR: Anterior urethral valves in children. J Urol 108:972, 1972.
8. Gonzales ET Jr: Posterior urethral valves and other urethral anomalies. In Walsh PC, Retik AB, Vaughan ED Jr., Wein AJ (eds): Campbell's Urology, 7th ed. Philadelphia, W. B. Saunders, 1998, p 2069.
9. Good CD, Vinnicombe SJ, Minty IL, et al: Posterior urethral valves in male infants and newborns: Detection with US of the urethra before and during voiding. Radiology 198:387, 1996.
10. Holmes N, Harrison MR, Baskin LS: Fetal surgery for posterior urethral valves: Long-term postnatal outcomes. Pediatrics 108:E7, 2001.
11. Hulbert WC, Duckett JW: Prognostic factors in infants with posterior urethral valves. J Urol 135:121A,1986.
12. Hutton KAR, Thomas DFM, Davies BW: Prenatally detected posterior urethral valves: Qaulitative assessment of second trimester scans and prediction of outcome. J Urol 158:1022, 1997.
13. Indudhara R, Joseph DB, Perez LM, et al: Renal transplantation in children with posterior urethral valves revisited: 10-year follow-up. J Urol 160:1201, 1998.
14. Krueger RP, Hardy BD, Churchill BM: Growth in boys with posterior urethral valves. Primary valve resection vs upper tract diversion. Urol Clin North Am 7:265, 1980.
15. Nakayama DK, Harrison MR, de Lorimier AA: Prognosis of posterior urethral valves presenting at birth. J Pediatr Surg 21:43, 1986.
16. Parkhouse HF, Barratt TM, Dillon MJ, et al: Long-term outcome of boys with posterior urethral valves. Br J Urol 62:59, 1988.
17. Rittenberg MH, Hulbert WC, Snyder HM, et al: Protective factors in posterior urethral valves. J Urol 140:993, 1988.
18. Rushton HG, Parrott TS, Woodard JR, et al: The role of vesicostomy in the management of anterior urethral valves in neonates and infants. J Urol 138:107, 1987.
19. Tietjen DN, Gloor JM, Husmann DA: Proximal urinary diversion in the management of posterior urethral valves: Is it necessary? J Urol 158:1008, 1997.
20. Whitaker TH, Sherwood T: An improved hook for destroying posterior urethral valves. J Urol 135:531, 1986.
21. Zaontz MR, Firlit CF: Percutaneous antegrade ablation of posterior urethral valves in infants with small-caliber urethras: An alternative to urinary diversion. J Urol 136:247, 1986.
22. Zaontz MR, Gibbons MD: An antegrade technique for ablation of posterior urethral valves. J Urol 132:982, 1984.

48. URETHRAL DIVERTICULUM IN FEMALES

Sandip P. Vasavada, MD

1. What is the reported incidence of female urethral diverticula?

It is estimated that 0.5 to 5% of the normal female population may have a diverticulum, but clearly, not all present for evaluation or management.

2. A urethral diverticulum is a defect in what anatomic layer?

Periurethral fascia. The leaves of the fascia form the outer portion of the envelope from within the diverticulum develops. Proper surgical repair requires fusion of this fascia to prevent recurrences.

3. What are the causes of urethral diverticula?

1. **Congenital**
2. **Acquired**
   Surgery/trauma
   Infection

If histologic sections contain smooth muscle, a congenital origin is inferred. However, most female diverticula are acquired.

4. Where are diverticula located? How do they form?

The diverticula always occur on the vaginal aspect of the urethra (anterior vaginal wall) on the distal two-thirds of the urethra where the periurethral glands are known to open. Infection and obstruction of the periurethral glands result in the formation of retention cysts, which rupture into the lumen and give rise to a diverticulum. These retention cysts progressively enlarge and entrap droplets of urine during voiding, and due to the lack of muscle in the diverticular sac, the contents remain stagnant and inflammation occurs. The most common offending organisms are gonococci, *Escherichia coli*, and *Chlamydia*.

5. What are the symptoms of a urethral diverticulum?

Symptoms may vary from mild occasional discomfort to severe pain frank urinary retention during acute infections. Most patients, however, present with non-specific irritative symptoms of the lower urinary tract similar to those of cystitis.

Clinical Symptoms and Signs of Urethral Diverticula

Symptoms
Classic 3 D triad (dribbling, dysuria, dyspareunia)
Urinary urgency
Hematuria
Recurrent urinary tract infection
Urinary incontinence
Urinary retention
Signs
None
Suburethral mass
Palpable stone
Expression of purulent material

6. Is a diverticulum always solitary?

No. Diverticula may be small or large, single or multiple, or multiloculated. Additionally, they may be circumferential and go all the way around the urethra, enveloping it.

185

7. Are any disease processes associated with diverticulum formation?

The stasis of urine and infection within the diverticulum provides an ideal condition for stone formation in some patients. In addition, urethral carcinoma may be discovered within the diverticulum.

8. What is the most common cancer found in a diverticulum?

Adenocarcinonoma represents the most common malignancy from within a diverticulum; however, squamous cell cancer and transitional cell cancer may also occur.

9. What signs are found on physical examination?

The classic physical finding is a **palpable suburethral mass** on vaginal examination, occasionally with expression of purulent material from the urethra when the mass is compressed. Often, however, no signs may be present and the diverticulum may go unrecognized on physical examination.

10. How is a urethral diverticulum diagnosed?

A high index of suspicion for the possibility of a urethral diverticulum is perhaps the most important factor in making the diagnosis. One must always consider the possibility of a urethral diverticulum in a female with persistent lower urinary tract symptoms resembling cystitis or with recurrent urinary tract infection. Often, the diagnosis is by exclusion of other common and easily treatable issues.

Confirming the diagnosis usually requires radiographic studies. **Voiding cystourethrography** depends on the filling of the diverticulum with contrast material when the patient is voiding. Filling the urethra with contrast while a balloon blocks the external urethral meatus and another at the bladder neck is called **positive-pressure retrograde urethrography. Magnetic resonance imaging (MRI)** represents the current gold standard for the diagnosis of suspect diverticula and is quite easily performed in most institutions. The study is usually performed using the T2-weighted sequences of the pelvis whereby the diverticulum and its corresponding fluid within it will light up on the MRI the same as the bladder with urine in it.

11. How are urethral diverticula treated?

There is no one operative procedure to correct all cases of urethral diverticula. If the diverticulum is very close to the external meatus, it may be incised through the urethra and vagina in a **marsupialization technique** (Spence procedure). On rare occasions, they may be managed **en-**

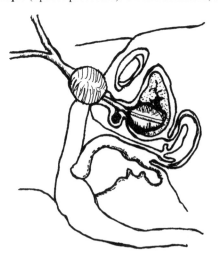

Positive-pressure uretherography allows filling of the diverticulum.

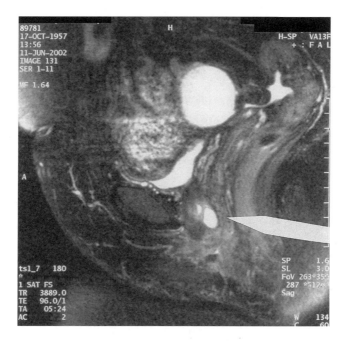

MRI mid-sagittal view of pelvis demonstrating urethral diverticulum. No contrast is given in this case, and the bladder and diverticulum both enhance on the T2-weighted study. Arrow points to diverticulum.

doscopically through a urethroscope using electrocautery to open the meatus of the diverticulum, which will allow it to drain better.

The standard approach is a **complete urethral diverticulectomy.** There are several approaches, but the essential idea is to expose and mobilize the diverticulum through an incision in the vagina and then excise the complete diverticulum. This must be done exposing sequentially each layer of the urethral wall until the diverticulum is exposed. It is then completely excised flush to the catheter. The small opening in the urethra is then closed with fine suture material. Each layer of the periurethral fascia is then reapproximated to avoid any overlapping suture lines and prevent a recurrent diverticulum.

BIBLIOGRAPHY

1. Nezu, FM, Vasavada, SP: Evaluation and management of female urethral diverticulum. Tech Urol 7(2):169–175, 2001
2. Pallapattu G, Vasavada SP, Comiter CV, Raz S: Repair of urethral diverticulum. In: S Raz, (ed): Atlas of the Urologic Clinics of North America—Vaginal Surgery. Williams & Wilkins, Baltimore, 61–70, Vol. 8, No. 1, 4/2000.
3. Appell RA: Urethral diverticulum and fistula. In Glenn JF (ed): Urological Surgery, 4th ed. Philadelphia, JB Lippincott, 1991, p 762.
4. Drutz HP: Urethral diverticula. Obstet Gynecol Clin North Am 16:923–929, 1989.
5. Leach GE, Bavendam TG: Female urethral diverticula. Urology 40:407–415, 1987.
6. Leach GE, Sirls LT, Ganabathi K, Zimmern PE: LNSC3: A proposed classification system for female urethral diverticula. Neurourol Urodyn 12:523–531, 1993.
7. Leng WW, McGuire EJ: Management of female urethral diverticula: A new classification. J Urol 160:1297–1300, 1998
8. Spence HM, Duckett JW: Diverticulum of the female urethra: Clinical aspects and presentation of a single operative technique for care. J Urol 104:432–437, 1970.
9. Spencer WF, Streem SB: Diverticulum of the female urethral roof managed endoscopically. J Urol 138:147–148, 1987.

49. HYPOSPADIAS

Robert Kay, M.D.

1. What is hypospadias?

Hypospadias refers to any condition in which the meatus, or opening of the urethra, occurs on the undersurface of the penis, rather than the tip. When it occurs on the dorsal side of the penis, it is referred to as epispadias.

2. Is hypospadias an inherited disorder?

In some cases, a genetic factor is involved, although most patients do not give a family history. In one series by Bauer, the father of the affected child had hypospadias in 7% of the cases. The brother was affected in 14% of cases of this series. If a child is born with hypospadias, the risk of the next child having hypospadias is 12% if there is no family history. This increases to 19% if another family member, such as a cousin or uncle, has hypospadias, and to 26% if the father and a sibling have hypospadias.

3. Do all children with hypospadias have a hooded foreskin?

Because of the embryologic development of the penis and urethra and the closure of lateral to medial tissues, the foreskin almost always fails to be complete in boys with hypospadias. Rarely, a variant of hypospadias with a large meatus, the megameatal hypospadias, does have an intact foreskin and usually is detected at the time of circumcision.

4. Do all children with a hooded foreskin have hypospadias?

No. Some children are born with a normal meatus, yet have a hooded foreskin. The penis should be carefully examined to exclude other penile abnormalities, such as chordee or atretic urethra. Hooded foreskin also may be seen in otherwise normal states and carries no significance other than a cosmetic factor.

5. What is the more common site for hypospadias, the penoscrotal junction or the distal portion of the penis?

The most common form of hypospadias is distal hypospadias. This is the most mild form of

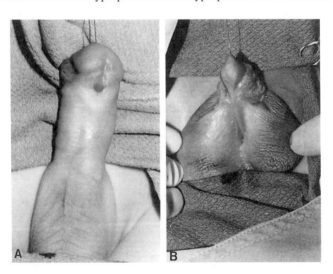

A. Distal hypospadias. **B.** Severe proximal hypospadias in the midscrotal area.

the disease and occurs in the subcoronal or glandular area in approximately 80–85% of all cases. Ten to fifteen percent of cases occur in the penile shaft, with only 5–10% occurring in the severe location of the penoscrotal or perineal location.

6. How often does hypospadias occur?
Recent studies indicate that the incidence of hypospadias is increasing. The incidence of hypospadias ranges from 5.2–8.2/1000 male births or approximately 1/200 male births.

7. Do boys with hypospadias need urologic evaluation to detect other anomalies?
Only boys with severe hypospadias and sexual ambiguity, which includes testicular abnormalities (e.g., undescended testis), need to be evaluated. Up to 25% of these patients have enlarged utricles or other female structures.

Routine evaluation of other forms of hypospadias is not needed because the incidence of abnormalities approximates the incidence in the general population.

8. What is the optimal age for hypospadias repair?
Emotional issues for both the child and family must be considered when determining the best age for surgical repair. When the factors of genital awareness, separation anxiety, ease of postoperative management, and technical aspects are considered, the ideal age is between 6 and 15 months.

9. How does one repair a severe hypospadias on a small penis?
Testosterone can be used in selective cases to induce growth of the penis. In complex cases, such as a small penis when early repair is desired, parenteral testosterone may be used preoperatively. Also, optical magnification is critical in the surgical repair of these cases.

10. Does the child need to be hospitalized for hypospadias repair?
The overwhelming majority of cases can be done on an outpatient basis. The medical advantage is the avoidance of communicable diseases, such as viral infections that are prevalent in the hospital. Cost savings are also dramatic as an outpatient. However, some of the major advantages are the emotional aspects of the surgery to both the child and family. The child prefers his own environment, the parents' lives are less disrupted, and other siblings are relieved. Postoperative care has become significantly easier with outpatient hypospadias surgery.

11. What is a hypospadias cripple?
A hypospadias cripple is an older term used for the male child or adult who has had numerous operations in attempts to repair the hypospadias defect. Once very common, this problem has been significantly reduced with technical advances and better understanding of hypospadias.

12. If hypospadias repair has been done several times with no success, what else can be done?
The failed hypospadias repair is a surgical challenge complicated by the presence of severe scar tissue and the lack of skin. (Material deleted—Often, skin must be imported to construct the urethra.) Although free skin grafts have been used in the past, other tissues such as buccal mucosa are preferred today, which give better results in both the short and long term. Exciting potential tissues include small intestine submucosa and tissue engineered urothelium.

13. List the most important factors for technical success of hypospadias surgery.
1. Use of vascularized tissues
2. Careful tissue handling
3. Tension-free anastomosis
4. Nonoverlapping suture lines
5. Meticulous hemostasis

6. Fine suture material
7. Adequate urinary diversion

14. What complications occur from hypospadias surgery?

Complications from any reconstructive surgery may occur and hypospadias is no exception. Complications may include urethrocutaneous fistulas, urethral strictures, meatal stenosis, urethral diverticulum, excess skin, persistent chordee, and persistent hypospadias.

15. Is urinary diversion required during hypospadias repair?

In most cases, urinary diversion is a preferred tool of management because it allows tissue healing and minimizes the risk of urethral cutaneous fistulas. Although some have advocated no diversions for distal repairs, urinary diversion offers advantages and, theoretically, fewer complications, particularly in complex repairs.

The use of an indwelling urethral stent has replaced a suprapubic cystotomy tube, even in severe cases. Although suprapubic diversion may have a limited role, urethral diversion is effective, serves as a stent, results in fewer bladder spasms, and is easier to manage than suprapubic tubes.

16. What is the best operation for hypospadias?

No single best operation for hypospadias repair exists. Over 150 operations have been described. Today, the most common operation for distal hypospadias includes tubularization of the incised urethral plate (Snodgrass), meatal advancement (MAGPI), and meatal-based flaps (Mathieu). Most proximal hypospadias repairs include tubularization of the incised plate (Snodgrass), onlay grafts, vascularized inner preputial transfer flaps (Duckett), free grafts (skin, buccal mucosa), or other variations of the above-mentioned repairs.

BIBLIOGRAPHY

1. Bauer SB, Retick AB, Colodny AH: Genetic aspects of hypospadias. Urol Clin North Am 8:559, 1981.
2. Belman AB: Hypospadias and other urethral abnormalities. In Kelalis PP, King LR, Belman AB (eds): Clinical Pediatric Urology, 3rd ed. Philadelphia, W. B. Saunders, 1992.
3. Belman AB, Kass EJ: Hypospadias repair in children under one year of age. J Urol 128:1273, 1982.
4. Duckett JW: MAGPI (meatoplasty and glanuloplasty): A procedure for subcoronal hypospadias. Urol Clin North Am 8:515, 1981.
5. Duckett JW: The island flap technique for hypospadias repair. Urol Clin North Am 8:503, 1981.
6. Duckett JW, Coplen D, Ewalt D, Baskin LS: Buccal mucosal urethral replacement. J Urol 153:1660–1663, 1995.
7. Hatch DA, Maizels M, Zaontz MR, et al: Hypospadias hidden by a complete prepuce. Surg Gynecol Obstet 169:233, 1989.
8. Kass EJ, Boling D: Single stage hypospadias reconstruction without fistula. J Urol 144:520, 1990.
9. Manley CB, Epstein ES: Early hypospadias repair. J Urol 125:698, 1981.
10. Paulozzi LJ, Erickson JD, Jackson RJ: Hypospadias trends in two U.S. surveillance systems. Pediatrics 100:831–834, 1997.
11. Rabinowitz R: Outpatient catheterless modified Mattieu hypospadias repair. J Urol 138:1074, 1987.
12. Retik AB, Keating M, Mandell J: Complications of hypospadias repair. Urol Clin North Am 15:223, 1988.
13. Ross JH, Kay R: Use of a de-epithelialized skin flap in hypospadias repairs accomplished by tubularization of the incised urethral plate. Urology 50:110–112, 1997.
14. Rushton HG, Belman AB: The split prepuce in situ onlay hypospadias repair. J Urol 160:1134–1137, 1998.
15. Snodgrass W, Koyle M, Manzoni G, et al: Tubularized incised plate hypospadias repair: Results of a multicenter experience. J Urol 156:839–841, 1996.
16. Sweet RA, Schrott HG, Kurland R, et al: Study of the incidence of hypospadias in Rochester, Minnesota, 1940–1970, and a case-controlled comparison of possible etiologic factors. Mayo Clin Proc 49:52, 1974.

50. EPISPADIAS

Jonathan H. Ross, M.D.

1. What is epispadias?

Epispadias is a penile anomaly in which the urethra opens on the dorsal aspect of the penis. The penis is generally foreshortened owing to separation of the pubic symphysis. Dorsal curvature of the penis and an incomplete foreskin dorsally are also characteristic. The glans generally has a flattened spade-like appearance, and the corporal bodies do not communicate.

2. What is "female epispadias"?

Females with epispadias have a bifid clitoris, patulous urethra, and unformed bladder neck. In addition to genitoplasty, they require bladder neck reconstruction in the same manner as girls with the complete exstrophy–epispadias complex.

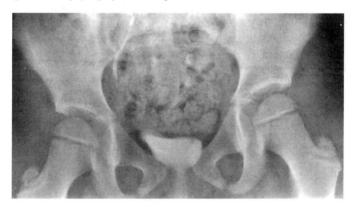

Bladder film of an intravenous urogram in a 6-year-old girl with epispadias demonstrates the typical findings of a small bladder, open bladder neck, and separation of the pubic symphysis.

3. Is epispadias closely related to hypospadias embryologically?

No. It is a form of the exstrophy–epispadias complex (see chapter 45). When caudal migration of the cloacal membrane fails, bladder exstrophy (which is always associated with epispadias) results. When partial migration occurs, then epispadias alone occurs. In fact, most patients with epispadias also have bladder exstrophy. The incidence of epispadias alone is approximately 1/100,000 male births, and 1/500,000 female births.

4. What abnormality on KUB examination is universally present in patients with epispadias?

Separation of the public symphysis.

5. Are most patients with epispadias incontinent?

Yes. Nearly all females and approximately 70% of males with epispadias are incontinent. Most males have penopubic epispadias, but those with penile shaft or glanular epispadias are usually continent.

6. Describe the bladder abnormalities found in most epispadias patients.

A small bladder capacity and vesicoureteral reflux (the latter being present in 90% of patients).

7. What are the three principles of epispadias repair?
- Penile lengthening
- Correction of chordee
- Urethroplasty

BIBLIOGRAPHY

1. Arap S, Nahas WC, Giron AM, et al: Incontinent epispadias: Surgical treatment of 38 cases. J Urol 140:577–581, 1988.
2. Borzi PA, Thomas DFM: Cantwell-Ransley epispadias repair in male epispadias and bladder exstrophy. U Urol 151:457–459, 1994.
3. Canning DA, Koo HP, Duckett JW: Anomalies of the bladder and cloaca. In Gillenwater JY, Grayhack JT, Howards SS, Duckett JW (eds): Adult and Pediatric Urology, 3rd ed. St. Louis, Mosby, 1996, pp 2445–2488.
4. Gearhart JP, Peppas DS, Jeffs RD: Complete genitourinary reconstruction in female epispadias. J Urol 149:1110–1113, 1993.
5. Kramer SA, Kelalis PP: Assessment of urinary continence in epispadias: Review of 94 patients. J Urol 128:290–293, 1982.
6. Kramer SA, Mesrobian HGJ, Kelalis PP: Long-term followup of cosmetic appearance and genital function in male epispadias: Review of 70 patients. J Urol 135:543–547, 1986.
7. Lemmers MJ, Tank ES: Epispadias. In Resnick MI, Kursh ED (eds): Current Therapy in Genitourinary Surgery. St. Louis, Mosby, 1992, pp 322–325.
8. Peters CA, Gearhart JP, Jeffs RD: Epispadias and incontinence: The challenge of the small bladder. J Urol 140:1199–1201, 1988.
9. Zaontz MR, Steckler RE, Shortliffe LM, et al: Multicenter experience with the Mitchell technique for epispadias repair. J Urol 160:172–176, 1998.

51. INTERLABIAL MASSES

Jeffrey S. Palmer, M.D. and Jack S. Elder, M.D.

1. What is the differential diagnosis of interlabial masses in young girls?

Urethral prolapse

Paraurethral cysts

Prolapsed ectopic ureterocele

Sarcoma botryoides

Imperforate hymen

Uterovaginal prolapse

2. What is urethral prolapse?

This condition refers to eversion of the urethral mucosa. It has the appearance of erythematous, inflamed mucosa protruding from and surrounding the urethral meatus. One theory of its pathogenesis is that urethral prolapse results from poor attachment between the smooth muscle layers of the urethra in association with episodic increases in intraabdominal pressure.

3. What is the typical presentation of a girl with urethral prolapse?

The disorder occurs predominantly in African-American girls between 1 and 9 years of age, with an average age of 4 years. The most common signs are bloody spotting on the underwear or diaper, dysuria, and perineal discomfort. Sexual abuse is suspected in many cases of urethral prolapse before the correct diagnosis is made. Urethral prolapse has also been reported in Caucasian girls with cystic fibrosis.

4. What is the treatment of urethral prolapse?

Initial management includes topical application of estrogen cream 2 or 3 times daily to the prolapsed urethra for 1–2 weeks as well as sitz baths. If intermittent bleeding persists, however, formal surgical excision is necessary. In general, surgical excision is recommended if the child is under anesthesia for examination because of suspected sexual abuse.

5. What is a paraurethral cyst?

Paraurethral cyst results from retained secretion in Skene's glands, secondary to ductal obstruction. Typically the cyst displaces the meatus in an eccentric manner.

6. How is a paraurethral cyst treated?

Most paraurethral cysts regress in size during the first 4–8 weeks of life, although occasionally, it is necessary to remove them.

7. What is a prolapsed ectopic ureterocele?

A ureterocele is a cystic dilatation of the distal ureter within the wall of the bladder. In girls, it almost always drains the upper pole of a completely duplicated urinary tract and usually is ectopic; that is, it extends beyond the bladder neck. In approximately 10% of girls with a ureterocele, the lesion may prolapse and appear as a cystic mass arising from the urethra. It may be erythematous or, if ischemic, purplish or even black.

8. What is the typical age of girls with an ectopic ureterocele? Are there other presenting symptoms or signs?

The typical age at presentation is 1 month to 3 years. Most girls with a ureterocele have a history of febrile urinary tract infection, unless the lesion was diagnosed by prenatal ultrasonography. Occasionally, the prolapsed ureterocele can cause bladder outlet obstruction.

9. How does the prolapsed ectopic ureterocele differ on examination from a paraurethral cyst?

A prolapsed ectopic ureterocele appears to arise from the urethra. It may be pale, erythematous, and purplish or even black, whereas the paraurethral cyst seems to arise from the wall of the urethra and usually is pale.

10. How is a ureterocele diagnosed?

The initial study in diagnosing a ureterocele is ultrasonography of the kidneys and bladder. Typically, a full bladder demonstrates the ureterocele in the bladder base. More than 90% of girls with a ureterocele have a complete duplication of the urinary tract, with the ureterocele draining the upper pole. A voiding cystourethrogram usually shows a filling defect in the base of the bladder. An intravenous urogram or renal scan usually shows a duplication anomaly on the affected side with nonfunction or diminished function in the hydronephrotic upper pole. A VCUG will determine if there is associated vesicoureteral reflux prior to treatment.

11. How is a ureterocele treated?

The short-term goal is to decompress the ureterocele that is protruding through the introitus. Insert an angiocath and aspirate fluid, or make a transverse incision in the ureterocele at the level of the vagina if the wall of the ureterocele is thick. Then, manually reduce the ureterocele back into the bladder. If one tries to reduce the ureterocele before decompressing it, the ureterocele is likely to recur. If the incision at the level of the vagina is not effective, endoscopic incision of the ureterocele in its intravesical portion may be necessary.

12. What is sarcoma botryoides?

This term refers to rhabdomyosarcoma of the vagina.

13. What is the appearance of this lesion? How is it diagnosed?

This lesion has the appearance of a firm grape-like mass protruding from the introitus, and often results in vaginal bleeding and sloughed tissue fragments from the vagina. The diagnosis is usually established by biopsy.

14. What is imperforate hymen?

Imperforate hymen refers to stenosis of the hymen, resulting in retained vaginal secretions that originate from stimulation by maternal estrogens.

15. How does imperforate hymen present?

It presents as a white bulging interlabial mass in the newborn.

16. How is an imperforate hymen treated?

Imperforate hymen is managed by hymenotomy, in which the hymen is incised, allowing release of retained vaginal secretions. Usually, signs of upper urinary tract obstruction resolve following decompression of the hydrocolpos.

17. Which type of patient is most likely to develop uterovaginal prolapse?

This condition usually occurs in the newborn and is most common in those with myelodysplasia. It was thought that this anomaly results from partial or complete denervation of the levator ani, which supports the uterus and vagina. Spontaneous resolution may occur, but temporary mechanical support with a rubber nipple or pessary may be necessary to restore the uterus to its normal position.

BIBLIOGRAPHY

1. Caldamone AA, Snyder HMcC III, Duckett JW: Ureteroceles in children: Followup of management with upper tract approach. J Urol 131:1130, 1984.
2. Carpenter SE, Rock JA: Procidentia in the newborn. Int J Obstet Gynecol 25:151, 1987.

3. Elder JS: Congenital anomalies of the genitalia. In Walsh PC, Retik AB, Vaughan ED Jr, Wein AJ (eds): Campbell's Urology, 7th ed. Philadelphia, W. B. Saunders, 1998, p 2120.

4. Elder JS: Interlabial masses. In Reece RM (ed): Manual of Emergency Pediatrics, 4th ed. Philadelphia, W. B. Saunders, 1992, p 448.

5. Klein FA, Vick CW III, Broecker BH: Neonatal vaginal cysts: Diagnosis and management. J Urol 135:371, 1986.

6. Lowe FC, Hill GS, Jeffs RD, Brendler CP: Urethral prolapse in children: Insights into etiology and management. J Urol 135:100, 1986.

7. McHenry CR, Reynolds M, Raffensperger JG: Vaginal neoplasms in infancy: The combined role of chemotherapy and conservative surgical resection. J Pediatr Surg 23:842, 1988.

8. Nussbaum AR, Bebowitz RL: Interlabial masses in little girls: Review and imaging considerations. Am J Radiol 141:65, 1983.

9. Richardson DA, Hajj SM, Herbst AJ: Medical treatment of urethral prolapse in children. Obstet Gynecol 59:69, 1982.

10. Rock JA, Azziz R: Genital anomalies in childhood. Clin Obstet Gynecol 30:62, 1987.

11. Wilson DA, Stacy TM, Smith EI: Ultrasound diagnosis of hydrocolpos and hydrometrocolpos. Radiology 128:451, 1978.

52. END-STAGE RENAL DISEASE AND RENAL TRANSPLANTATION

Charles S. Modlin, Jr., M.D.

END-STAGE RENAL DISEASE

1. What are the causes of end-stage renal disease?

Diabetes has become the most common overall cause of end-stage renal disease (ESRD). Glomerulonephritis ranks as the number 1 cause in children. Diabetes is the second leading cause of end-stage renal disease in African-Americans. The various etiologies and frequency for patients presenting with end-stage renal disease are listed below:

Cause and Frequency of End-stage Renal Disease

ADULT		PEDIATRIC	
Diabetes	34.2%	Glomerulonephritis	37.6%
Hypertension	29.4%	Congenital/other hereditary diseases	19.1%
Glomerulonephritis	14.2%	Collagen vascular diseases	9.9%
Cystic kidney diseases	3.4%	Obstructive nephropathy	6%
Interstitial nephritis	3.4%	Cystic kidney diseases	4.3%
Obstructive nephropathy	2.3%	Interstitial nephritis	4.2%
Collagen vascular diseases	2.2%	Hypertension	4.2%
Malignancies	1.3%	Diabetes	1.4%
		Malignancies	0.4%

2. What is the incidence and prevalence of end-stage renal disease?

The incidence of end-stage renal disease in the United States is 315 new cases per million population as of 1999. Currently, more than 340,000 patients require treatment for end-stage renal disease, approximately 70% of whom are receiving dialysis; 30% are receiving kidney transplantation.

3. How does the incidence of end-stage renal disease vary with age?

There is an age-dependent increase in the incidence of end-stage renal disease, including 33 cases per million population for the pediatric age group (ages 0–15 years), 147 cases per million for patients 35–39 years, 201 cases for patients age 40–44 years, and 1198 cases per million population for patients age 65–69 years. African-Americans have an incidence of 953 cases per million compared with 237 cases in whites.

4. How does end-stage renal disease affect life expectancy?

Life expectancy of patients with end-stage renal disease is significantly worse (70–80%) than the general population. In the United States, life expectancy is 29.8 years for individuals 49 years of age and 21.6 years for those 59 years of age, while it is 7.0 and 4.5 years, respectively, for patients with end-stage renal disease. In the dialysis population, approximately 22% of patients die in the first year, 50% after 3 years, and 67% 5 years after developing end-stage renal disease. There are significant differences, however, when patient survival is categorized by patient age, diagnosis, and race. The current annual mortality rate of ESRD patients in the U.S. is about 24%, but it varies according to ESRD cause, patient age, and treatment modality, with diabetics faring worse.

5. What is the major cause of death in patients with end-stage renal disease?

The primary cause of death in patients with end-stage renal disease is cardiovascular disease. Infectious complications are the second leading cause of death.

6. How do patients with end-stage renal disease typically present?

End-stage renal disease patients often present with vague symptoms such as general fatigue, anorexia, nausea and vomiting, and sometimes pruritus with advanced uremia. Patients may present with congestive heart failure or pulmonary edema from fluid overload.

7. To what degree must renal impairment exist before symptoms of uremia develop?

The degree of renal impairment required before symptoms develop is variable. The majority of patients, however, have lost greater than 90% of renal function before significant symptoms occur and have creatinine clearances of 10–15 ml/min.

8. Which electrolyte disturbances are associated with end-stage renal disease?

Renal failure patients have varying degrees of metabolic acidosis with decreased serum bicarbonate levels. The most dangerous electrolyte imbalance seen in patients with end-stage renal disease is hyperkalemia, which can most effectively be treated with hemodialysis. Kayexalate orally or per rectum may be administered to lower serum potassium levels. Kayexalate should not be administered to patients taking cyclosporine because this combination has been associated with rectal necrosis. Other measures to acutely lower serum potassium levels, such as calcium, insulin, and glucose, are only temporary measures.

9. Describe the clinical findings commonly noted in patients with end-stage renal disease.

Anemia, often profound, is usually present and contributes to symptoms such as fatigue. The use of synthetic erythropoietin has markedly diminished problems associated with anemia. **Hypertension** is almost a universal finding and is usually related to fluid and sodium retention. **Peripheral neuropathy** accompanies more advanced stages of uremia. Uremic pericarditis, although not common, is a potentially life-threatening complication. **Renal osteodystrophy** results from altered calcium and phosphorus metabolism (secondary and tertiary hyperparathyroidism). Young children with end-stage renal disease exhibit a marked retardation in growth that is often alleviated following successful transplantation.

10. Which patients should be screened for the development of end-stage renal disease?

Those individuals with family histories of familial renal cystic diseases or systemic diseases, such as diabetes, that lead to renal failure should undergo routine physical examination (blood pressure, etc.) and laboratory monitoring (urinalysis to screen for microscopic hematuria and/or proteinuria) to aid in detection of intrinsic renal disease. Renal ultrasonography and chromosome analysis are reserved for selected situations.

11. In what manner are sexual and fertility problems associated with end-stage renal disease?

Many patients suffer from diminished libido. Women are often anovulatory and unable to conceive. Men commonly have low sperm counts and erectile dysfunction.

12. Can the development of end-stage renal disease be prevented?

Several measures appear to retard the progression of renal failure, especially in high-risk patients such as diabetics. Aggressive control of high blood pressure is mandatory. Medications found to be useful to control blood pressure include angiotensin-converting enzyme (ACE) inhibitors and calcium channel blockers. Dietary protein restriction and adherence to other dietary restrictions, especially salt and water intake, are other steps taken to retard the progression of renal insufficiency to end-stage renal disease.

13. How is end-stage renal disease treated?

The therapeutic options for patients with end-stage renal disease include hemodialysis, peritoneal dialysis, and transplantation. In 1997, 60% of patients with end-stage renal disease were on hemodialysis, 30% had a functioning transplanted kidney, and 10% were managed with peritoneal dialysis.

14. What complications do patients commonly experience that are related to dialysis?

Thrombosis and vascular access infection are frequent complications related to hemodialysis. Complications related to electrolyte abnormalities and fluid overload may ensue or progress between dialysis sessions. Complications of peritoneal dialysis include peritonitis, catheter site infection, and mechanical failure related to occlusion of the dialysis catheter.

15. What is the cost for treatment of end-stage renal disease and who pays?

The Medicare cost of treating end-stage renal in the United States in 1999 was 11.3 billion dollars and continues to increase significantly each year. Dialysis accounts for the majority of expenditures. In 1973, the End-Stage Renal Disease Medicare Act was passed, and 80% of the costs are paid by the federal government. The remainder is paid for by patients and insurance, including state-funded Medicaid programs.

RENAL TRANSPLANTATION

16. What are the results of renal transplantation?

In 2000, 13,258 kidney transplants were performed. In contrast, as of January 2001, 47,831 individuals were actively awaiting transplantation in the United States (58% males, 38% 50–64 years old, 55% white vs. 36% black). An estimated 10,000 to 14,000 people who die each year meet the criteria for organ donation, but less than half of that number become actual organ donors. In 2000, 2806 patients died awaiting a kidney transplant. In 2000, of the 13,258 kidney-only transplants performed, 5292 were from living donors and 7966 patients received kidneys from cadaveric donors. The median waiting time to transplant in 2000 was 1131 days. Current overall, 1-, 3-, and 5-year patient and allograft (living donor vs. cadaver donor) survival are demonstrated below:

Overall Patient and Allograft Survival Following Transplantation

	LIVE DONOR	CADAVERIC DONOR
Patient Survival		
One year	97.8%	95.0%
Three years	95.2%	89.2%
Five years	90.5%	81.3%
Allograft Survival		
One year	94.7%	89.2%
Three years	87.4%	77.7%
Five years	76.0%	61.3%

Graft and patient survival have been demonstrated to vary depending on various factors, such as recipient age (worse in those at extremes of age) and etiology of end-stage renal disease (worse in diabetics). Other factors found to impact graft and patient survival include delayed graft function, number of rejection episodes, prior transplantation, and pre-existing co-morbidities (cardiovascular disease, obesity), as well as donor factors such as ischemia time, cause of donor death, and donor age.

17. Is transplantation superior to dialysis in the treatment of patients with end-stage renal disease?

Most studies, even those correcting for sex, age, and etiology of renal failure, demonstrate both improved survival and improved quality of life following renal transplantation compared to dialysis. However, patients selected for transplantation are usually healthier patients than those maintained on dialysis. Many of the complications of chronic renal failure (e.g., anemia, metabolic difficulties including bone disease, sexual dysfunction, infertility, neuropathy) are reversed following successful transplantation.

18. How are donor kidneys allocated?

If a patient has a live donor (living related or living unrelated) who is ABO blood-type compatible, medically suitable, and has a negative "crossmatch" with the recipient, then the patient may receive a kidney from that individual. However, in the absence of a suitable living donor, patients are placed on the United Network for Organ Sharing (UNOS) national cadaveric kidney waiting list. Kidneys are allocated on a local geographic basis to patients based upon a point system that takes into account waiting time and HLA match (degree of match between donor and recipient). In cases of "perfect matches," kidneys are allocated on a national level (zero mismatch or 6-antigen match).

19. What evaluation process must potential renal transplant candidates undergo?
To be a candidate for transplantation, renal failure must be of a permanent nonreversible nature. All potential transplant recipients undergo a thorough medical evaluation in an effort to identify in the pretransplant period any correctable conditions or medical contraindications to transplantation. Risk factors for transplantation are included in the following table:

Risk Factors for Transplantation

Extremes of recipient age (>55 years or <1 year old)
Prior failed transplants
Obesity (body mass index >30 kg/m^2)
Diabetes
African-American race
Coronary artery disease
Donor age >50 years or <2 years of age (if transplanted as single pediatric donor kidneys)

Significant disease in other organ systems also adversely affects the results of transplantation, and patients who have evidence of coronary artery disease, and peptic ulcer disease require correction of these problems before transplantation. Patients with anatomic **abnormal lower urinary tracts** (e.g., neurogenic bladder, bladder outlet obstruction, previous urinary diversion), those with **anuria** or **severe oliguria,** and those patients with history or symptoms suggesting abnormal voiding require thorough urologic evaluation and possible intervention before being accepted for transplantation, although they are at higher risk for urinary tract infections. Existing infections must be erradicated before transplantation. Patients requiring urinary diversion should have the diversion created at least six weeks before transplantation.

Pretransplantation Evaluation, Screening Tests, and Vaccinations

Nephrology and Transplant Surgeon Evaluation
History and physical examination
Hemoccult
Chest x-ray
EKG (with exercise male >35, or all patients > 50 years)
Social worker consultation
Laboratory evaluation
CBC & automated differential
PT/PTT
Immunoglobulins
Lipid-lipoprotein profile I
Parathyroid hormone
SMA-16 (serum chemistries)
Liver function tests
Cold agglutinins
Type and cross (2 units leukocyte poor, CMV-negative packed red blood cells)
Tissue-typing specimens
Panel reactive activity determination (PRA)
PSA—if male age 40 years and older
Beta HCG-female of childbearing age
Urinalysis/ urine culture
Serologies
Hepatitis B virus (HBV)
  Hepatitis B surface antigen, HbcIgM and IgG hepatitis surface antibody (HBV-DNA where appropriate)

Pretransplantation Evaluation, Screening Tests, and Vaccinations (Continued)

Hepatitis C virus (HCV)
  Serologic testing (HCV-RNA where appropriate)
Cytomegalovirus (CMV) titer (IgG and IgM)
CMV buffy coat culture/ CMV-DNA
Syphilis (rapid plasma reagin, [RPR])
Epstein-Barr virus (IgG and IgM)
HSV titer (IgG) herpes simplex virus
Human immunodeficiency virus (HIV) antibody
  Enzyme-linked immunoadsorbent assay (ELISA)
  Western Blot for seropositive patients
Human T-cell leukemia virus 1 (HTLV-1)
Toxoplasma (IgM and IgG)
Tuberculosis (purified protein derivative and anergy panel)
Varicella-zoster virus (VZV) IgG
Vaccinations
Pneumococcal polysaccharide vaccine (if not given within 6 years)
Influenza vaccine (yearly)
Hepatitis B series (0, 1, and 6 months)
Varicella vaccine (for seronegative patients)
Tetanus/diphtheria toxoid (if needed)
Polio booster if needed (use inactivated injection, not live oral vaccine if taking immunosuppressive medications)
Measles-mumps-rubella, if needed (not for patients taking immunosuppressive medications)

20. What are the contraindications to renal transplantation?

Active malignancy is one of the few absolute contraindications to transplantation because immunosuppressive medications can enhance progression of cancer. However, many cancers such as squamous and basal cell cancer of the skin and in situ carcinoma of the cervix carry much less risk and no mandatory waiting time to transplantation. Patients treated for incidentally diagnosed renal cell carcinoma with no evidence of metastatic disease require no waiting period to transplantation. Patients who have had appropriate treatment of their malignancy and remain cancer-free for some of time (usually 1–2 years) are candidates for transplantation. Additional contraindications are listed below:

- Active systemic renal disease (e.g., active lupus; active antiglomerular basement membrane disease; active antinuclear cytoplasmic antibody-positive glomerulonephritis)
- Oxalosis (combined liver-kidney transplant recommended)
- Active infection
- Recently treated or uncontrolled/disseminated malignancy (except certain skin cancers)
- Severe extrarenal disease patient that makes the high surgical risk
- Active intravenous drug abuse or alcohol abuse
- Repeated noncompliance
- Uncontrolled psychiatric disorders

21. How is organ preservation accomplished following procurement?

Kidneys are transplanted with the minimal ischemic time possible (i.e., time that the kidney is removed from circulation). In the case of cadaveric renal transplantation, kidneys are ideally transplanted by 24–36 hours; however, there have been reports of successful kidney transplantation with ischemic times up to 72 hours.

In the case of living donor transplantation, the donor and the recipient surgery occur simultaneously, and consequently, ischemic times are rarely longer than 1 hour. The incidence of delayed graft function or primary nonfunction of the kidney increases with increasing ischemic times beyond 24–36 hours.

Following kidney procurement, the kidney is flushed with a cold intracellular-like solution that rapidly cools the kidney (to prevent cellular death and decrease cellular metabolic requirements) and also flushes out blood to prevent allograft clotting.

From this point, two alternatives for preservation exist: cold slush storage and and pulsatile perfusion. **Cold slush storage** is accomplished after the initial flushing of the kidney by placing it into a sterile bag that contains a similar solution (University of Wisconsin Solution); this bag is in turn placed into a container of ice solution. In **pulsatile perfusion** perservation, following initial flushing, the kidney is placed in an incubator with a pulsatile pump that perfuses the kidney at 4°C with a denatured plasma solution. Pulsatile perfusion is more expensive and technically more cumbersome. Pulsatile perfusion remains the preferred mode of preservation for kidneys from elderly donors (> 55 years) and those kidneys considered potentially high-risk or marginal (e.g., prolonged ischemic times, donors treated with high doses of vasopressors, significant percentages of glomerulosclerosis on biopsy, poor backtable flush, vascular plaque). The use of the perfusion pump allows one to assess flow (> 100 ml/min), pressure (<40/25 systolic/diastolic mm Hg), and renal vascular resistance (<0.30) characteristics of the donor kidneys that assist in determining the suitability of the donor kidney for transplantation.

22. What are the current indications for pretransplant nephrectomy?

Routine pretransplant nephrectomy is no longer performed. Specific indications for pretransplant nephrectomy exist and are listed below. Many patients, especially those with polycystic kidney disease, appear to do better with their native kidneys preserved, because the native kidneys often continue to produce erythropoietin and contribute to improved fluid dynamics. Indications for pretransplant native nephrectomy are as follows:

- Chronically infected pyelonephric kidneys
- Massively enlarged polycystic kidneys
- Kidneys with stones
- High-grade reflux (grade 3 or 4 reflux with or without bacteriuria)
- Acquired renal cystic disease
- Renal malignancy or suspicious renal mass
- Hemorrhagic kidneys
- Obstructed kidneys
- Poorly controlled renin-mediated hypertension
- Nephrotic range proteinuria
- Kidneys diverted into conduits or cutaneous ureterostomies

23. Why do transplants fail?

Rejection is mediated by both the humoral and cellular arms of the immune system. The various forms are discussed below:

Chronic rejection accounts for the majority of graft losses (90%). This usually occurs late after transplantation and is believed to be humorally mediated and a result from allograft injury caused by repeated episodes of acute rejection, although mechanisms for nonimmunologically mediated "chronic rejection" have been proposed. Chronic rejection is often suspected clinically with a slowly progressive deterioration of renal function accompanied by hypertension and proteinuria. It is confirmed on renal biopsy that demonstrates vascular changes (intimal proliferation, glomerulosclerosis) and interstitial fibrosis, as well as tubular atrophy. Chronic rejection is not responsive to antirejection therapy.

Hyperacute rejection occurs within the first 24 hours following transplantation, but usually occurs intraoperatively within minutes following revascularization. It is irreversible, activates the clotting system, and results in intrarenal thrombosis and renal infarction. Hyperacute rejection is humorally mediated by preformed cytotoxic antibodies that result from previous antigen exposure via blood transfusion, previous transplant, or pregnancy.

Accelerated rejection usually occurs within 4–7 days and is mediated by both the humoral and cellular components of the immune system. It can occasionally be reversed with antirejection treatment.

Acute rejection occurs at any time after transplant but usually within the first 3–6 months. It has a varible presentation and is usually suspected owing to a decrease in urine output, low-grade fever, weight gain, hypertension, allograft swelling, and tenderness with an associated rise in serum creatinine above baseline values. Patients often are asymptomatic and present with only creatinine elevation. Allograft biopsy is the gold standard for diagnosis of rejection. Histologically, the kidney usually reveals a mononuclear lymphocyte and plasma cell interstitial and tubular infiltrate with more severe cases demonstrating lymphocytosis of blood vessel walls— "vasculitis." Acute rejection is graded by the Banff classification. It is typically responsive to antirejection therapy (see question 10).

Technical complications such as renal artery or venous thrombosis, renal artery stenosis, or ureteral obstruction are another cause of graft loss, although these technical causes of graft loss are rare and account for less than 5% of allograft losses. A small percentage of kidneys are lost because of other problems such as **infectious complications, recurrent or de novo medical renal disease,** and **drug toxicity** (e.g., cyclosporine toxicity).

24. What is the role of tissue typing and cross-matching in renal transplantation?

Tissue typing of potential donor and recipients is performed to identify specific human leukocyte antigens (HLAs) located in the major histocompatibility complex on chromosome 6. There are six major loci (three each on the maternally and paternally derived chromosomes). The major HLA loci tested for include HLA-A, HLA-B, and HLA-DR, although a number of other "minor" loci exist. The goal of tissue typing is to select the donor/recipient with the most HLA in common. In cadaver and living unrelated renal transplantation, the best match occurs when the donor and recipient have all 6-HLA in common (or have zero mismatches detected). Living, related renal transplantation matches may be zero haplotype, 1-haplotype, or 2-haplotye.

Recipients of a 2-haptotype "perfectly matched" kidney experience superior allograft survival than that noted following transplantion of a lesser matched family member. However, data have shown that zero-antigen matched living unrelated donor kidney transplants have superior graft survival compared to 6-antigen–matched cadaver transplants (because of shorter preservation periods).

Immediately before transplantation, lymphocytotoxic crossmatches are performed between donor lymphocytes and recipient sera to detect the presence of preformed cytotoxic antibodies that may preclude transplantation, thus preventing hyperacute rejection. In addition to lymphocytotoxicity crossmatching, some histocompatibility laboratories also perform sensitive T- and B-cell flow cytometry analysis to detect preformed antibodies.

25. How is rejection prevented and treated?

The mainstay of rejection prevention and treatment is immunosuppressive medication. The principal immunosuppressive medications used for the prevention of rejection include triple therapy with **corticosteroids, mycophenolate mofetil (azathioprine),** and **cyclosporine (FK506).** Recently, a nonnephrotoxic immunosuppressive medication (Rapamycin) has been used for maintenance with or without calcineurin inhibitors (cyclosporine or tacrolimus). For the treatment of established rejection, initial therapy usually consists of corticosteroid pulses with antilymphocyte preparations (polyclonal or monoclonal) reserved for steroid-resistant cases. In living-unrelated and cadaver transplantation, induction antilymphocyte preparations (ATG, OKT3, Thymoglobulin) or IL-2 receptor blockers (basiliximab or daclizumab) are used before beginning maintenance immunosuppression (as listed above) in an attempt to reduce rejection and delay the introduction of nephrotoxic calcineurin inhibitor immunosuppression until adequate graft function has ensued.

The ultimate goal of transplantation is induction of a state of tolerance, in which the recipient immune system fails to recognize the transplanted organ as foreign after transplantation. With tolerance, rejection does not occur and immunosuppression is not required. Research is currently focused in this area. A number of procedures used to manipulate the immune system, including splenectomy, total lymphoid irradiation, thoracic duct drainage (depletion of lymphocytes), and donor-specific blood transfusions, have not been successful in inducing tolerance, have had adverse side effects, and have been abandoned in clinical transplantation.

26. What are the side effects of immunosuppressive medications?

Immunosuppressive medications make patients more susceptible to infection (bacterial, viral, fungal, opportunistic infections) as well as malignancies, particularly lymphoproliferative disorders and skin cancers. The following table indicates specific toxicities of the commonly used immunosuppressive agents:

Side Effects of Immunosuppressive Medications

Corticosteroids	**Azathioprine**
Diabetes	Bone marrow suppression (pancytopenia)
Lipid disorders	Gastrointestinal disturbances
Cushingoid features	Hepatotoxicity
Obesity	Hair loss
Poor wound healing	**Antilymphocytic agents**
Avascular necrosis (bone)	**Polyclonal**
Cataracts	Fever, chills
Hypertension, coronary artery disease (CAD)	Leukopenia, thrombocytopenia
Peptic ulceration, gastritis, bowel perforation	Serum sickness
Growth retardation	Local phlebitis
Pancreatitis	**Monoclonal**
Cyclosporine	Flulike syndrome:
Nephrotoxicity	Fever, chills, tremors, headache, nausea,
Hypertension, CAD	vomiting, and diarrhea
Hyperkalemia	Aseptic meningitis
Hyperuricemia	Hyptotension
Heptatotoxicity	Pulmonary edema
Hirsutism	**FK506 (Prograf/Tacrolimus)**
Gingival hyperplasia	Nephrotoxicity
Tremors/seizures	Diabetes
Pancreatitis	Neurotoxicity
Hemolytic-uremic syndrome	**Interleukin Inhibitor**
Mycophenolate Mofetil (CellCept)	Simulect
Leukopenia	**Rapamune (Rapamycin)**
Gastrointestinal disturbances	Bone marrow suppression
GI bleeding, diarrhea, ulceration,	GI toxicity
esophagitis, gastritis	Skin rash
	Hyperlipidemia

27. What complications are commonly encountered after renal transplantation?

Complications commonly encountered after transplant are medical versus surgical complications. **Medical complications** generally relate to preoperative existing co-morbidities, such as coronary artery disease, hypertension, and diabetes, but they also result from the use of immunosuppressive medications as indicated above (e.g., lipid abnormalities, infection, progressive cardiovascular disease, posttransplant induced diabetes, bone marrow suppression, deep venous thrombosis). **Surgical complications** are grouped into early versus late complications. Early complications are related to vascular catastrophies, urinary fistulization, wound infection, or pelvic lymphocele. Later surgical complications include urinary obstruction and renal artery stenosis.

28. Is routine anticoagulation required during transplantation?

No. Patients are not routinely anticoagulated for transplantation. Patients are however maintained on antiplatelet medications (baby aspirin or Persantine) after transplant.

29. How does a cytomegaloviral (CMV) infection typically present, and how is it treated?

CMV infection generally occurs within the first 2–3 months after transplant, at the time the patient is maximally immunosuppressed, and also during periods of treatment of acute rejection, especially with antilymphocyte agents. Patients may present with a variety of symptoms, from fever, malaise, and weakness to gastrointestinal bleeding, gastritis, esophagitis, hepatitis, pneumonia, allograft dysfunction, retinitis, cerebritis, and sepsis. Most often, the diagnosis is suspected when the patient presents with neutropenia. The diagnosis is confirmed on blood DNR detection by polymerase chain reaction (PCR), or it is suggested by CMV IgM serology. Treatment consists of either intravenous or oral ganciclovir or valganciclovir depending on the severity of the disease. Patients particularly at risk for developing CMV disease are those transplant recipients with negative CMV serology before transplant who receive kidneys from CMV-positive donors. These patients receive prophylaxis with oral ganciclovir or oral acyclovir with or without the addition of hyperimmune CMV immunoglobulin.

BIBLIOGRAPHY

Contemporary Results of Transplantation
1. Annual report of the U.S. Scientific Registry for Organ Transplantation and the Organ Procurement and Transplantation Network, 1991–2000. Richmond, VA, UNOS, 2001.
2. Cecka MJ: The United Network for Organ Sharing (UNOS) Scientific Renal Transplant Registry. In Cecka MJ, Terasaki PI (eds): Clinical Transplants. UCLA Tissue Typing Laboratory, Los Angeles, California, 1996.
3. Christensen AJ, Holman JM, Turner CW, Slaughter JR: Quality of life in end-stage renal disease. Influence of renal transplantation. Clin Transplant 3:46–53, 1989.
4. Health Care Financing Research Report, End Stage Renal Disease 1999–2001. Department of Health and Human Services, Health Care Financing Administration, HCFA Pub. No. 03393. Baltimore, MD, October 2001.
5. Hobart MG, Modlin CS, Kapoor A, et al: Transplantation of pediatric en bloc cadaver kidneys into adult recipients. Transplantation 66:1689–1694, 1998.
6. Hodge EE: End-stage renal disease. In Resnick MI, Novick AC (eds.): Urology Secrets. Philadelphia, Hanley & Belfus, 1995, pp 165–171.
7. Hutchinson TA, Thomas DC, Lemieux JC, Harvey CE: Prognostically controlled comparison of dialysis and renal transplantation. Kidney Int 26:44–51, 1984.
8. Modlin, CS, Novick AC, Goormastic M, Hodge EE: Long-term results using single pediatric donor allografts in adult recipients. J Urol 156:885–888, 1996.
9. Modlin, CS, Novick AC. Renal transplantation. In Weiss G, O'Reilly (eds): Comprehensive Urology 2001. St. Louis, Mosby, 2001.
10. Morris PT: Kidney Transplantation: Principles and Practice, 4th ed. Philadelphia, W. B. Saunders, 1994.
11. Rigg KM: Renal transplantation: Current status, complications and prevention. J Antimicrob Chemother 36(suppl B):51–57, 1995.

Contraindications and Adverse Factors for Renal Transplantation
1. Braun WE, Marwick TH: Coronary artery disease in renal transplant recipients. Cleveland Clin J Med 61:370–385, 1994.
2. Briggs JD: Patient selection for renal transplantation. Nephrol Dial Transplant 10 (suppl 1):10–13, 1995.
3. Hunt J: Pretransplant evaluation and outcome. Semin Nephrol 12:227–233, 1992.
4. Modlin CS, Flechner SM, Goormastic M, et al: Should obese patients lose weight prior to receiving a kidney transplant? Transplantation 64:599–604, 1997.
5. Nossent HC, Swaak TJ, Berden JH: Systemic lupus erythematosus after renal transplantation: Patient and graft survival and disease activity. Ann Intern Med 114:183–188, 1991.
6. Waiser J, Budde K, Bohler T, Neumayer HH: The influence of age on outcome after renal transplantation. Geriatr Nephrol Urol 7:137–146, 1997.

Pretransplant Urologic Evaluation
1. Barnett M, Reginald B, Glass N, et al: Long-term clean intermittent self-catheterization in renal transplant recipients. J Urol 134:654–657, 1985.
2. Barry JM, Lemmers MJ: Update on renal transplantation. Monogr Urol 10:5–14, 1989.
3. Bretan PNJ, Busch PM, Hricak H, Williams RD: Chronic renal failure: A significant risk factor in the development of acquired renal cysts and renal cell carcinoma. Case reports and review of the literature. Cancer 57:1871–1879, 1986.
4. Bretan PN, Novick AC, Steinmuller DR, et al: Ultrasonographic prospective pretransplant screening in 100 patients for acquired renal cysts and renal cell carcinoma. Transplant Proc 21:1974–1975, 1989.
5. Flechner SN, Conley SB, Bluer ED, et al: An alternative to diversion in continent transplant recipients with lower urinary tract dysfunction. J Urol 130:878–881, 1993.
6. Hatch DA, Belitsky P, Barry JM, et al: Fate of renal allografts transplanted in patients with urinary diversion. Transplantation 56:838–842, 1993.

7. McGuire EJ, Woodside JR, Borden TA, Weiss RM: Prognostic value of urodynamic testing in myelodysplastic patients. J Urol 126:205, 1981.
8. Reinberg Y, Bumgartner GL, Alibadi H: Urological aspects of renal transplantation. J Urol 143:1087–1091, 1990.
9. Schneidman RJ, Pulliam JP, Barry JM: Clean intermittent self-catheterization in renal transplant recipients. Transplantation 38:312–314, 1984.
10. Serrano, DP, Flechner SM, Modlin CS, et al: Transplantation into the long-term defunctionalized urinary bladder. J Urol 156: 885–888, 1996.
11. Waltzer WC: The preoperative evaluation of the urinary tract for adults and children undergoing solid-organ transplantation. Seminars Urol 12:84–88, 1994.
12. Zaragoza MR, Ritchey ML, Bloom DA, McGuire EJ: Enterocystoplasty in renal transplantation candidates: Urodynamic evaluation and outcome. J Urol 150:1463–1466, 1993.

Bone Disease and Renal Transplantation
1. Chestnut CH: Osteoporosis and its treatment. N Eng J Med 326:406–407, 1992.
2. Pickette Y, Prud'homme L, Gagne M, et al: Osteopenia in kidney transplant recipients: Prevalence and risk factors. J Am Soc Nephrol 4:955(Abstract), 1993.

Preoperative Living Donor Evaluation
1. Shokeir AA, Gad HM, Shaaban AA, et al: Differential kidney scans in preoperative evaluation of kidney donors. Transplant Proc 25:2327, 1993.

Preoperative Living Donor Evaluation
1. Shokeir AA, Gad HM, Shaaban AA, et al: Differential kidney scans in preoperative evaluation of kidney donors. Transplant Proc 25:2327, 1993.

Perioperative Care
1. Dawidson I, Peters P, Sagalowsky A, et al: The effect of intraoperative fluid management on the incidence of acute tubular necrosis. Transplant Proc 19: 2056, 1987.
2. Dawidson I, Rooth P, Lu C, et al: Verapamil improves the outcome after cadaver renal transplantation. J Am Soc Nephrol 2:983, 1991.
3. Dawidson I, Sandor ZF, Coorpender L, et al: Intraoperative albumin administration affects the outcome of cadaver renal transplantation. Transplantation 53:774, 1992.
4. Willms CD, Dawidson I, Dickerman D, et al: Intraoperative blood volume expansion induces primary function after renal transplantation: A study of 96 paired cadaver kidneys. Transplant Proc 23:1338, 1991.

The Donor Evaluation
1. Jones J, Payne WD, Matas AJ: The living donor: Risks, benefits, and related concerns. Transplant Rev 7:115–128, 1993.
2. Lowell JA, Taylor RJ: The evaluation of the living renal donor, surgical techniques and results. Semin Urol 12:102–107, 1994.
3. Ringden O, Friman L, Jundgren G, et al: Living related kidney donors: Complications and long-term renal function. Transplantation 25:221–223, 1978.

Living Donor Nephrectomy
1. Frisk B, Persson H, Wedel N, et al: Study of 172 patients at 10 to 21 years after renal transplantation. Transplant Proc 19:3769–3771, 1987.
2. Najarian JS, Chavers BM, McHugh LE, Matas AJ: Twenty years or more of follow-up of living kidney donors. Lancet 340:807–810, 1992.
3. Reinberg Y, Bumgartner GL, Alibadi H: Urologic aspects of renal transplantation. J Urol 143:1087–1091, 1990.
4. Ringden O, Friman L, Lundgren G, et al: Living related kidney donors: Complications and long-term renal function. Transplantation 25:221–223, 1978.
5. Serrano DP, Flechner SM, Modlin CS, et al: The use of kidneys from living donors with renal vascular disease: Expanding the donor pool. J Urol 157:1587–1591, 1997.

Immunosuppression
1. Cosimi AB: The future of monoclonal antibody immunosuppression in solid organ transplantation. Transplant Sci 2:28–31, 1992.
2. Cosimi AB, Burton RC, Colvin RB, et al: Treatment of acute renal allograft rejection with OKT3 monoclonal antibody. Transplantation 32:535–539, 1981.
3. Eugui EM, Mirkovich A, Allison AC: Lymphocyte-selective antiproliferative and immunosuppressive effects of mycophenolic acid in mice. Scand J Immunol 33:175, 1991.
4. Sablinski T, Hancock WW, Tilney NL, et al: CD4 monoclonal antibodies in organ transplantation—A review of progress. Transplantation 52:579–589, 1991.

5. Sollinger HW: Mycophenolate mofetil for the prevention of acute rejection in primary cadaveric renal allograft recipients. Transplantation 60:225–232, 1995.

Assessment of Allograft Dysfunction

1. D'Alessandro AM, Lorentzen DF, Pirsch JD, et al: Cadaveric renal transplantation in the cyclosporine and OKT3 eras: An update of the University of Wisconsin-Madison experience. In Terasaki PI (ed): Clinical Transplants 1989. Los Angeles, UCLA Tissue Typing Laboratory, 1989, pp 239–251.
2. Dunn J, Golden D, Van Buren CT, et al: Causes of graft loss beyond two years in the cyclosporine era. Transplantation 49:349–353, 1990.
3. Modlin CS, Goldfarb DA, Novick AC: Hyperfiltration nephropathy as a cause of late graft loss in renal transplantation. World J Urol 14:256–264, 1996.

Evaluation and Treatment of Acute and Chronic Rejection

1. Flechner SM, Modlin CS, Serrano DP, et al: Determinants of chronic renal allograft rejection in cyclosporine-treated recipients. Transplantation 62:1235–1241, 1996.
2. Solez K, Axelsen RA, Benediktsson H, et al: International standardization criteria for the histologic diagnosis of renal allograft rejection. Kidney Int 44:411–412, 1993.
3. Thistlethwaite JR, Gaber AO, Stuart FP, et al: OKT3 treatment of steroid-resistant renal allograft rejection. Transplantation 43:176, 1982.

Indications and Timing of Allograft Nephrectomy

1. Hansen BL, Rohr N, Starklint H, et al: Indications for and timing of removal of non-functioning kidney transplant. Scand J Urol Nephrol 20:217–220, 1986.
2. O'Sullivan DC, Murphy DM, McLean P, Donovan MG: Transplant nephrectomy over 20 years: Factors involved in associated morbidity and mortality. J Urol 151:855–858, 1994.
3. Sharma DK, Pandey AP, Nath V, Gopalakrishnan G: Allograft nephrectomy-A 16-year experience. Br J Urol 64:122, 1989.
4. Toledo-Pereyra LH, Gordon C, Kaufmann R, et al: Role of immediate versus delayed nephrectomy for failed renal transplants. Am Surg 53:534, 1987.
5. Vanrenterghem Y, Khamis S: The management of the failed renal allograft. Nephrol Dial Transplant 11:955–957, 1996.

Posttransplant Infections: Prophylaxis and Treatment

1. Avery R: Infections in transplantation. Cleveland Clin J Med 65:305–314, 1998.
2. Hans Sollinger (ed): Transplantation Drug Pocket Reference Guide. Austin, Texas, R.G. Landes Co, 1994.
3. Rubin-Tolkoff NE, Rubin RH: Clinical approach to viral and fungal infections in the renal transplant patient. Semin Nephrol 12:364–375, 1992.
4. Rubin RH, Wolfson JS, Cosimi AB, et al: Infection in the renal transplant recipient. Am J Med 70:405–411, 1981.

Urinary Tract Infections Posttransplant

1. Cho D, Jackson DA, Cheigh J, et al: Urinary calculi in renal transplant recipients. Transplantation 45:899–902, 1988.
2. Dempsey J, Scott R: Duplex Doppler examination of a perinephric abscess in a renal transplant. Southern Med J 83:1213–1215, 1990.
3. Ellis E, Wagner C, Arnold W, et al: Extracorporeal shock-wave lithotripsy in a renal transplant patient. J Urol 141:98–99, 1989.
4. Franz M, Klaar U, Hofbauer H, et al: Incidence of urinary tract infections and vesicorenal reflux: A comparison between conventional and antirefluxive techniques of ureter implantation. Transplant Proc 24:2773–2774, 1992.
5. Hamshere RJ, Chisholm GD, Shackman R: Late urinary tract infection after renal transplantation. Lancet 2:793–794, 1974.
6. Hulbert JC, Reddy P, Young AT, et al: The percutaneous removal of calculi from transplanted kidneys. J Urol 134:324–326, 1985.
7. Gottesdiener KM: Transplaned infections: Donor-to-host transmission with the allograft. Ann Intern Med 110:1001–1013, 1989.
8. Grunberger T, Gnant M, Sautner T, et al: Impact of vesicoureteral reflux on graft survival in renal transplantation. Transplant Proc 25:1058–1059, 1993.
9. Lapchik MS, Castelo Filho A, Pestana JOA: Risk factors for nosocomial urinary tract and postoperative wound infections in renal transplant patients: A matched-pair case-control study. J Urol 147:994–998, 1992.
10. Levy DA, Seftel A, Schulak JA: Acute focal bacterial nephritis in a kidney transplant. Clin Tranpl 6: 325–327, 1992.

11. Lobo PI, Rudolf LE, Krieger JN: Wound infections in renal transplant recipients—a complication of urinary tract infections during allograft malfunction. Surgery 92:491–496, 1982.
12. Mahon FB, Malek GH, Uehling DT: Urinary tract infection after renal transplantation. Urology 1:579–581, 1973.
13. Mastrosimone S, Pignata G, Maresca MC, et al: Clinical significance of vesicoureteral reflux after kidney transplantation. Clin Nephrol 40:38–45, 1993.
14. Nicholson ML, Veitch PS, Donnelly PK, et al: Urological complications of renal transplantation: The impact of double J ureteric stents. Ann R Coll Surg Engl 73:316–321, 1991.
15. Nicol DL, P'ng K, Hardie DR, et al: Routine use of indwelling ureteral stents in renal transplantation. J Urol 150:1375–1379, 1993.
16. Ramsey DE, Finch WT, Birtch WT: Urinary tract infections in kidney transplant recipients. Arch Surg 114:1022–1025, 1979.
17. Rubin RM, Tolkoff-Rubin NE: Antimicrobial strategies in the care of organ transplant recipients. Antimicrob Agents Chemother 37:619–624, 1993.
18. Simmons RL, Weil R, Tallent MB, et al: Do mild infections trigger the rejection of renal allografts? Transplant Proc 2:419–423, 1970.
19. Walter S, Pedersen FB, Vejlsgaard R: Urinary tract infection and wound infection in kidney transplant patients. Br J Urol 47:513–517, 1975.
20. Wyner LM: The evaluation and management of urinary tract infections in recipients of solid-organ transplants. Semin Urol 12:134–139, 1994.

Posttransplant Hypertension

1. Curtis JJ, Lucas BA, Kotchen TA, Luke RG: Surgical therapy for persistent hypertension after renal transplantation. Transplantation 31:125–128, 1981.
2. Dubovsky EV, Curtis JJ, Luke RG, et al: Captopril as a predictor of curable hypertension in renal transplant recipients. Controv Nephrol 56:117–123, 1987.
3. Pollini J, Guttmann RD, Beaudoin JG, Morehouse DD, Klassen J, Knaack J. Late hypertension following renal allotransplantation. Clin Nephrol 11:202–212, 1979.
4. Rao TKS, Gupta SK, Butt KHM, et al: Relationship of renal transplantation to hypertension in end-stage renal failure. Arch Intern Med 138:1236–1241, 1978.

Posttransplant Diabetes

1. Freidman EA, Shyh Tai-ping, Beyer MM, et al: Posttransplant diabetes in kidney transplant recipients. Am J Nephrol 5:196–202, 1985.
2. Hariharan S, Schroder TJ, Weiskittel P, et al: Prednisone withdrawal in HLA identical and one haplotype-matched live related donor and cadaver renal transplants. Kidney Int 44:S30–S35, 1993.
3. Sumrani NB, Delaney V, Ding Z, et al: Posttransplant diabetes. Transplantation 51:343, 1991.

Posttransplant Malignancies

1. Modlin CS, Flechner SM, Penn I: Testicular seminoma in a renal allograft recipient originating in an undescended testis. Urology 48:145–148, 1996.
2. Nalesnik M, Makowka L, Starzl T: The diagnosis and treatment of posttransplant lymphoproliferative disorders. Curr Probl Surg 25:371–472, 1988.
3. Penn I: Cancers complicating organ transplantation. N Engl J Med 323:1767–1769, 1990.
4. Penn I: The effect of immunosuppression on pre-existing cancers. Transplantation 55:742–747, 1993.
5. Pirsch JD, Stratta RJ, Sollinger HW, et al: Treatment of severe Epstein-Barr virus–induced lymphoproliferative syndrome with ganciclovir: Two cases after solid organ transplantation. Am J Med 86:241–244, 1989.
6. Smith JL, Wilkinson AH, Hunsicker LG, et al: Increased frequency of posttransplant lymphomas in patients treated with cyclosporin, azathioprine, and prednisone. Transplant Proc 21:3199–3200, 1989.

Early Graft Dysfunction

1. Cacciarelli T, Sumrani N, Delaney V, et al: The influence of delayed graft renal allograft function on long-term outcome in the cyclosporin era. Clin Nephrol 39:335–339, 1993.

Recurrent Renal Disease Posttransplant

1. Braun WE: Long-term complications of renal transplantation. Kidney Int 37:1363–1378, 1990.
2. Cameron JS: Glomerulonephritis in renal transplants. Transplantation 34:237–245, 1982.
3. Cosyns JP, Pirson Y, Squifflet JP, et al: De novo membranous nephropathy in human renal allografts: Report of nine patients. Kidney Int 22:177–183, 1982.
4. Mathew TH: Recurrent disease in renal allografts. Am J Kidney Dis 12:85–96, 1988.

Vascular Complications Posttranspant

1. Chiu AS, Landsberg DN: Successful treatment of acute transplant renal vein thrombosis with selective streptokinase infusion. Transplant Proc 23:2297–2300, 1991.

2. Dodd GD, Tublin ME, Shah A, Zajko AB: Imaging of vascular complications associated with renal transplants. Am J Radiol 157:449–459, 1991.

Renal Artery Stenosis

1. Benoit G, Moukarzel M, Hiesse C, et al: Transplant renal artery stenosis: Experience and comparative results between surgery and angioplasty. Transplant Int 3:137–140, 1990.
2. Erley CM, Duda SH, Wakat J-P, et al: Noninvasive procedures for diagnosis of renovascular hypertension in renal transplant recipients: A prospective analysis. Transplantation 54:863–867, 1992.
3. Fauchald P, Vatne K, Paulsen D, et al: Long term clinical results of percutaneous transluminal angioplasty in transplant renal artery stenosis. Nephrol Dial Transplant 7:256–259, 1992.
4. Gray DWR: Graft renal artery stenosis in the transplanted kidney. Transplantation Rev 8:15–21, 1994.
5. Grossman RA, Dafoe DC, Shoenfeld RB, et al: Percutaneous transluminal angioplasty treatment of renal transplant artery stenosis. Transplantation 34:339–343, 1982.
6. Idrissi A, Fournier H, Renaud B, et al: The captopril challenge test as a screening test for renovascular hypertension. Kidney Int 34(suppl 25):138–141, 1988.
7. Kuo PC, Peterson J, Semba C, et al: CO2 angiography: A technique for vascular imaging in renal allograft dysfunction. Transplantation 61:652–654, 1996.
8. Merkus JWS, Huymans FTM, Hoitsma AJ, et al: Renal allograft artery stenosis: Results of medical treatment and intervention: A retrospective analysis. Transplant Int 6:111–115, 1993.
9. Newman-Sander APG, Gedroyc WG, Al-Kutouby MA, et al: The use of expandable metal stents in transplant renal artery stenosis. Clin Radiol 50:245–250, 1995.
10. Rubin GD, Dake MD, Napel SA, et al: Three-dimensional spiral CT angiography of the abdomen: Initial clinical experience. Radiology 186:147–152, 1993.
11. Shamlou KK, Drane WE, Hawkins IF, Fennell RS: Captopril renogram and the hypertensive renal transplantation patient: A predictive test of therapeutic outcome. Radiology 190:153–159, 1994.
12. Smith RB, Cosimi AB, Lordon R, et al: Diagnosis and management of arterial stenosis causing hypertension after successful renal transplantation. J Urol 115:639–642, 1976.
13. Sutherland RS, Spees EK, Jones JW, Fink DW: Renal artery stenosis after renal transplantation: The impact of the hypogastric artery anastomosis. J Urol 149:980–985, 1993.

Urologic Complications Posttransplant

1. Bennett LN, Voegeli DR, Crummy AB, et al: Urologic complications following renal transplantation. Role of interventional radiologic procedures. Radiology 160:531, 1986.
2. Benoit G, Alexander L, Moukarzel M, et al: Percutaneous antegrade dilations of ureteral strictures in kidney transplants. J Urol 150:37, 1993.
3. Caldwell TC, Burns JR: Current operative management of urinary calculi after renal transplantation. J Urol 140:1360–1363, 1988.
4. Lieberman RP, Glass NR, Crummy AB, et al: Nonoperative percutaneous management of urinary fistulas and strictures in renal transplantation. Surg Gynecol Obstet 155:667, 1992.
5. Pardalidis NP, Waltzer WC, Tellis VA, et al: Endourologic management of complications in renal allografts. J Endourol 8:321–327, 1994.
6. Schiff M Jr, McGuire EJ, Weiss RM, Lytton B: Management of urinary fistulas after renal transplantation. J Urol 115:251–255, 1976.
7. Streem SB: Endourological management of urological complications following renal transplantation. Semin Urol 12:123–133, 1994.
8. Streem SB, Novick AC, Steinmuller DR, et al: Percutaneous techniques for the management of urological renal transplant complications. J Urol 135:456, 1986.
9. Swierzewski SJ III, Konnak JW, Ellis JH: Treatment of renal transplant ureteral complications by percutaneous techniques. J Urol 149:986, 1993.

Infertility and Impotence Posttransplant

1. Barry JM: The evaluation and treatment of erectile dysfunction following organ transplantation. Semin Urol 12:147–153, 1994.
2. Baumgarten SR, Lindsay GK, Wise GJ: Fertility problems in the renal transplant patient. J Urol 118:991–993, 1977.
3. Mancini R, Lavieri J, Muller F, et al: Effect of prednisolone upon normal and pathologic human spermatogenesis. Fertil Steril 17:500–513, 1996.
4. Phadke AG, MacKinnon KJ, Dossetor JB: Male fertility in uremia: Restoration by renal allografts. CMA J 102:607–608, 1970.
5. Reinberg Y, Bumgardner GL, Aliabadi H: Urological aspects of renal transplantation. J Urol 143:1087–1092, 1990.
6. Rodrigues Netto N, Pecoraro G, Sabbaga E, et al: Spermatogenesis before and after renal transplant. Int J Fertil 25:131–133, 1980.

7. Seethalakshmi L, Diamond D, Malhotra R, et al: Cyclosporine-induced testicular dysfunction: A Separation of the nephrotoxic component and an assessment of a 60-day recovery period. Transplant Proc 10:1005–1010, 1988.

8. Seethalakshmi L, Menon M, Pallias J, et al: Cyclosporine: Its harmful effects on testicular function and male fertility. Transplant Proc 21:928–930, 1989.

Pregnancy Posttransplantation

1. Killion D, Rajfer J: The evaluation and management of male infertility following solid-organ transplantation. Semin Urol 12:140–146, 1994.

2. Penn I, Makowski E, Harris P: Parenthood following renal and hepatic transplantation. Transplantation 30:397–400, 1980.

53. RENAL ARTERY DISEASE

Andrew C. Novick, M.D.

1. What are the causes of renal artery disease (RAD)?

RAD is most commonly characterized by stenosis of the renal artery from atherosclerosis or fibrous dysplasia. These diseases account for approximately **75%** and **25%**, respectively, of all such lesions. The three different varieties of fibrous dysplasia are termed *intimal fibroplasia, medial fibroplasia,* and *perimedial fibroplasia.* Each fibrous lesion has distinctive histologic and arteriographic features and a different biologic history. Other less common disorders that can cause RAD include an arterial aneurysm, arterial-venous fistula, neurofibromatosis, arteritis, Takayasu's disease, and renal artery thrombosis or embolism.

2. What is the difference between renovascular disease and renovascular hypertension (RVH)?

RVH is an important correctable cause of hypertension with an estimated prevalence of approximately 0.5% among all patients with hypertension. It is important to differentiate between renovascular disease and RVH, because occlusive lesions of the renal artery do not always result in hypertension. The diagnosis of renovascular disease depends on angiographic demonstration of a stenotic lesion in the renal artery or its branches, whereas the diagnosis of RVH can only be confirmed in retrospect, and implies permanent relief of hypertension after revascularization or removal of the affected kidney. The simultaneous occurrence of essential hypertension and coincidental renovascular disease is, in fact, more frequent than the occurrence of true RVH.

3. What are the clinical manifestations of RVH?

No single clinical manifestation can reliably distinguish RVH from essential hypertension. Nevertheless, when taken in the aggregate, certain clinical manifestations are helpful in making this differential diagnosis. Patients with RVH are much more likely to have a short duration of hypertension, advanced retinopathy, azotemia, hypokalemia, alkalosis, or a bruit auscultated in the abdomen or flank. RVH is much less common in African-Americans than Caucasians. In general, the most helpful clues to the diagnosis of RVH, in descending order of importance, have been:

1. An abdominal bruit with both systolic and diastolic components.
2. An abrupt onset or exacerbation of hypertension with rapid progression.
3. Onset of hypertension before age 30 or after age 55.
4. Retinal vascular changes.

4. What are the most useful screening tests for RVH?

Several screening tests are available for establishing the diagnosis of RVH in patients with suggestive clinical features.

1. The **rapid sequence intravenous pyelogram** (IVP) is still occasionally used as a screening test for the disease. Findings that suggest significant renal artery obstruction include delay in the function of one kidney, a decrease in renal length of > 1.5 cm on the right or 1 cm on the left, late hyperconcentration of contrast medium in one kidney, or the presence of ureteral notching due to collateral vessels. The utility of the rapid sequence IVP as a screening test for RVH is limited by a high rate of false-positive and false-negative studies.

2. **Isotope renography** with technetium or hippuran has not been a useful diagnostic test for RVH owing to a large number of false-positive results. However, when an angiotension-converting enzyme inhibitor (such as captopril) is added to the standard isotope renogram, the sensitivity and specificity increase considerably, especially for unilateral renal artery stenosis.

3. **Duplex ultrasound scanning** of the renal arteries has become a useful noninvasive screening test for significant renal artery stenosis. When the arterial segment is stenotic, there are

alterations in laminar blood flow and the Doppler signal changes. Although this technique is operator-dependent and time consuming, initial reports indicate sensitivity and specificity rates of 80–90% in patients with renal artery stenosis

4. **Magnetic resonance angiography** is another useful noninvasive technique for imaging the aorta and renal arteries.

5. **Renal arteriography** remains the gold standard for establishing the diagnosis of renal artery stenosis, and **intra-arterial digital subtraction arteriography** is the preferred method.

5. How useful are plasma renin assays?

Differential renal vein plasma renin assays were formerly a popular test; the diagnosis of RVH can be made with 90% accuracy when the renin level from the stenotic kidney is two or more times higher than the renin level from the normal contralateral kidney. However, the finding of nonlateralization with this test is very unreliable, because more than 50% of such patients have ultimately proved to have RVH. In patients with bilateral renal artery stenosis, renal vein renin ratios may be helpful in indicating which kidney is more severely affected.

Measurement of the peripheral plasma renin level is not reliable in identifying patients with RVH. However, the utility of this test can be significantly enhanced by administering an oral dose of captopril and obtaining a repeat plasma renin measurement 1 hour later. Captopril-stimulated peripheral plasma renin activity has become a useful noninvasive test for demonstrating the presence of renin-mediated or renovascular hypertension.

6. How often does RAD cause renal failure?

It is now believed that RAD from atherosclerosis is an important cause of chronic renal failure, and this has been termed *ischemic nephropathy*. Epidemiologic studies have shown that atherosclerotic RAD is quite common in patients with generalized atherosclerosis obliterans, regardless of whether or not RVH is present. Studies on the natural history of atherosclerotic RAD have made it possible to identify patients in whom this disease poses a significant threat to overall renal function. This designation applies to patients with high-grade arterial stenosis affecting both kidneys or a solitary kidney. Intervention to restore normal renal arterial blood flow is indicated in such patients to prevent deterioration of renal function that may culminate in the need for dialytic replacement therapy.

7. What are the treatment options for patients with RAD?

Currently, **four** treatment options are available for patients with severe hypertension, renal insufficiency, or both, resulting from RAD: (1) medical antihypertensive therapy; (2) surgical revascularization or nephrectomy; (3) percutaneous transluminal angioplasty (PTA); and (4) endovascular stenting.

8. What is the appropriate treatment for RVH due to fibrous dysplasia?

In patients with fibrous dysplasia and suspected RVH, the need for interventive treatment (surgery or PTA) is guided by the specific type of disease based on angiographic findings and the associated natural history. **Medical management** of hypertension is the preferred initial treatment for patients with medial fibroplasia because loss of renal function from progressive obstruction is uncommon with this disease. **Interventive treatment** in the latter category is reserved for patients whose blood pressure is difficult to control with multidrug antihypertensive therapy. Conversely, renal artery stenosis due to intimal fibroplasia or perimedial fibroplasia generally progresses and often eventuates in ischemic renal atrophy. Furthermore, these lesions tend to occur in younger patients and cause hypertension that may be difficult to control. Early interventive therapy in these groups is therefore indicated both to preserve renal function and to minimize the need for long-term antihypertensive medication.

The results of **PTA** in patients with main renal artery stenosis due to fibrous dysplasia are excellent and equivalent to those obtained with surgical revascularization. Therefore, PTA is the treatment of choice in such cases. However, as many as 30% of patients with fibrous dysplasia have branch renal arterial involvement, which increases the technical difficulty of PTA and often renders this difficult or impossible to perform. Surgical renal revascularization remains the primary interventive treatment for such patients with branch renal artery disease.

9. What is the appropriate treatment for RVH due to atherosclerosis?

In patients with atherosclerosis and suspected RVH, the indications for interventive therapy (surgery or endovascular stenting) are more restrictive because of their older age and the frequent presence of extrarenal vascular disease. In this group, more vigorous attempts at medical management are warranted and multidrug regimens that control the blood pressure are often the preferred approach, particularly in patients with generalized atherosclerosis. Surgical revascularization or endovascular stenting is more appropriately reserved for patients whose hypertension cannot be controlled or when renal function is threatened by severe stenosis involving both kidneys or a solitary kidney.

In patients with atherosclerotic RAD who require intervention, endovascular stenting has become the initial treatment approach in most cases. The early results of stenting are satisfactory, but recurrent renal artery stenosis ultimately develops in 25–30% of patients due to neointimal hyperplasia. Surgical renal revascularization remains the gold standard for interventive management. However, this is now reserved for patients in whom endovascular stenting is not possible or has failed.

BIBLIOGRAPHY

1. Debatin JJ, Spritzer CE, Grist TM, et al: Imaging of the renal arteries: Value of MR angiography. Am J Radiol 157:981–990, 1991.
2. Fergany A, Kolettis P, Novick AC: The contemporary role of extra-anatomic surgical renal revascularization in patients with atherosclerotic renal artery disease. J Urol 153:1798, 1995.
3. Hansen KJ, Tribble RW, Reavis SW, et al: Renal duplex sonography: Evaluation of clinical utility. J Vasc Surg 12:227–236, 1990.
4. Hayes J, Risius B, Novick AC, et al: Experience with percutaneous transluminal angioplasty for renal artery stenosis at The Cleveland Clinic. J Urol 139:488–492, 1988.
5. Kaylor W, Novick AC, Ziegelbaum M, Vidt D: Reversal of end-stage renal failure with surgical revascularization in patients with atherosclerotic renal artery occlusion. J Urol 141:486–488, 1989.
6. Libertino JA, Bosco PJ, Ying CY, et al: Renal revascularization to preserve and restore renal function. J Urol 147:1485–1487, 1992.
7. Nally JV, Black HR: State-of-the art review: Captopril renography—pathophysiological considerations and clinical observations. Semin Nucl Med 22:85–97, 1992.
8. Novick AC: Surgical correction of renovascular hypertension. Surg Clin North Am 68:1007, 1988.
9. Novick AC, Ziegelbaum M, Vidt DG, et al: Trends in surgical revascularization for renal artery disease: Ten years' experience. JAMA 257:498–501, 1987.
10. Deletion Novick AC, Fergany A: Renal vascular hypertension and ischemic nephropathy. In Walsh P, Wein A, Retik A, Vaughan D (eds): Campbell's Urology, 8th ed, Philadelphia, W.B. Saunders, 2002.
11. Schreiber MJ, Pohl MA, Novick AC: The natural history of atherosclerotic and fibrous renal artery disease. Urol Clin North Am 11:383–392, 1984.
12. Sos TA, Pickering PG, Sniderman KW, et al: Percutaneous transluminal renal angiography in renovascular hypertension due to atheroma or fibrous dysplasia. N Engl J Med 309:274–279, 1983.
13. Steinbach F, Novick AC, Campbell S, Dykstra D: Long-term survival after surgical revascularization for atherosclerotic renal artery disease. J Urol 158:38, 1997.
14. Svetky LP, Himmelstein SL, Dunnick NR, et al: Prospective analysis of strategies for diagnosing renovascular hypertension. Hypertension 14:247–257, 1989.

54. AMBIGUOUS GENITALIA

Robert Kay, M.D.

1. How does the indifferent gonad become the testis or ovary?

The indifferent gonad begins at 6 weeks to become differentiated. The presence of the Y chromosome and genetic material in the short arm of the Y chromosome direct the gonad toward the testis. The absence of the Y chromosome directs the gonad into an ovary.

2. What hormones does the testis produce that are important in sexual differentiation?

Testosterone and müllerian-inhibiting substance.

3. How does testosterone affect sexual differentiation?

Testosterone stimulates the internal genitalia and the wolffian duct to develop. In the male, the wolffian duct becomes the epididymis, vas, and seminal vesicles. In the female, the wolffian duct becomes Gartner's duct at one end and the epoophoron at the other end near the ovary.

4. What is the müllerian-inhibiting substance?

The müllerian-inhibiting substance is a hormone produced by the testis that suppresses the müllerian ducts. The müllerian structures in the female become the fallopian tube of the uterus and the upper third of the vagina. In the male, the müllerian duct regresses to the appendix testis on one end and the prostatic utricle on the other end.

5. What hormones in females lead to sexual differentiation?

In the female, androgen and müllerian-inhibiting factor are not produced. Therefore, the wolffian duct structures do not develop and the müllerian structures do develop. In a child who has no ovaries or testes, they will phenotypically develop as a female and the internal genitalia will be that of a female.

6. What is the most common cause of ambiguous genitalia in the newborn?

Congenital adrenal hyperplasia is the most common cause of ambiguous genitalia in the newborn, and it is the only cause that is potentially life-threatening (due to salt-wasting).

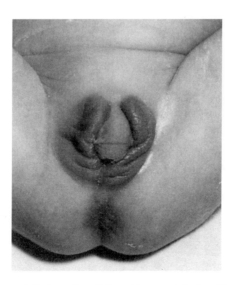

Ambiguous genitalia in newborn infant with congenital adrenal hyperplasia.

7. Describe the evaluation of ambiguous genitalia.

Evaluation of Ambiguous Genitalia

History	Genetic determination
Family history	Karyotype
Pregnancy (drugs, illness)	Biochemical
Physical examination	Plasma 17-OH progesterone
Phallus size	Genitogram
Location of urethra	Ultrasound of pelvis
Labio-scrotal folds	Endoscopy
Palpable gonads	Laparoscopy
Excessive pigmentation	Gonadal biopsy
Rectal (presence of cervix)	

8. What causes masculinization of the male external genitalia?

Testosterone is converted by the enzyme 5 α-reductase to become the active androgen, 5α-dihydrotestosterone. This androgen stimulates the indifferent external genitalia toward the male external genitalia.

9. At what gestational age does the male external genitalia develop?

By the end of the third month, the development is complete, with further growth of the phallus shortly before birth.

10. Which physical characteristic helps assess male differentiation in the newborn?

The palpable gonad is usually a testis and suggests male differentiation. Rarely, an ovary can be palpated with a large inguinal hernia, but in general, if a gonad is palpated, it is a testis.

11. What is the most common enzymatic defect in congenital adrenal hyperplasia?

21-Hydroxylase deficiency accounts for 90% of cases of congenital adrenal hyperplasia.

12. Can a blood test confirm congenital adrenal hyperplasia?

Plasma 17-hydroxyprogesterone is a sensitive marker for congenital adrenal hyperplasia.

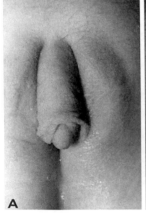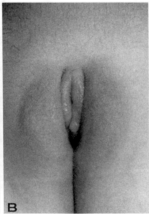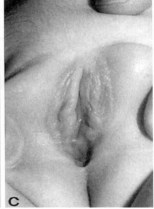

External genitalia of a child with late-onset congenital adrenal hyperplasia. Note virilization. **B** and **C,** External genitalia of the child following surgical repair.

13. How do children with 21-hydroxylase deficiency and 11β-hydroxylase deficiency differ clinically?

Children with 11β-hydroxylase deficiency may have hypertension secondary to a buildup of deoxycorticosterone (DOCA).

14. Are there nonadrenal factors that lead to virilization of the female newborn?

Yes. Maternal progestational agents taken in the first trimester of life or virilizing tumors in the mother may lead to virilization of the child.

15. Define true hermaphroditism.

True hermaphroditism is defined as having the presence of both ovarian and testicular tissue.

16. What is the karyotype of true hermaphroditism?

Although there is some geographical variation, approximately 50% of all true hermaphrodites are 46XX, and 50% are divided between a mosaicism and 46XY.

17. What tumors are most often seen in the gonads of intersexual patients?

Gonadoblastoma and dysgerminoma.

18. How do children with complete testicular feminization come to attention?

Patients with complete testicular feminization or total androgen insensitivity present either with a testis found during inguinal surgery or, more likely, during an evaluation of primary amenorrhea.

19. How are testosterone and luteinizing hormone levels affected in patients with complete testicular feminization?

Both are significantly elevated. Because the pituitary cannot detect testosterone owing to total androgen insensitivity, gonadotropins are increased and stimulate the testis to release testosterone.

20. What do Reifenstein, Gilbert-Dreyfus, Lubs, and Rosewater have in common?

All are syndromes seen in patients with partial androgen insensitivity.

21. What is the second most common cause of ambiguous genitalia in the newborn?

Mixed gonadal dysgenesis.

22. What is the classic karyotype for mixed gonadal dysgenesis?

45XO/46XY.

23. Describe the internal genitalia in mixed gonadal dysgenesis.

The internal genitalia in mixed gonadal dysgenesis is almost always a testis on one side and a streak gonad on the other. On the side of the testis, the vas and epididymis may be normal, while on the side of the streak gonad (usually a fallopian tube and uterus are present).

24. Describe the Denys-Drash syndrome.

Denys-Drash syndrome refers to children with ambiguous genitalia, glomerulonephritis or other renal abnormalities, and Wilms tumor.

BIBLIOGRAPHY

1. Aaronson IA: Sexual differentiation and intersexuality. In Kelalis PP, King LR, Belman AB (eds): Clinical Pediatric Urology, 3rd ed. Philadelphia, W. B. Saunders, 1992.
2. Allen TD: Disorders of sexual differentiation. Urology 7:1, 1976.

3. Donahoe PK: The diagnosis and treatment of infants with intersex abnormalities. Pediatr Clin North Am 34:1333, 1987.
4. Donahoe PK, Ito Y, Morikawa Y, Hendren WH: Müllerian inhibiting substance in human testes after birth. J Pediatr Surg 12:323, 1977.
5. Federman D, Donahoe P: Ambiguous genitalia—Etiology, diagnosis, and therapy. Advances in Endocrinology and Metabolism, vol 6. St. Louis, Mosby–Year Book Inc, 1995, pp 91–117.
6. Gosalbez R, Castellan M, Kim C: The use of ureter for vaginal reconstruction. J Urol 160:2143, 1998. In Walsh PC, Retik AB, Vaughan ED Jr, Wein AJ (eds): Campbell's Urology, 7th ed. Philadelphia, W.B. Saunders, 1998, pp 2145–2154.
7. Howe EG: Intersexuality: What should careproviders do now. J Clin Ethics 9:337, 1998.
8. Jensen JC, Ehrlich RM, Hanna MK, et al: A report of 4 patients with Drash syndrome and a review of the literature. J Urol 141:1174, 1989.
9. Mandell J: Sexual differentiation: Normal and abnormal.
10. Pagan RA: Diagnostic approach to the newborn with ambiguous genitalia. Pediatr Clin North Am 34:1019, 1987.
11. Sloan WR, Walsh PC: Familial persistent müllerian duct syndrome. J Urol 115:459, 1976
12. Shobert JM: Sexual behaviors, sexual orientation and gender identity in adult intersexuals. J Urol 165:2350–2353, 2001.
13. Walsh PC, Madden JD, Harrod MJ, et al: Familial incomplete male pseudohermaphroditism, type 2: Reversed dihydrotestosterone formation in pseudovaginal perineoscrotal hypospadias. N Engl J Med 291:944, 1974.
14. White PC, New MI, Dupont B: Congenital adrenal hyperplasia. N Engl J Med 316:1519, 1987.

55. CRYPTORCHIDISM

Jonathan H. Ross, M.D.

1. Explain the difference between a cryptorchid testis and an ectopic testis.

A cryptorchid testis is a testis that is located along the normal path of descent but has failed to reach a dependent position in the scrotum. Ectopic testes are misdirected to an ectopic site. Possible locations for ectopic testes include perineal, prepenile, contralateral scrotal, femoral, and umbilical sites.

2. Where are most undescended testes located?

The inguinal canal.

3. What is the incidence of cryptorchidism at birth?

In term infants, 3.4%; in premature infants, 30%.

4. Can an undescended testis descend spontaneously?

Yes, but only in the first year of life (and most descend in the first 3 months). Approximately 74% of undescended testes in term infants and 95% of undescended testes in premature infants will descend spontaneously.

5. What is the normal mechanism of testicular descent?

Several theories exist, and normal descent may indeed be multifactorial. The most commonly proposed factors include:

1. Downward traction by the gubernaculum.
2. Differential growth of the body relative to the spermatic cord and gubernaculum.
3. Increased intraabdominal pressure pushing the testis through the internal ring.
4. Development and maturation of the epididymis.
5. Endocrinologic factors.

6. Why is the finding of hypospadias in association with cryptorchidism significant?

It raises the possibility of intersex. A female with congenital adrenal hyperplasia may present with hypospadias and bilateral impalpable gonads, and a male with mixed gonadal dysgenesis may present with hypospadias and unilateral or bilateral undescended gonads. Of course, many children with hypospadias and cryptorchidism are not intersex patients.

7. What is a retractile testis?

A retractile testis is a normal testis. The term really describes a finding artificially created by the environment of the doctor's office. When a child is cold and frightened, the cremasteric reflex is activated, and the testis may be pulled out of the scrotum temporarily. Children with particularly active cremasteric reflexes (or children who are especially cold and frightened) may appear to have an undescended testis.

8. How can one distinguish a retractile testis from an undescended testis?

The following suggest the testis is retractile:

1. The parents report that when the child is relaxed (particularly in a warm bath), the testis is in the scrotum.
2. The testis can be milked into the scrotum and remains there, at least temporarily, without tension.
3. The hemiscrotum is well developed on the side in question.
4. Serial examination several months apart may clarify an equivocal case.
5. Hormonal therapy.

9. What is the most common treatment for an undescended testicle?
Orchiopexy.

10. What is hormonal therapy?
The administration of human chorionic gonadotropin (hCG), 5,000–10,000 units given in several injections over a period of 2–4 weeks, is used to stimulate descent without an operation. Gonadotropin-releasing hormone (GnRH) nasal spray has been used in Europe but is not approved for use in the United States.

11. How successful is hormonal therapy?
There is widespread disagreement on this point. Reported success rates range from 6–70%. The true efficacy is probably in the range of 10–20%. Series reporting higher success rates probably include a large number of patients with retractile testes that are known to "descend" in response to hCG.

12. What are the roles of MRI, CT, and ultrasound in localizing an impalpable testis?
Very limited. The differential diagnosis of an impalpable testis is an intraabdominal testis or an absent testis. If an imaging study identifies an intraabdominal testis, then an operation is indicated. Because of a significant false-negative rate with each of these studies, failure to demonstrate a testis does not prove that it is absent. Therefore, patients with a negative imaging study also require an operation. Because the imaging study will not alter the management of the patient, it is not indicated. The rare exception is an obese boy with an impalpable testis. Inguinal ultrasound may identify a testis, precluding the need for laparoscopy.

13. What biochemical test can be used to prove anorchia in a patient with bilateral impalpable testes?
Elevated baseline serum gonadotropin levels and castrate levels of serum testosterone after hCG stimulation.

14. How do you definitively locate an impalpable testis?
Surgical exploration is the gold standard. This can be accomplished laparoscopically, though occasionally a high intraabdominal testis may not be visualized.

15. If an intraabdominal testis is discovered at laparoscopy, what are the options for management?
1. Immediate orchiopexy, if the vessels are thought to be long enough to allow it.
2. Laparoscopic ligation of the testicular artery, which stimulates enlargement of collateral vessels. Six months later, the testicular artery is divided and the testis brought down on a pedicle of collateral vessels (Fowler-Stephens orchidopexy).
3. Laparoscopic orchiectomy, if the testis is grossly abnormal, or if the patient is postpubertal and has a normal contralateral testis.

16. If blind-ending vessels and vas are discovered at laparoscopy, what should be done?
The finding of blind-ending vessels confirms anorchia, and nothing further need be done.

17. If a blind-ending vas is discovered at laparoscopy and the vessels are not identified, what should be done?
A blind-ending vas does not confirm the diagnosis of anorchia. The vessels must be identified. If they cannot be, then an exploration is indicated to rule out a high intraabdominal testis that was missed laparoscopically.

18. On laparoscopy, the vas and vessels are seen to enter the internal ring. Describe the management options.

If a hernia is present, then the patient probably has an undescended testis at the internal ring. These can move into and out of the abdomen (so-called **peeping** testis), accounting for the failure to palpate them on physical examination. Palpation over the inguinal canal during laparoscopy may push the testis into the abdomen where it can be seen. An inguinal exploration or laparoscopic orchidopexy should be performed.

If the testis is impalpable and the internal ring is closed, then the patient probably has a **vanishing** testis. This occurs when a testis descends beyond the internal ring and then is lost, probably to prenatal torsion. Some pediatric urologists believe that in this circumstance, no exploration is needed. Others claim that an inguinal exploration is required to excise an atrophic remnant that may contain some viable seminiferous tubules with malignant potential and to rule out an inguinal testis missed on physical exam.

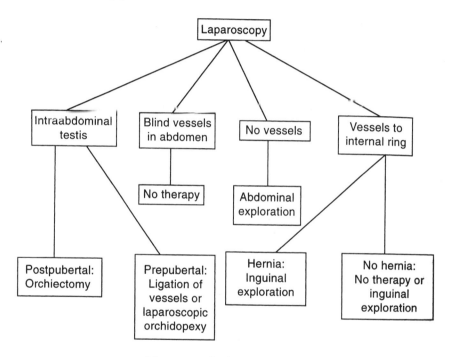

Management of an impalpable testis.

19. List four complications of an undescended testis.

1. **Testicular cancer** is approximately 5–10 times more common in undescended testes. The risk is greatest for intraabdominal testes.

2. **Torsion** is more common in undescended testes.

3. A **patent processus vaginalis** (hernia) is present in nearly all cases, although it is rarely a clinical problem.

4. **Infertility** may occur, particularly in patients with bilateral undescended testes, of whom approximately 50% are infertile.

20. What is the most common tumor in a cryptorchid testis?

Seminoma.

21. Is the contralateral testis at risk for tumor?

Yes. Twenty percent of tumors in patients with unilateral cryptorchidism occur in the contralateral testis. In a patient with bilateral cryptorchidism and a testis tumor, there is a 15% chance that a contralateral tumor will develop. If both testes are intraabdominal, the risk is 30%.

22. What is the significance of testicular torsion of a cryptorchid testis in an adult?

More than 50% will be found to have a tumor. This diagnosis should be considered in a man with abdominal pain and an empty hemiscrotum.

23. Do patients with unilateral cryptorchidism have a normal contralateral testis?

No. There is a significant decrease in sperm density of the contralateral testis with a mild decrease in clinical fertility.

BIBLIOGRAPHY

 1. Andrews PE, Malek RS: Unilateral cryptorchidism in adults. In Resnick MI, Kursh ED (eds): Current Therapy in Genitourinary Surgery. St. Louis, Mosby, 1992, pp 339–344.
 2. Cendron M, Huff D, Keating MA, et al: Anatomical, morphological and volumetric analysis: A review of 759 cases of testicular maldescent. J Urol 149:570–573, 1993.
 3. Hrebinko RL, Bellinger MF: The limited role of imaging techniques in managing children with undescended testes. J Urol 150:458–460, 1993.
 4. Joseph DB, Bauer SB: Bilateral cryptorchidism. In Resnick MI, Kursh ED (eds): Current Therapy in Genitourinary Surgery. St. Louis, Mosby, 1992, pp 344–346.
 5. Kaplan GW: Unilateral cryptorchidism in children. In Resnick MI, Kursh ED (eds): Current Therapy in Genitourinary Surgery. St. Louis, Mosby, 1992, pp 336–339.
 6. Kogan S, Hadziselimovic, Howards SS, et al: Pediatric andrology. In Gillenwater JY, Grayhack JT, Howards SS, Duckett JW (eds): Adult and Pediatric Urology, 3rd ed. St. Louis, Mosby, 1996, pp 2629–2634, 2749–2752.
 7. Moore RG, Peters CA, Bauer SB, et al: Laparoscopic evaluation of the nonpalpable testis: A prospective assessment of accuracy. J Urol 151:728–731, 1994.
 8. Rajfer J, Handelsman DJ, Swerdloff RS, et al: Hormonal therapy of cryptorchidism. N Engl J Med 314:466–470, 1986.
 9. Tennenbaum SY, Lerner SE, McAleer IM, et al: Preoperative laparoscopic localization of the nonpalpable testis: A critical analysis of a 10-year experience. J Urol 151:732–734, 1994.
10. Turek PJ, Ewaslt DH, Synder HM III, et al: The absent cryptorchid testis: Surgical findings and their implications for diagnosis and etiology. J Urol 151:718–721, 1994.

56. SCROTAL MASS IN ADULTS

J. Patrick Spirnak, M.D.

1. What is the most common malignant scrotal mass?
Testicular cancer. It is the most common solid cancer in young adult males between ages 15 and 34 years.

2. What is the most common benign scrotal mass?
Hydrocele, occurring in an estimated 1% of adult males.

3. Define a hydrocele.
A hydrocele is a collection of serous fluid between the two layers of the tunica vaginalis.

4. What causes a hydrocele to form?
Any process that acts to stimulate increased production of serous fluid (e.g., tumor, inflammation, trauma) by the tunica vaginalis or to decrease the resorption of this fluid (e.g., inguinal surgery) by the scrotal lymphatics or venous system will result in hydrocele formation.

5. What is the characteristic physical finding of a hydrocele?
A smooth, cystic-feeling mass completely surrounding the testicle and not involving the spermatic cord is typical of a hydrocele. In addition, it readily transilluminates.

6. When is scrotal ultrasonography indicated in the evaluation of suspected hydrocele?
When a hydrocele is large and testicular palpation is not possible.

7. How are hydroceles treated?
Small asymptomatic hydroceles require no treatment other than patient reassurance. Surgical excision is recommended when the hydrocele is large and symptomatic.

8. Is aspiration ever indicated as a means of treatment?
Needle aspiration is a treatment option usually reserved for individuals who are poor surgical candidates. Unfortunately, fluid usually reaccumulates and the hydrocele recurs.

9. What is a spermatocele?
It is a sperm-containing cyst that usually arises from the head of the epididymis.

10. What causes a spermatocele to form?
A spermatocele may be idiopathic or due to ductal obstruction, usually caused by trauma or inflammation.

11. How does one differentiate a spermatocele from a hydrocele on physical examination?
A spermatocele is palpable as a cystic, nontender nodule, usually arising superior to the testicle. Unlike a hydrocele, a spermatocele allows complete palpation of the entire testis.

12. When is surgical excision indicated?
Surgical excision is indicated when the spermatocele is large and symptomatic, or when it is socially embarrassing to the individual.

13. What is a varicocele?
A varicocele is an abnormal dilation of the veins of the pampiniform plexus. It is present in

about 15% of adult men. It may be primary and due to a congenital anomaly of the venous valves, or secondary and due to any abdominal or retroperitoneal process obstructing the venous system.

14. Do varicoceles occur equally on right and left sides?
No. Clinical varicoceles occur more commonly on the left side.

15. Why are varicoceles more common on the left side?
The left testicular vein drains into the left renal vein and inserts at a 90° angle, whereas the right testicular vein inserts obliquely into the inferior vena cava.

16. Describe the physical findings of a large varicocele.
With the patient standing, a large varicocele appears as an irregular, worm-like mass beneath the scrotal skin overlying the spermatic cord. It is cystic on palpation and increases in size with a Valsalva maneuver. Primary varicoceles disappear when the patient is supine. Testicular atrophy may also be present.

17. Can a hernia ever present as scrotal mass?
Yes. A large, indirect inguinal hernia may contain small bowel located within the scrotum.

18. How can one differentiate an indirect inguinal hernia from other common causes of scrotal swelling?
Small, indirect inguinal hernias are typically palpated when the patient coughs or performs a Valsalva maneuver. Large hernias can usually be reduced with the patient supine. Hydroceles, spermatoceles, and testicular tumors do not change with a Valsalva maneuver and cannot be reduced.

19. What is the treatment of an inguinal hernia?
Surgical repair.

20. How does a testicular cancer usually present?
The typical patient presents with a painless testicular mass.

21. What is the treatment of a solid testicular mass?
Inguinal exploration with orchiectomy.

22. Is scrotal ultrasound ever indicated in the evaluation of a solid testicular mass?
Ultrasound is performed when the physical findings are inconclusive and one is unable to determine whether the mass is rising from the epididymis or from the testis.

BIBLIOGRAPHY

1. Donohue JP (ed): Testes Tumors. Baltimore, Williams & Wilkins, 1983.
2. Fournier GR, Laing FC, Jeffrey B, et al: High resolution scrotal ultrasound. J Urol 134:490, 1985.
3. Papanicolaou N: Urinary tract imaging and intervention: Basic principles. In Walsh PC, Retik AB, Vaughan ED Jr, Wein AJ (eds): Campbell's Urology, 7th ed. Philadelphia, W.B. Saunders, 1998, pp 170–260.
4. Spirnak JP: Adult scrotal mass. In Resnick MI, Caldamone AA, Spirnak JP (eds): Decision Making in Urology. Toronto, B. C. Decker, 1985, p 184.
5. Spirnak JP, Resnick MI: Hydrocele repair, the Lord procedure. Contemp Urol 1989, p 55.
6. Zornow DH, Landes RR: Scrotal palpation. Am Fam Physician 23:150, 1981.

57. VARICOCELE

James A. Daitch, M.D., and Anthony J. Thomas, Jr., M.D.

1. What is a varicocele?

A varicocele is a dilatation of the veins of the pampiniform plexus of the spermatic cord. The engorgement is caused by a lack of valves within the vein(s). The condition is apparent when the affected man is in the upright position. Varicoceles are present in approximately 15% of men, and about 30% of subfertile men have a varicocele. Varicoceles usually become apparent at puberty. Most affect the left testis, but they may be found on both sides or occasionally on the right side only.

2. What is the clinical significance of a varicocele?

In men with either unilateral or bilateral varicoceles, sperm quality may range from an azoospermic state to minimal or no abnormality in the semen. Some men with a unilateral varicocele may exhibit a measurable ipsilateral loss in testicular size. A varicocele rarely causes discomfort, but men who complain of testicular pain associated with this condition often describe it as a "heaviness or dull ache" on the affected side, particularly evident after long periods of standing or heavy exercise. Assuming the supine position and elevating the scrotum should quickly resolve pain due to a varicocele.

3. What methods are useful to identify a varicocele?

The most common method of identifying a varicocele is direct examination of the patient's scrotum when he is standing upright in a warm, well-lighted room. The veins of a moderate or large varicocele bulge outward above and often behind the affected testis. Smaller varicoceles may be palpable and increase in size when the patient performs a Valsalva maneuver. Using a simple, 5.3-MHz Doppler stethoscope over the suspected varicocele, the examiner can hear an audible rush of blood when the patient performs a Valsalva maneuver. When the patient is recumbent, the varicocele should collapse as the testis is elevated. If the varicocele does not collapse in the recumbent position, an underlying retroperitoneal process impairing spermatic vein drainage should be suspected (i.e., neoplasm). Color Doppler ultrasound has been used to identify smaller, so-called subclinical varicoceles that are difficult to palpate. Some investigators question the clinical significance of this "subclinical" entity.

4. What causes the alterations in sperm quality associated with a varicocele?

Many theories have been proposed, including increased testicular temperature, reflux of adrenal/renal metabolites into the spermatic vein, testicular hypoxia due to venous stasis, small vessel occlusion leading to Leydig and germinal cell dysfunction, and depressed androgen secretion. Of the many theories, the most widely accepted is increased testicular temperature. The temperature in both testicles increases, even in the presence of a unilateral varicocele. Recent studies have demonstrated higher reactive oxygen species (hydrogen peroxide and highly unstable oxygen free radicals) levels in men with varicoceles. High levels of reactive oxygen species may damage sperm.

5. Is any risk other than infertility or pain associated with varicocele?

No specific health risks are associated with a varicocele other than the possibility of impaired sperm quality, which does not affect all men with varicoceles. Some men have a smaller testis on the ipsilateral side, and an increased incidence of sperm antibodies has been noted in men with varicoceles. Sperm quality may gradually diminish over time in some men. Varicoceles have been noted to be a prominent finding in men who seek medical attention for secondary infertility.

6. If not all men with varicoceles are infertile, what are the indications for recommending correction?

1. **Impaired sperm quality.** Impairment may range from azoospermia associated with maturational arrest to mild impairment in concentration or motility. In a small percentage of non-obstructive azoospermic or severely oligospermic men with atrophic, scarred testes or testicles that demonstrate Sertoli Cells Only by biopsy, correction of the varicocele(s) may improve sperm production to a mild degree.

2. **Pain.** Although relatively uncommon, a "dull ache" is highly characteristic. A careful and thorough history should differentiate men who stand a good chance of pain relief from men with other causes of testicular pain.

3. **Cosmetic indications,** particularly in the presence of a large varicocele in an adolescent, most of whom are particularly conscious of their genitals and have a great desire to be "like everyone else."

4. **Failure of the affected testis to grow** compared with its contralateral partner in the young adolescent (see question 11).

7. Is there an optimal method or surgical approach to correct a varicocele?

Five techniques are used to obliterate a varicocele: (1) retroperitoneal approach; (2) inguinal approach; (3) subinguinal incision; (4) laparoscopic clipping; and (5) transvenous embolization. Each method can be effective in the proper hands. Most urologists are familiar with the inguinal incision and ligation. Special training is required for the laparoscopic technique because it pre-

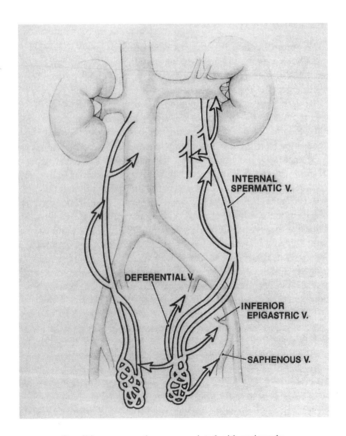

Possible venous pathways associated with varicocele.

sents greater risks to the patient than the standard surgical approaches. Unless laparoscopy is done with sufficient frequency to maintain proficiency, it is not recommended to be used for varicocele obliteration. Inguinal and subinguinal incisions seem to provide the surgeon with the best chance of ligating all the major venous channels and collaterals (see figure below). The authors prefer a subinguinal microsurgical approach that facilitates identification of all the spermatic cord structures while minimizing operative morbidity. Transvenous embolization, when done by a skilled interventional radiologist, may be as effective and safe as surgery and may allow a faster return to full activity.

8. Why do some varicoceles persist after surgery or embolization?

The estimated failure rate of varicocele surgery is 0–10%, depending on the series. The most obvious explanation is a missed vein that was not ligated or embolized. A number of collateral channels may be associated with the varicocele, and the spermatic cord must be scrutinized carefully at the time of surgery. Particularly large varicoceles often have posterior collateral veins that traverse the floor of the inguinal canal and enter the iliac vein below. Careful dissection of the cord, preserving the testicular artery, the vas deferens with its associated vessels, and the lymphatics, minimizes failure. It is also helpful to place a Penrose drain beneath the cord and to lift upward, pulling the testis toward the incision to identify and ligate any perforating veins that travel toward the iliac or hypogastric veins. Failure of embolization procedures usually is due to the inability of the radiologist to catheterize a collateral vein because of the angle at which it branches from the main vein or because of its proximity to the testis.

9. What is the anticipated rate of improvement in sperm quality and fertility?

Rates of improvement in sperm quality and subsequent fertility vary depending on the investigator and the series size. Some report no improvement, whereas others report improvement in as many as 75% of patients. The true rate is probably somewhere between the two extremes. When the statistics from many large studies are combined, approximately two-thirds of patients showed some improvement in some of their semen parameters, and 40% established pregnancies with their partners. Statistics vary with factors such as the partner's fertility potential, sperm–cervical mucus interaction, and frequency of intercourse.

In addition, pregnancy rates of 20–30% have been achieved after varicocele repair among subfertile men who could not achieve a pregnancy by coitus and in whom intrauterine insemination or in vitro fertilization was unsuccessful.

10. What are the potential complications of varicocele surgery or embolization?

Major complications are rare with surgery but may include wound infection, hematoma, hydrocele, and even testicular atrophy. Hydroceles can be prevented by carefully preserving the lymphatic vessels that parallel the testicular artery and veins. Testicular atrophy may occur as a consequence of inadvertent or intentional ligation and division of the testicular artery. Of note, some investigators report routine ligation of the artery and vein in the retroperitoneum without subsequent atrophy. Routine ligation is not recommended, however, because the vasal artery and other small branches may be insufficient to sustain normal testicular function, even with no measurable change in size of the testis. Laparoscopy, particularly in less experienced hands, involves the risk of bowel injury by perforation or coagulation, major vascular injury, and even inadvertent ligation of the ureter, which may be mistaken for the spermatic vein. In experienced hands, laparoscopy appears as safe and effective as open surgery. Complications during and after percutaneous embolization are also related to the experience of the interventional radiologist. Occlusive balloons involve the risk of migration to the pulmonary arteries, but because of their small size, they may be tolerated without sequelae. Stainless steel coils, hot contrast, and concentrated dextrose solutions (70% dextrose) are suitable alternatives that remain popular and equally safe with some radiologists. Other complications of the percutaneous technique relate to venous access, which may result in deep vein thrombosis, venous perforation, adverse reaction to contrast material, or hematoma at the site of puncture.

11. If a varicocele is discovered during a routine school physical in an adolescent boy, should anything be done?

There is considerable controversy about whether to recommend correction or observation. Most urologists favor correction of the varicocele if the involved testis is significantly smaller ($\geq$ 20% reduction) than its contralateral mate, or if the involved testis fails to grow normally as the boy is followed from year to year. Some evidence suggests that compensatory growth may occur after obliteration of the varicocele; for this reason alone, fertility potential may be greater if correction is immediate rather than delayed until the young man is trying to father children. Whether immediate correction alters fertility is yet to be completely proved, but at this point it seems a reasonable approach. It is not appropriate to request a semen sample from adolescent boys, nor is it wise to focus so much attention on scrotal contents that they perceive themselves as "sexually abnormal." If the testes are of equal size and growing normally, the young man needs to be seen only on a yearly basis to ensure that atrophy does not occur; if it does, correction is recommended. Prospective studies of boys and young men with varicoceles are in progress; it will be some time before an optimal answer is available.

BIBLIOGRAPHY

 1. Ashkenazi J, Dicker D, Feldberg D, et al: The impact of spermatic vein ligation on the male factor in in vitro fertilization—embryo transfer and its relation to testosterone levels before and after operation. Fertil Steril 51:471–474, 1989.
 2. Comhaire F: The pathogenesis of epididymo-testicular dysfunction in varicocele: Factors other than temperature. Adv Exp Med Biol 286:281–287, 1991.
 3. Constabile RA, Skoog S, Radowich M: Testicular volume assessment in the adolescent with a varicocele. J Urol 147:1348–1350, 1992.
 4. Dewire DM, Thomas AJ Jr, Falk RM, et al: Clinical outcome and cost comparison of percutaneous embolization and surgical ligation of varicocele. J Androl 15:38s–41s, 1994.
 5. Gorelick JI, Goldstein M: Loss of fertility in men with varicocele. Fertil Steril 59:613–616, 1993.
 6. Howards SS: Subclinical varicocele [editorial]. Fertil Steril 57:725–726, 1992.
 7. Kondoh N, Meguro N, Matsumiya K, et al: Significance of subclinical varicocele detected by scrotal sonography in male infertility: A preliminary report. J Urol 150:1158–1160, 1993.
 8. Laven JS, Haans LC, Mali WP, et al: Effects of varicocele treatment in adolescents: A randomized study. Fertil Steril 58:756–762, 1992.
 9. Lemack GE, Uzzo RG, Schlegel PN, et al: Microsurgical repair of the adolescent varicocele. J Urol 160: 179–181, 1998.
10. Marmar JL, Corson SL, Batzer FR, et al: Insemination data on men with varicoceles. Fertil Steril 57: 1084–1090, 1992.
11. Matthews GJ, Matthews ED, Goldstein M: Induction of spermatogenesis and achievement of pregnancy after microsurgical varicocelectomy in men with azoospermia and severe oligoasthenospermia. Fertil Steril 70:71–75, 1998.
12. McClure RD, Khoo D, Jarvi K, et al: Subclinical varicocele: The effectiveness of varicocelectomy. J Urol 145:789–791, 1991.
13. Mehan DJ, Andrus CH, Parra RO: Laparoscopic internal spermatic vein ligation: Report of a new technique. Fertil Steril 58:1263–1266, 1992.
14. Sharma RK, Agarwal A: Role of reactive oxygen species in male infertility. Urology 48:835–850, 1996.
15. Takihara H, Sakatoku J, Cockett AT: The pathophysiology of varicocele in male infertility. Fertil Steril 55:861–868, 1991.
16. Thomas AJ, Geisinger MA: Current management of varicoceles. Urol Clin North Am 17:893–907, 1990.
17. Witt MA, Lipshultz LI: Varicocele: A progressive or static lesion. Urology 42:541–543, 1993.

58. PELVIC ORGAN PROLAPSE

Raymond R. Rackley, MD

1. What is pelvic organ prolapse?

Pelvic organ prolapse is a commonly occurring condition in women that may involve a single or multiple pelvic organ structure such as the urethra (urethrocele), bladder (cystocele), uterus, small bowel (enterocele), or rectum (rectocele). Some degree of pelvic organ prolapse is estimated to occur in 50–100% of multiparous women, 20% of whom are usually symptomatic. Pelvic organ prolapse may produce symptoms reflecting a minimal effect on the supportive structures of the genitourinary and bowel system or major effects on the function of normal urinary, bowel, and sexual physiology. Typical presenting symptoms of patients with pelvic organ prolapse may be irritative and obstructive voiding, recurrent urinary tract infections due to elevated postvoid residuals in individuals susceptible to infections, defecating dysfunction, pelvic or lower back and abdominal pain, and dyspareunia. Recent epidemiologic studies reveal variations in the incidence, symptoms, and pathogenesis of prolapse in different ethnic groups.

2. How does pelvic organ prolapse occur?

The female pelvic organs are supported within the pelvis by a complex array of fascial and muscular structures. Prolapse occurs when a breakdown or weakness occurs in one or more areas of the musculofascial support system. Most women may have multiple etiologic factors that can be identified as potential causes of musculofascial injury, such as vaginal delivery, straining due to chronic constipation, or pulmonary disease, pelvic surgery, advancing age (maturational changes of collagen, elastin, muscle), connective tissue disorders, and menopause (estrogen deficiency). Many of these causes of musculofascial injury may be due to direct ruptures of support or an indirect result of pelvic or pudendal nerve injury that leads to loss of muscle support of fascia with resultant fascial tearing and stretching. For the minority of women without identifiable causes of musculofascial or nerve injury, biomechanical analyses of motion and molecular analyses of changes in collagen, elastin, and muscle composition may explain the development of laxity in pelvic organ support.

3. What are the grading systems for pelvic organ prolapse?

The interposition of the vaginal vault between pelvic organs has been historically characterized in terms of the anterior, apical, and posterior compartments. Within these compartments, various defects of pelvic organ support can occur. The defects encountered in the anterior vaginal vault are urethral hypermobility and cystocele formation; the defects in the apical vaginal vault are uterine prolapse and enterocele formation; and the defects of the posterior vaginal wall are rectocele formation and perineal body laxity. More recently, the compartmental description of pelvic organ prolapse has been replaced by using the levels of vaginal vault support as a means to better conceptualize the defects of the supportive structures of the pelvic organs.

Vaginal Vault Support

LEVELS	MUSCULOFASCIAL SUPPORT STRUCTURES	COMPARTMENTAL FINDINGS
Level I	Uterosacral, broad, cardinal ligaments	Uterine prolapse, enterocele
Level II	Pubocervical and perirectal fascia	Cystocele, rectocele
Level III	Pubourethral complex, perineal body	Urethrocele, perineal body laxity

Grading pelvic organ prolapse can be used to longitudinally follow the magnitude of site-specific change, to determine treatment options, and to monitor the outcome of interventions selected. Although while (Material Deleted) the International Continence Society System has recently been (Material Deleted) introduced the pelvic organ prolapse quantification (POP-Q) system as a reproducible method of grading specific sites of pelvic organ prolapse, the favored method of grading prolapse remains the practical "halfway system" of Baden and Walker. With the patient straining in the lithotomy position, the grade of prolapse using the halfway system is determined by the level of descent for each of the pelvic organs separately within the vaginal vault in relation to the fixed reference point of the hymenal ring. The higher grade is always chosen when an intermediate level of descent is found.

Halfway System of Grading Prolapse with Patient Straining

GRADE OF PROLAPSE	FINDINGS OF PELVIC ORGAN POSITION
0	Normal position for each site
1	Descent halfway to hymen
2	Descent to hymen
3	Descent halfway past hymen
4	Maximum possible descent for each site

For the POP-Q system, specific sites are defined separately on the anterior, posterior, and apical vaginal compartments and are measured with respect to the fixed reference point, the hymen. These measurements can then be catergorized into an ordinal staging system ranging from 0–4.

POP-Q Staging System

STAGE OF PROLAPSE	FINDINGS OF VAGINAL POSITION
0	No prolapse (descent of the apex is allowed as far as 2 cm relative to total vaginal length)
1	Most distal portion of the prolapse descends to a point that is farther than 1 cm above the hymen
2	The most maximal extent of the prolapse is within 1 cm of the hymen (outside or inside the vagina)
3	The prolapse extends more than 1 cm beyond the hymen but no farther than within 2 cm of the total vaginal length
4	Complete vaginal eversion defined as extending to within 2 cm of total vaginal length

4. How does one evaluate pelvic organ prolapse?

The evaluation of the patient with pelvic organ prolapse begins by focusing on the review of systems from the urinary, bowel, sexual function, and neurologic aspects of a thorough history. A detailed obstetric/gynecologic history and history of prior interventions are needed in order to understand the context of the patient's symptom complex.

A careful and systematic pelvic examination should be performed in which each level of vaginal vault support is evaluated at rest and with straining. If prolapse is found, it should be graded. Patients may need to be evaluated in the standing position to accentuate the degree of pelvic organ prolapse. A postvoid residual should be checked and a provocative stress test for urinary incontinence is routinely performed.

5. What are the effects of pelvic prolapse on lower urinary tract function?

The most common form of prolapse affecting the lower urinary tract function is cystocele formation. Urinary incontinence, bladder outlet obstruction, and urinary retention can occur with pelvic organ prolapse as well as result from the various medical treatments and surgical procedures chosen to treat these disorders. Therefore, urodynamic evaluation plays an important role in the assessment of a patient before recommending specific management and treatment options.

In patients with large cystocele formation that is often associated with prolapse of other pelvic organs, the ureters also tend to prolapse outside of the pelvis, which may lead to ureteral obstruction and hydronephrosis. Increasing grades of prolapse (grades 3 and 4) are associated with an increasing incidence of hydronephrosis.

In addition to cystocele formation, prolapse of other pelvic organs independent or in conjunction with bladder prolapse can cause irritative and obstructive symptoms as well as urinary retention. In addition to pudendal nerve stretching and its irritative effect on the bladder from rectal fullness due to constipation, a large rectocele can compress the urethra and bladder neck from below, causing obstruction and urinary retention. Uterine prolapse and enterocele formation may cause similar findings due to direct external compression or kinking of the bladder neck and urethra during organ descent. In patients with impaired detrusor contractility due to medical illnesses, maturation changes, or polypharmacy, less compression or distortion is needed to effect the function of the lower urinary tract.

6. What are the treatments for pelvic organ prolapse?

Treatment of pelvic organ prolapse is usually reserved for the symptomatic patient. Conservative therapies consist of options designed to maximize the physiology of the prolapsed organ. These choices, often considered management options, may consist of behavior and diet modifications of urinary and bowel function, incorporating forms of pelvic floor biofeedback, use of vaginal pessaries, performing intermittent straight catheterization of the bladder, and manual repositioning of the prolapsed pelvic organ. More definitive treatment involves the surgical repair of all the prolapsing components combined with the conservative management options just described.

Techniques for repairing urethrocele formation and anatomic stress urinary incontinence are described in chapter 43. Cystocele repairs depend upon the grade and type (central, lateral, or combination) of defects detected and are often combined with procedures for anatomic stress urinary incontinence. Uterine prolapse is most commonly treated by hysterectomy (abdominal or vaginal approach) because uterine suspension procedures have a high failure rate. Enteroceles that may form after a hysterectomy may be repaired by a transvaginal or abdominal approach. Rectocele repair is easily performed as an isolated procedure or in conjunction with other prolapse procedures and perineal body repair. Advances in technology and surgical training allow many of these procedures to be performed with minimally invasive techniques and less potential of surgical morbidity.

The ultimate goals of surgery are the restoration of pelvic organ support while maintaining vaginal axis and depth for preservation of sexual function. Combining medical management options after establishing a foundation of pelvic organ support has evolved through the recognition that repairing anatomic support alone will not address the loss of physiologic organ function because of the etiology of pelvic organ prolapse, such as pudendal or pelvic nerve neuropathy, medical illness, or maturational changes.

BIBLIOGRAPHY

1. Mallet VT, Bump RC: The epidemiology of female pelvic floor dysfunction. Curr Opin Obstet Gynecol 6:308, 1994.
2. Baden WF, Walker T: Fundamentals, symptoms, and classification. In Baden WF, Walker T (eds): Surgical Repair of Vaginal Defects. Philadelphia, J.B. Lippincott, 1992.
3. Mostwin JL: Current concepts in female pelvic anatomy and physiology. Urol Clin North Am 2:175, 1991.
4. Benson JT, McClellan E: The effect of vaginal dissection on the pudendal nerve. Obstet Gynecol 82:387, 1993.
5. Nichols DH: Vaginal prolapse affecting bladder function. Urol Clin North Am 12:329, 1985.
6. McGuire EJ, Gardy M, Elkins T, Delancey JO: Treatment of incontinence with pelvic prolapse. Urol Clin North Am 18:349, 1991.

59. PROSTATE BIOPSY

J. Stephen Jones, M.D.

1. What are the indications for prostate biopsy?

An elevated prostate-specific antigen (PSA) or a suspicious abnormality on physical examination usually leads to biopsy. This should be reserved for men likely to live long enough to benefit from cure, which is usually regarded as having at least 10 years of life expectancy. Men with a shorter life expectancy might be biopsied if symptomatic from local disease (obstruction or bleeding) or metastatic disease that may benefit from therapy if the diagnosis is confirmed.

2. How is prostate biopsy performed?

A rectal ultrasound probe is placed with the patient in the left lateral decubitus position. A spring-loaded 18-gauge biopsy needle is inserted through a guide and aimed at the area of interest. A marker on the screen corresponding to the needle tract is used to direct the needle appropriately. These needles provide consistent cores of tissue for pathologic examination. A rarely needed alternative is transperineal biopsy using a Tru-Cut or similar biopsy needle under rectally placed digital guidance. These needles are more difficult to use and localization is less exact. Transurethral biopsies are usually not recommended for the diagnosis of prostate cancer but are reserved for staging of urothelial cancer.

3. How many cores should be taken?

Recent evidence points to a 10–12 core sampling in most men. Additional biopsies may be needed if there are abnormalities on rectal examination or ultrasound that require specific evaluation.

4. From where are the cores taken?

The sextant biopsy described by Stamey originally was done in the parasagittal plane, but recent evidence makes it clear that laterally based biopsies are more likely to find cancer.

5. Does it hurt?

That depends on whom you ask. Urologists have traditionally felt that anesthesia was unnecessary. However, up to 96% of patients report pain with the procedure.

6. Is anesthesia possible?

Yes, about 5 cc of a local anesthetic can be injected into the area where the nerves enter the prostate.

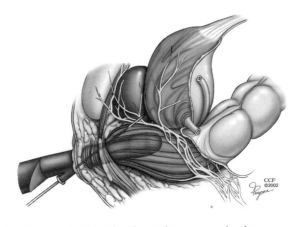

Needle placement to block periprostatic nerves entering the prostate.

7. How do you know where to inject the local anesthetic?

The correct location on each side is identified under ultrasound guidance in the sagittal plane just lateral to the junction of the prostate and seminal vesicle. This ultrasound finding is called the "Mount Everest sign" because it appears white (hyperechoic from fat) and peaked like the famous summit. When lidocaine is injected into this site with a 7-inch .22-gauge spinal needle placed through the biopsy guide, an ultrasonic wheal causes the prostatic base and seminal vesicles to separate from the rectal wall. This gives immediate anesthesia to each half of the prostate. Biopsy can proceed with essentially no sensation in the prostate.

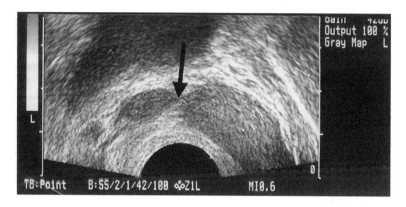

The "Mount Everest sign" shows the pyramidal site for lidocaine injection.

8. Why do apical biopsies hurt more?

Before we were able to anesthetize the prostate, it was assumed that the apex was more sensitive. However, it has now become clear that apical biopsies hurt more because the needle traverses the rectal mucosa below the dentate line. Above that line, there are no rectal pain fibers. Therefore, the apex isn't actually more sensitive; rather, the needle passing through the rectal mucosa below the dentate line causes rectal pain even with the prostate anesthetized. Often the needle can be brought through the rectal mucosa above the dentate line and then angled anteriorly to biopsy the apex without pain.

9. How should patients be prepared for biopsy?

There is no consensus in the literature regarding the use of enemas to prevent infection. Some clinicians feel that removal of feces enhances ultrasound visualization. Nonsteroidal anti-inflammatory drugs (NSAIDs) and other blood thinners should be stopped 5–7 days before biopsy to minimize bleeding.

10. Should antibiotics be given?

Antibiotics appropriate for urinary tract pathogens should be provided. The simplest regimen is to give a single fluoroquinolone orally 30 minutes before biopsy. This may be continued for one or more days after the procedure, especially if the patient is at risk of infectious complications. Parenteral antibiotics might be appropriate if the patient has had recent bacterial prostatitis, or if a catheter or other any prosthesis is in use. American Heart Association (AHA) guidelines also should be followed when indicated by cardiac conditions.

11. What are potential complications of prostate biopsy?

Assuming that pain is adequately prevented with local anesthetic injection, the most common complication is minor bleeding (hematuria, hematochezia, or hematospermia) in most patients. This is almost always self-limiting. Prostatitis occurs less than 1% of the time if antibiotics are given.

12. When should biopsy be repeated?

Data from the 1990s showed that a second biopsy was positive about 20% of the time if the PSA remained elevated. However, with the increased yield of laterally based biopsies using a 10–12 core technique, a second biopsy may not be necessary. This technique appears to give biopsies that replicate repeat biopsy in the first setting. Thus, if a thorough biopsy is performed initially, a repeat may be required only if clinical suspicion rises. This might involve a progressive rise in PSA or a suspicious change in physical examination.

13. What is a "saturation biopsy"?

Several centers have shown an increased yield for repeat biopsies when 18–24 cores are obtained. Although most reports in the literature have involved patients who had this performed under anesthesia, we have found no difficulty performing these saturation biopsies in the office, using local anesthesia as described earlier. At this time, the exact role of saturation biopsy is undefined in that the increased yield may not be significant. However, there is no increased morbidity in adding these additional cores unless anesthetic risks are encountered.

14. What does PIN or atypia mean on the biopsy report?

PIN stands for *Prostatic Intraepithelial Neoplasia*. About half of men with high-grade PIN are eventually found to have prostate cancer. Atypia is even more of a concern, and many pathologists believe that atypia is likely to be associated with cancer. Cytokeratin staining often identifies malignancy in these specimens. If the final pathologic interpretation is either high-grade PIN or atypia, repeat biopsy should be strongly considered if any clinical suspicion persists on follow-up rectal or PSA testing 3–6 months later.

BIBLIOGRAPHY

1. Gore JL, Shariat SF, Miles BJ, et al: Optimal combinations of systematic sextant and laterally directed biopsies for the detection of prostate cancer. J Urol 165:1554–1559, 2001.
2. Bauer JJ, Zeng J, Weir J, et al: Three-dimensional computer simulated prostate models: Lateral prostate biopsies increase the detection rate of cancer. Urology 53:961–967, 1999.
3. Zisman A, Leibovich D, Kleinmann J, et al: The impact of prostate biopsy on patient well-being: A prospective study of pain, anxiety, and erectile dysfunction. J Urol 165:445–454, 2001.
4. Kaver I, Mabjeesh NJ, Matzkin H: Randomized prospective study of periprostatic local anesthesia during transrectal ultrasound-guided biopsy. Urology 59:405–408, 2002.
5. Catalona WJ, Beiser JA, Smith DS: Serum free prostate specific antigen and prostate specific antigen density measurements for predicting cancer in men with prior negative prostatic biopsies. J Urol 158:2162–2167, 1997.
6. Jones JS, Oder M, Zippe CD: Saturation prostate biopsy with periprostatic block can be performed in the office. J Urol (in press).
7. Bostwick DG: Prostatic intraepithelial neoplasia is a risk factor for cancer. Semin Urol Oncol 17:187–198, 1999.

60. VASECTOMY

J. Stephen Jones, M.D.

1. How does vasectomy produce sterilization?

Interruption of the vas deferens prevents sperm from reaching the seminal vesicles, where they would normally complete maturation. Thus, the semen appears visibly normal but contains no sperm.

2. Who should have a vasectomy?

Men who desire permanent sterilization. If they aren't sure permanent sterility is desirable, temporary contraception is preferable. Unfortunately, despite proper counseling to this effect, about 5% of men request vasectomy reversal.

3. What happens to the sperm?

Like almost all other cells in the body, sperm naturally die and are reabsorbed if not released through emission. This can occur even if the patient hasn't had a vasectomy. There is no known harm to this, although it may lead to the formation of antisperm antibodies. (See Chapter 15, Infertility.)

4. When is the patient considered sterile?

Only after semen analysis confirms the complete absence of sperm in the ejaculate. Most physicians prefer to see two successive specimens clear before being comfortable that sterility is assured. This usually occurs within the first 2–3 months, but it may take up to 1 year in some patients. Until sterility is confirmed, the patient must absolutely use alternative birth control to prevent undesired pregnancy.

5. Does vasectomy always result in sterilization?

Almost, although the failure rate is somewhere between 1/200 and 1/1000. This is believed to result from recanalization, whereby a microscopic channel forms between the two divided ends of the vas. This compares very favorably with annual pregnancy rates with other birth control methods, as is shown in the following table.

Yearly Failure (Pregnancy) Rates of Contraceptive Methods

Implant	2%
Female hormonal injection	4%
Birth control pill	8–9%
Diaphragm	13%
Cervical cap	13%
Condom	15%
Rhythm (periodic abstinence)	22%
Withdrawal	26%
Spermicides	28%
Tubal ligation	1–2%
Vasectomy	0.5–0.1%

6. Compare vasectomy to tubal ligation.

Tubal ligation is the female alternative for permanent surgical sterilization. However, because the fallopian (ovarian) tubes are intraabdominal, they can realistically be divided only through abdominal surgery under anesthesia. This not only increases the risk and cost manifold, but it also means that there is much greater opportunity to cut the wrong tubular structure, leading to a failure rate of approximately 1 in 100.

7. Will vasectomy affect potency?

Not at all. Because the only thing cut is the vas, there is no change in male sexual function other than the desired result of sterilization. In fact, many men report improved sexual function after removing the worry about pregnancy.

8. Does vasectomy cause prostate cancer or heart disease?

Over the years, there have been rare reports of minimal increases of these diseases in men who have had vasectomy. They appear to be misleading, in that multiple further studies have shown absolutely no long-term health risks. These findings appear to actually reflect the generally excellent health of men who have vasectomies. In other words, they live long enough to develop these diseases of old age instead of dying young. They are also usually health-conscious men who undergo health screening. Therefore, if these diseases develop, they are usually identified early and managed appropriately.

9. What other complications are possible?

Minor swelling, bleeding, and pain occasionally occur. Very rarely, an infection will develop that may require antibiotics or drainage. A small swelling at the site of the vasectomy, called a *sperm granuloma,* is a nodular tissue reaction to the irritating nature of the sperm at the transection site.

10. How is a vasectomy performed?

Two main options exist. A **traditional vasectomy** is performed through either one or two incisions using standard surgical instruments. A **"no-scalpel vasectomy"** is performed through a small "keyhole" puncture, as is the newer **percutaneous vasectomy.** The no-scalpel vasectomy is performed by grasping the vas through the skin using a special ringed clamp before making the incision. After a puncture wound is made, the vas is speared with a sharp clamp, which is rotated 180 degrees. While this is being done, the ringed clamp is released and the vas regrasped, divided, and ligated.

11. Why don't all physicians perform the no-scalpel vasectomy?

Less than one third of vasectomies in America are the no-scalpel type. Despite its speed and less invasive nature, the learning curve of the above maneuvers is steep. Because most physicians already have a procedure that works well for them, there may be no good reason to change.

The third option, percutaneous vasectomy, uses similar instruments, but the vas is exposed through the puncture before it is grasped. The difficult maneuvers that have kept most physicians from adopting the Li (no-scalpel) technique are avoided, so this procedure can be learned in only a few sessions. A recent study at our institution found that the percutaneous vasectomy is performed in an average time of less than 10 minutes, with results comparable to those of the no-scalpel option. Patients reported 100% recovery and return to normal activities an average of 9.7 days postoperatively.

12. What method of vasal closure is best?

The best method is probably the method each individual surgeon has developed confidence and success in using. Although the literature shows some advantages to simply placing two clips on either end of the severed vas, comparative studies are lacking. Suture ligature is the most common method, although there are reports of vasal sloughing and recanalization. A needle electrocautery placed in the lumen theoretically scars the vas beyond its direct contact. Some authors also advocate separation of the two severed ends into different tissue planes.

13. Does vasectomy prevent AIDS and other sexually transmitted diseases?

No. Vasectomized men have been shown to have less HIV titer in semen than controls, but they are still capable of transmitting HIV and all other forms of sexually transmitted disease.

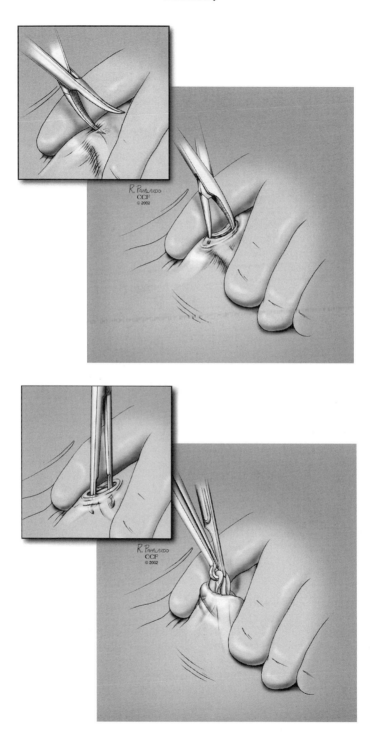

The vas is secured to skin using the "tripod grasp." The curved sharp hemostat punctures and opens the skin. Then the ringed clamp grasps the vas and pulls it out in order to expose for excision and ligation.

BIBLIOGRAPHY

1. Fu H, Darroch JE, Haas T, Ranjit N: Contraceptive failure rates: New estimates from the 1995 national survey of family growth. Fam Plann Perspect 31:56–63, 1999.
2. Sokal D: A comparative study of the no scalpel and standard incision approaches to vasectomy in 5 countries. The Male Sterilization Investigator Team. J Urol 163:1892–1893, 2000.
3. Jones JS: Percutaneous vasectomy: A simple modification eliminates the steep learning curve of no-scalpel vasectomy. In press.

IV. Inflammation and Infection

61. ACUTE PYELONEPHRITIS

Bashir R. Sankari, M.D.

1. What is acute pyelonephritis?

Acute pyelonephritis is an acute infection of the renal parenchyma and collecting system. It is most commonly caused by a bacterial pathogen. *Escherichia coli* and other Enterobacteriaceae account for over 90% of infections. Acute pyelonephritis is sometimes referred to as **upper urinary tract system infection** and should be differentiated from the more common, uncomplicated lower urinary tract infections such as cystitis.

2. What is the route of infection?

Two routes of infection exist. Ascending uriniferous spread is the most common and is caused by retrograde ascent of bacteria from the bladder through the ureter to the renal pelvis and parenchyma. Colonization of the perineum with gut enterobacteria precedes the episode of acute pyelonephritis. The second route of infection, hematogenous spread, is less common. It is usually associated with other extrarenal foci of infection such as tuberculosis and staphylococcal septicemia.

3. Do any conditions predispose to acute pyelonephritis?

- Obstruction of the urinary collecting system
- Vesicoureteral reflux
- Renal calculi
- Neurogenic bladder
- Diabetes mellitus
- Altered host resistance (immunosuppression)
- Congenital anomalies
- Pregnancy
- Prolonged catheter drainage

4. Describe the clinical presentation in acute pyelonephritis.

Because acute pyelonephritis is a parenchymal infection, it is most frequently associated with fever, chills, malaise, and flank pain, with or without radiation to the groin. Gastrointestinal symptoms are often present with nausea and vomiting and are mainly secondary to paralytic ileus. Lower urinary tract symptoms such as dysuria, urgency, and frequency are present in 50% of the cases. On physical examination, the hallmark finding is the presence of costovertebral angle tenderness on the affected side. Concurrent abdominal pain and tenderness and paralytic ileus also may occur, adding to the confusion and prompting consideration of other intraabdominal processes such as appendicitis, diverticulitis, pancreatitis, and cholecystitis in the differential diagnosis.

5. What are the laboratory findings?

The urinalysis shows pyuria, bacteriuria, and gross or microscopic blood. The complete blood count reveals leukocytosis with predominance of neutrophils. The serum creatinine may be elevated due to the transient renal dysfunction and/or dehydration. Urine cultures are diagnostic, and the sensitivity study will identify the appropriate antibiotic therapy.

6. What is the spectrum of the disease?

Infectious Disease Processes in the Kidney

Acute pyelonephritis
Focal bacterial nephritis (lobar nephronia)
Multifocal bacterial nephritis
Renal abscess, perinephric abscess
Emphysematous pyelonephritis
Xanthogranulomatous pyelonephritis

Acute pyelonephritis may take a more or less complicated course, depending on the severity of infectious process, the time of presentation, predisposing conditions, and the promptness of effective therapy. Because the route of infection is mostly ascending, many renal infections follow the lobar and lobular distribution of renal parenchyma and remain confined within the rigid capsule of the kidney. In the classic presentation of **acute pyelonephritis,** the whole kidney is enlarged, with generalized inflammation and swelling. **Urosepsis** can result from the associated bacteremia. In its severe form, acute renal infection with heavy leukocyte infiltrate may be confined to a single renal lobe or multiple lobes, resulting in **acute focal** or **multifocal bacterial nephritis. Renal abscesses** can evolve from such lesions with progressive suppuration of the renal parenchyma. Rupture outside the renal capsule can result in perinephric abscess collection.

In diabetic patients, fermentation of sugar by gas-forming organisms (such as *E. coli*) will result in carbon dioxide production that is visualized as air in the renal parenchyma, a condition referred to as emphysematous pyelonephritis. Patients with associated chronic infectious stones (ammonium-magnesium-phosphate or struvite stones) related to infection with urea-splitting organisms such as *Proteus* and *E. coli* can develop **xanthogranulomatous pyelonephritis,** an atypical form of renal infection characterized by a cellular infiltrate of lipid-laden mononuclear macrophagias (foam cells) on microscopic examination. Grossly, it has the shape of a mass lesion, which could be localized or diffuse depending on the severity and the extent of the disease, and is confused commonly with renal cell carcinoma.

7. Is radiologic investigation needed in the patient with acute pyelonephritis?

Radiologic investigation is important in acute pyelonephritis to rule out associated anomalies that have predisposed the patient to the infectious process, and to define the pathologic process in complicated cases. Imaging studies become essential if the infectious process fails to improve despite appropriate therapy.

8. What is the best radiologic test in acute pyelonephritis?

No single study provides a uniformly diagnostic picture under all circumstances. The work-up must be tailored to the anticipated abnormality and the clinical outcome of treatment, and should be adjusted when further study is expected to provide additional useful information.

1. A simple **plain film** of the abdomen is useful to rule out air in the renal parenchyma and also may show radiopaque stones or shadowing of psoas muscle in perinephric or renal abscess.

2. **Intravenous pyelogram** (IVP) is usually negative in acute pyelonephritis or may show only some delay in visualization and excretion of the contrast and swelling of renal parenchyma. IVP is very important to rule out congenital anomalies, such as ureteropelvic junction obstruction or an obstructing stone in the ureter. The bladder film will help assess the wall of the bladder and rule out neurogenic bladder, and the postvoid film will rule out bladder outlet obstruction.

3. **Computed tomography** (CT) scan with intravenous contrast offers excellent images of the renal parenchyma and surrounding tissues. CT scan defines the renal parenchyma involvement in the infectious process to a better extent. It also helps in the diagnosis of renal abscess, perinephric abscess, focal bacterial nephritis, and xanthogranulomatous pyelonephritis. Helical

CT is a new technology that is replacing conventional CT in imaging renal parenchyma due to its higher sensitivity and speed of image acquisition.

4. **Ultrasonography** is helpful in the diagnosis of obstructive uropathy and stone disease and in the follow-up of renal abscess and focal bacterial nephritis.

5. **Renal nuclear scan** with mercaptoacetyltriglycine (MAG-3) or diethylenetriamine pentaacetic acid (DTPA) is important to assess residual renal function when clinical conditions warrant surgical intervention or ablation. Dimercaptosuccinic acid (DMSA) renal scan concentrates in the renal cortex and is a highly effective study in assessing cortical scar when indicated, such as in the follow-up of children with vesicoureteral reflux.

In general, most uncomplicated cases of acute pyelonephritis in adults do not require imaging for diagnosis and treatment. When imaging is indicated, contrast-enhanced CT scan is the study of choice. In diabetic patients, a plain abdominal radiograph is recommended to screen for emphysematous pyelonephritis.

9. How does acute pyelonephritis affect renal function?

With each kidney infection, a variable degree of structural damage occurs, depending on the severity of infection and the promptness of therapy. Residual scarring with some loss of functioning tissue is the rule and depends upon the severity and the chronicity of the infection.

10. Explain the treatment of acute pyelonephritis.

Treatment is usually indicated upon clinical suspicion and should be prompt, preferably in a hospital with intravenous antibiotics. Some uncomplicated cases can be treated as outpatients. The antibiotics used should cover the prevalent gram-negative pathogens (*Escherichia coli, Proteus, Pseudomonas,* and *Klebsiella*) and other common gram-positive pathogens (Enterococcus, and coagulase-negative Staphylococcus).

Empirically, one-drug therapy with a third-generation cephalosporin or ureido penicillin is usually effective. Fluoroquinolones are good alternative agents and can be continued orally as outpatient therapy. In severe cases, two-drug therapies should be considered for synergistic effect. Aminoglycosides can be added for synergistic coverage against gram-negative bacteria as well as that *Enterococcus* and *Staphylococcus* infection. Once cultures and sensitivities become available, the antibiotic therapy can be adjusted accordingly. If the patient does not improve within an acceptable time frame (3–5 days), despite appropriate therapy, further investigation should be done to rule out associated anomalies and conditions that require intervention, such as obstruction and renal abscess.

Acute pyelonephritis requires 2 weeks of combined intravenous and oral antibiotics. Focal and multifocal bacterial nephritis requires up to 6 weeks of combined therapy depending on response. Emphysematous pyelonephritis requires an aggressive intravenous antibiotic course. If symptoms persist, percutaneous drainage and/or nephrectomy should be considered. Xanthogranulomatous pyelonephritis requires surgical intervention through either total or partial nephrectomy.

BIBLIOGRAPHY

1. Conway J: The role of scintigraphy in urinary tract infection. Semin Nucl Med 18:308–319, 1988.
2. Dembry LM, Andriole VT: Renal and perirenal abscesses. Infect Dis Clin North Am 11:663–680, 1997.
3. Hill GS: Renal infection. In Hill GS (ed): Uropathology. New York, Churchill Livingstone, 1989, pp 333–429.
4. Kaplan DM, Rosenfield AT, Smith RC: Advances in the imaging of renal infection: Helical CT and modern coordinated imaging. Infect Dis Clin North Am 11:681–705, 1997.
5. Schaeffer AJ: Urinary tract infections. In Gillenwater JY, Grayhack JT, Howards SS, Duckett JW (eds): Adult and Pediatric Urology, 3rd ed. St. Louis, Mosby, 1996, pp 289–351.
6. Stamm WE, Hooton TM: Management of urinary tract infections in adults. N Engl J Med 329:1328–1334, 1993.

62. RENAL AND PERIRENAL ABSCESS

Nehemia Hampel, M.D.

1. What is an abscess?

An abscess is a focus of suppuration within an organ, tissue, or region of the body; it may be microscopic or macroscopic. Most abscesses are acute, but some may be chronic. Renal abscesses are located within the renal parenchyma, whereas perirenal abscesses are located within the perirenal fascia (Gerota's fascia).

2. What is the difference between renal and perirenal abscess?

Renal abscesses are localized kidney lesions that are either intraparenchymal (cortical, medullary, or infected renal cyst) or confined to an obstructed renal calyx. Perirenal abscesses involve the perirenal space surrounded by the perirenal fascia of Gerota. Most perinephric abscesses are associated with renal abscess.

3. What is the significance of renal and perirenal abscesses?

The major risk is life-threatening urosepsis and septicemia. Because they are located in the retroperitoneum, they are difficult to diagnose. Poor prognosis is related to delay in diagnosis and to associated medical problems.

4. What is the pathogenesis?

In the past, the majority of renal and perirenal abscesses were caused by hematologic spread from skin or respiratory infections. Today, a majority result from ascending infections from the lower urinary tract. Perinephric abscesses develop mainly from rupture of an renal abscess. Usually Gerota's fascia confines abscess formation to the perinephric space, but the process may extend to adjacent cavities and structures. Preexisting renal disease is present in the majority of cases. Gram-negative abscesses are commonly associated with pyelonephritis and renal calculus disease. Vesicoureteral reflux and urinary tract infections in children as well as adults may result in renal or perirenal abscesses. Predisposing conditions include diabetes mellitus, urinary tract infection, urinary tract obstruction, nephrolithiasis, intravenous drug use, and immunosuppressive conditions.

5. What are the significant symptoms and signs?

Renal abscess has an abrupt onset. Chills, fever, and localized costovertebral angle pain and tenderness are typical features. When the etiology is associated with lower urinary tract infection, symptoms include frequency of urination, urgency, and dysuria. Nausea and vomiting may be present, often causing the clinician to suspect intraperitoneal disease. Perinephric abscesses are often insidious in nature. Usually they are symptomatic for several weeks before the patient seeks medical attention, resulting in a confusing clinical presentation. Fever and malaise are usually present. Most renal and perirenal abscesses are unilateral. Physical examination findings include flank and costovertebral angle tenderness. Scoliosis with concavity toward the side with abscess is common. In extensive renal abscesses or perirenal abscesses, flank or abdominal mass and edema of the flank skin may be evident. Extension of the thigh increases the pain owing to stretching of the psoas muscle.

6. What microorganisms are involved in renal and perirenal abscesses?

The infective organisms of renal and perirenal abscesses are the same. Hematogenous spread involves gram-positive organisms, most commonly *Staphylococcus aureus*. Ascending infection usually involves gram-negative organisms, mainly strains of *Escherichia coli, Klebsiella,* and *Proteus*. Other bacteria, including *Pseudomonas,* obligatory anaerobic bacteria, fungi, and *My-*

cobacterium tuberculosis, are sometimes responsible. In about 25% of cases, cultures are polymicrobial.

7. Which laboratory tests are helpful in evaluation?

Complete blood count usually shows marked leukocytosis with shift to the left in the acute abscess; however, in longstanding infection, leukocytosis may be moderate. When there is communication between the abscess cavity and the renal collecting system, urinalysis reveals leukocytes, and urinary culture is usually positive. This is true for renal and perirenal abscesses secondary to urinary tract infections. In hematogenous infection, urinalysis may be negative. Depending on the associated renal involvement and abnormalities, serum urea nitrogen and creatinine levels may be normal or elevated. Patients with diabetes who have an abscess often have hyperglycemia, ketoaciduria, and glycosuria. In addition to urine culture, blood cultures should be obtained to identify bacteremia.

8. What imaging studies are most helpful?

Plain radiography of the abdomen often shows a mass effect, and scoliosis with concavity toward the affected side is usually present. The renal size may be enlarged, and if the inflammation is extrarenal, the shadow of the psoas muscle is lost. Intravenous urography may suggest the pathology, but ultrasonography and particularly CT scanning are fundamental in the diagnosis of all retroperitoneal abscesses and in establishing the location, size, and extension of the abscess. CT scan is more helpful than ultrasonography and should be obtained in every patient with suspected retroperitoneal abscess. Renal arteriography and radionuclide scanning are seldom indicated or diagnostic.

9. What is the treatment of renal and perirenal abscesses?

Until culture and sensitivity test results are available, parenteral broad-spectrum antimicrobial therapy should be initiated and directed against the wide range of parenteral pathogens. Usually a combination of aminoglycoside and broad-spectrum penicillin is a proper initial treatment. If staphylococcal infection is suspected, therapy should include a beta-lactamase–resistant penicillin. Antibacterial therapy should be adjusted according to culture results and clinical response. Parenteral therapy should be continued for 7–14 days and followed by several weeks of oral therapy. As a general rule, abscesses must be drained; only small, localized lesions with prompt response to antibiotic therapy can be managed conservatively. CT scan–guided or ultrasonography-guided percutaneous drainage can be used when the abscess is not loculated. If drainage appears to be inadequate, open surgical drainage should be performed promptly. Perirenal abscesses should always be treated with early and thorough drainage. Open drainage has traditionally been advocated, but recently appropriate percutaneous drainage has been reported in selected cases. Rarely, nephrectomy may be required to control extensive renal involvement.

10. What are the treatment outcomes?

In treatment experiences reported several decades ago, the mortality rate was about 50%. Early diagnosis with CT scan and ultrasonography has led to prompt treatment and improved survival. More effective antimicrobial therapy and better supportive care also have contributed to the improvement. Currently, survival is expected to be 90% or better. Patients with less extensive renal abscesses have a better prognosis than patients with extensive renal or perirenal abscesses.

BIBLIOGRAPHY

1. Dalla Palma L, Pozzi-Mucelli F, Ene V: Medical treatment of renal and perirenal abscesses: CT evaluation. Clin Radiol 54:792–797, 1999.
2. Fowler JE Jr, Perkias T: Presentation, diagnosis and treatment of renal abscesses: 1972–1988. J Urol 151:847–851, 1994.
3. Gerzof SG: Percutaneous drainage of renal and perirenal abscess. Urol Radiol 2:171, 1981.

4. Gerzof SG, Gale ME: Computed tomography and ultrasonography for the diagnosis and treatment of renal and retroperitoneal abscesses. Urol Clin North Am 9:185–193, 1982.
5. Gillenwater JY, Gryhack JT, Howards SS, Duckett JW: Adult and Pediatric Urology, 3rd ed. St. Louis,
   Mosby, 1996.
6. Edelstein H, McCabe R: Perinephric abscess: Modern diagnosis and treatment in 47 cases. Medicine
   67:118–131, 1988.
7. Schaeffer AJ: Infections of the urinary tract.In Walsh PC, Retik AB, Vaughan ED Jr, Wein AJ (eds):
   Campbell's Urology, 7th ed. Philadelphia, W.B. Saunders, 1998, pp 533–614.
8. Thornbury JR: Acute renal infections. Urol Radiol 12:209–213, 1991.

63. RENAL TUBERCULOSIS

Lawrence M. Wyner, M.D.

1. How many people worldwide are infected with the tubercle bacillus?

Approximately 1.9 billion, or one-third of humanity, of whom 19 million are Americans.

2. How many people worldwide develop clinical tuberculosis (TB) each year?

Approximately 10 million, of whom roughly 20,000 are Americans. The vast majority of cases arise from reactivation, often many years after the initial exposure.

3. How common is extrapulmonary TB in patients who have already been diagnosed with pulmonary TB?

About one-sixth of patients with pulmonary involvement develop tuberculous disease in other organs. The risk is doubled in patients with compromised immune function, poor nutrition, or poor living conditions.

4. Is there a relationship between clinical TB and human immunodeficiency virus (HIV) disease?

Yes. Pulmonary TB often occurs early in the course of HIV disease, and in fact may be the first indication that a patient is HIV-positive. In contrast, extrapulmonary TB is more common in the later stages of HIV. The World Health Organization estimates that "Material Deleted" 15 million HIV-positive people worldwide are coinfected with TB.

5. What organs are most commonly involved in extrapulmonary TB?

Lymph nodes, intestine, bone, and kidneys.

6. Renal TB cases represent what percentage of extrapulmonary TB?

Roughly 20%.

7. Do any symptoms suggest a diagnosis of renal TB?

Early in the disease process, patients present with vague, nonspecific symptoms, such as lethargy, malaise, low-grade fever, and weight loss. Urinary seeding of the bladder gives rise to frequency and dysuria. Flank pain and hematuria usually take years to develop, after considerable renal destruction and stricture formation have occurred.

8. What are the characteristic physical findings in renal TB?

Urinary seeding may affect any genitourinary organ: In males, look for thickening or coarseness of the epididymides or prostate, or a "beaded" vas deferens. Upper abdominal bruits may indicate advanced renal destruction, with obliterative changes of the renal artery and its branches.

9. What does the urinalysis show in renal TB?

About 50% of patients have microscopic hematuria, and almost all have pyuria. Proteinuria is common also.

10. What does the phrase *sterile pyuria* mean?

Actually, this is a misnomer, because the urine of patients with renal TB is loaded with tubercle bacilli! The phrase reminds us that a routine culture will not detect the tubercle bacillus, and that special media are required in order to grow this organism. Remember also that at least 20% of patients with renal TB have a superimposed bacterial urinary tract infection, so that a positive routine urine culture does not rule out coexisting renal TB. Moreover, tetracycline and sulfa are bacteriostatic for the tubercle bacillus, and ofloxacin and ciprofloxacin are mycobactericidal; thus, their use may result in false-negative urinary acid-fast bacteria (AFB) cultures. A minimum of three early morning urine specimens are recommended in order to culture AFB successfully.

11. What blood work is helpful in managing patients with renal TB?
Baseline renal and hepatic function should be assessed, because antibiotic therapy may cause liver toxicity, and doses may need to be adjusted for renal insufficiency. The erythrocyte sedimentation rate also is useful in monitoring the response to treatment.

12. Is the tuberculin skin test usually positive in patients with renal TB?
Yes, in greater than 90%.

13. What are the characteristic intravenous pyelogram (IVP) findings of renal TB?
About half of the patients have renal calcifications on the KUB film. Although renal TB is a bilateral disease, typically one kidney is affected more severely. Contrast excretion is poor on the more-involved side. The parenchyma is deformed and may be completely destroyed (autonephrectomy). The minor calyces are dilated and irregular, and intrarenal fistulae may be seen. The ureters may be straightened or strictured, and the bladder capacity is diminished. Infundibular stenosis is pathognomonic of renal TB. In children and in patients whose disease is diagnosed early, however, the IVP may be normal.

14. What are the characteristic ultrasound findings of renal TB?
A nonfunctioning kidney on IVP, with a normal appearance on ultrasound, should at least raise the suspicion of early renal TB, because diffuse parenchymal tuberculomas can account for this scenario. Later, with the development of profound calyectasis and contraction of the renal pelvis, the so-called "daisy sign" is seen—a ring of dilated calyces, often without a demonstrable renal pelvis.

15. What are the characteristic pathologic features of renal TB?
Hematogenous spread of tubercle bacilli to the kidneys from a primary infection site, usually the lungs, causes tuberculomas to develop in the glomerular capillaries. The organisms then spread along the nephron to the loop of Henle. Granuloma formation ensues, with caseous necrosis of the renal papillae and deformity of the collecting system.

16. What are two consequences of the chronic inflammation on the urothelium?
1. Stricture formation.
2. Squamous metaplasia, with resultant squamous cell carcinoma.

17. How is renal TB treated?
Isoniazid and rifampin are administered for 9 months. If the organism is resistant to one of these agents, either streptomycin and pyrazinamide, or ethambutol, is added. Always obtain a chest x-ray and sputum for AFB before beginning treatment. If concomitant pulmonary tuberculosis is found, the 9-month course of therapy should be adequate to treat both sites of infection.

18. What are the side effects of the antituberculous drugs?

Side Effects of Antituberculous Drugs

DRUG	SIDE EFFECTS
Isoniazid	Hepatotoxicity; urticaria; fever; neurotoxicity (may be alleviated by pyridoxine)
Rifampin	Hepatotoxicity; may decrease serum levels of other drugs that undergo hepatic metabolism (e.g., estrogens, warfarin, digoxin, oral hypoglycemics); orange discoloration of body fluids; thrombocytopenic purpura; flulike syndrome; gastrointestinal upset
Streptomycin	Ototoxicity
Pyrazinamide	Gastrointestinal upset; gouty arthralgias
Ethambutol	Optic neuritis; gouty arthralgias

19. Is surgery ever indicated in the treatment of renal TB?

Very rarely; effective antibiotics alone cure more than 95% of patients. However, for patients with intractable pain or hypertension or with chronic bacterial infection proximal to a strictured ureteral segment, partial or total nephrectomy may be needed.

20. How are patients with renal TB followed up?

Compliance with the antibiotic regimen is crucial to ensure proper treatment and to prevent resistant organisms from developing. The problem of drug-resistant TB is worsening worldwide, with up to 40% of TB-infected patients resistant to at least one of the antituberculous drugs in some regions. A medical social worker should be involved early, and the local public health department must be notified. Patients are no longer contagious after 2–3 weeks on antituberculous therapy. Urine for AFB should be obtained at 2–3 months intervals in order to assess both the adequacy of therapy and the possible emergence of resistant organisms.

21. What is the most common iatrogenic cause of TB?

BCG bladder instillation for treatment of superficial bladder cancer.

22. What is BCG?

BCG is short for bacilli Calmette-Guérin, a live-attenuated TB vaccine that produces intense urothelial inflammation when administered intravesically, sometimes leading to granulomatous prostatitis. Acute BCG sepsis occurs when the tubercle bacillus enters the bloodstream (e.g., from an unrecognized traumatic catheterization).

23. What is the key drug to use in the treatment of acute BCG sepsis?

Cycloserine. It inhibits growth of the tubercule bacillus within 24 hours, and is used in combination with isoniazid, rifampin, and ethambutol.

24. What is the major side effect of cycloserine?

It lowers the seizure threshold.

BIBLIOGRAPHY

1. Association for Professionals in Infection Control and Epidemiology Guidelines Committee: 1998 APIC position paper. Responsibility for interpretation of the PPD tuberculin skin test. Am J Infect Control 27:56–58, 1999.
2. Bradford WZ, Daley CL: Multiple drug-resistant tuberculosis. Infect Dis Clin North Am 12:157–172, 1998.
3. Cegielsk JP, et al: The global tuberculosis situation: Progress and problems in the 20th century, prospects for the 21st century. Infect Dis Clin North Am 16:1–5, 2002.
4. Centers for Disease Control: Tuberculosis Control Laws—United States, 1993. MMWR 42 (No. RR-15), 1993.
5. Cox LR, Cockett ATK: Genitourinary tuberculosis revisited. Urology 20:111–117, 1982.
6. Dutt AK, Moers D, Stead WW: Short-course chemotherapy for extrapulmonary tuberculosis: Nine years' experience. Ann Intern Med 104:7–12, 1986.
7. Dye C, et al: Global burden of tuberculosis. JAMA 282:677–686, 1999.
8. Ehrlich RM, Lattimer JK: Urogenital tuberculosis in children. J Urol 105:461–465, 1971.
9. Gow JG: Genitourinary tuberculosis. In Walsh PC, Tetik AB, Vaughan ED, Wein AJ (eds): Campbell's Urology, 7th ed. Philadelphia, W.B. Saunders, 1998, pp 807–836.
10. Kaufman JJ, Goodwin WE: Renal hypertension secondary to renal tuberculosis. Am J Med 38:337–344, 1965.
11. Lamm DL: Complications of bacillus Calmette-Guérin immunotherapy. Urol Clin North Am 19:565–572, 1992.
12. National Institute of Allergy and Infectious Disease Office on Communications, Bethesda, MD: Fact sheet, March 1997.
13. O'Sullivan DC, Murphy D, Conlon P, Walshe J: Hypercalcemia due to squamous cell carcinoma in a tuberculous kidney: Case report and review of pathogenesis. Br J Urol 73:106–107, 1994.

14. Pitchenik AE, Fertel D: Tuberculosis and nontuberculous mycobacterial disease. Med Clin North Am 76:121–171, 1992.
15. Scott RF, Engelbrecht HE: Ultrasonography of the advanced tuberculous kidney. S Afr Med J 75:371–372, 1989.
16. Seaworth BJ: Multidrug-resistant tuberculosis. Infect Dis Clin North Am 16:73–106, 2002.
17. Simon HB, Weinstein AJ, Pasternak MS, et al: Genitourinary tuberculosis—Clinical features in a general hospital population. Am J Med 63:410–420, 1977.
18. Snider DE: Introduction. In Fogarty International Center Workshop, National Institutes of Health, Bethesda, Md. Research towards global control and prevention of tuberculosis with emphasis on vaccine development. Rev Infect Dis (suppl 2):S336–S338, 1989.
19. Weinberg AC, Boyd SD: Short course chemotherapy and role of surgery in adult and pediatric genitourinary tuberculosis. Urology 31:95–102, 1988.

64. RETROPERITONEAL FIBROSIS

Mark J. Noble, M.D.

1. What is retroperitoneal fibrosis?

Retroperitoncal fibrosis is the formation of a fibrotic plaque that is usually centered over L4 and L5 and extends caudally to the sacral promontory and cephalad to the renal hilum. The lateral margins of extent are typically the outer edges of the psoas muscle. Occasionally, the fibrotic plaque extends caudally along the iliac vessels. Rarely, the process may be more localized and focally surround a ureter and/or other retroperitoneal structures.

2. Does retroperitoneal fibrosis extend to other areas?

Yes. It has been associated with mediastinal fibrosis, mesenteric fibrosis, sclerosing cholangitis, Reidel's fibrosing thyroiditis, and fibrotic orbital pseudotumors.

3. What are the causes of retroperitoneal fibrosis?

Retroperitoneal fibrosis is idiopathic in two-thirds of cases. Numerous causes have been reported for the other one-third of patients, including drugs (an example is methysergide—Sansert—which 20 years ago was used to treat migraine headaches and formerly accounted for nearly 10% of all cases), malignancies, infections, radiation, and other inflammatory conditions.

Causes of Retroperitoneal Fibrosis

Idiopathic	Malignancies
Drugs	Primary (e.g., lymphoma, sarcoma)
Amphetamines	Metastatic
Analgesics (phenacetin)	Inflammatory lesions
Beta blockers	Inflammatory bowel disease
Methyldopa (Aldomet)	Other GI tract infections (e.g., diverticulitis)
Lysergic acid diethylamide (LSD)	Biliary tract disease
Methysergide (Sansert)	Endometriosis
Other ergot alkaloids (e.g., bromocriptine)	Sarcoidosis
Reserpine	Periarteritis
Haloperidol	Perianeurysms (aortic or iliac)
Infections	Collagen vascular disease
Chronic urinary tract infections	Autoimmune diseases
Gonorrhea	Urinary extravasation
Syphilis	Hemorrhage (e.g., trauma, Schönlein-Henoch purpura)
Tuberculosis	Previous intraabdominal surgery
Radiation	

4. Is there an explanation for idopathic retroperitoneal fibrosis?

Many believe that it is the result of an immunologic response to the leakage of material from diseased (atherosclerotic) blood vessels, although the true etiology is unknown.

5. How often does retroperitoneal fibrosis occur?

Retroperitoneal fibrosis is uncommon, with a prevalence of approximately 1/200,000 population. It is usually diagnosed between ages 30 and 60, and idiopathic retroperitoneal fibrosis occurs twice as commonly in males as females.

6. Name the consequences of retroperitoneal fibrosis.

The most common sequela is obstructive uropathy secondary to ureteral compression. However, intestinal, venous, and less commonly, arterial and biliary obstruction may also occur.

7. What clinical symptoms do patients experience?

Most patients generally present with vague symptoms, including low back pain, malaise, anorexia, and weight loss. Occasionally, patients may exhibit low-grade fever and symptoms specifically related to areas of obstruction, e.g., lower extremity edema from venous obstruction.

8. Are any abnormal laboratory values associated with retroperitoneal fibrosis?

Although are no specific laboratory values are associated with retroperitoneal fibrosis, approximately 60–90% of patients have an elevated erythrocyte sedimentation rate, a nonspecific indicator of inflammation. Anemia and leukocytosis also may be present, as well as varying degrees of azotemia.

9. Which radiographic studies best demonstrate retroperitoneal fibrosis? What are the findings?

Historically, the **intravenous urogram** has been used to identify the findings of retroperitoneal fibrosis, which include long narrowed segments of the ureter with medial deviation of the middle third of the ureters and hydronephrosis. If a kidney has suffered damage or has high-grade obstruction, a **retrograde pyelogram** may be performed to visualize the ureter and renal pelvis. However, the medial deviation is not always present in retroperitoneal fibrosis, and as many as 20% of individuals with normal urinary tracts have medial deviations of the ureters on an intravenous urogram or retrograde pyelogram. Recently, **computed tomography** (CT) and **magnetic resonance imaging** (MRI) have been used to better delineate retroperitoneal fibrosis, which is seen as a mass encompassing the vena cava and aorta.

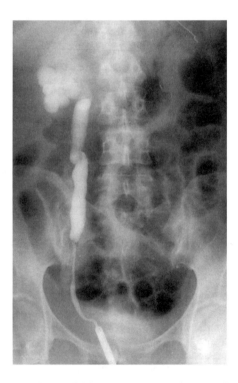

Note the long, tapered distal narrowing, medial deviation, and proximal dilation of the right ureter demonstrated by retrograde pyelography. This particular patient had pelvic malignancy with obstruction of the right distal ureter; this typifies the radiographic appearance of retroperitoneal fibrosis involving the distal right ureter.

10. Are the radiographic findings sufficient to diagnose the cause?

No. Although MRI may be sufficient in a few cases, current radiographic techniques do not permit differentiation between malignant and benign causes of retroperitoneal fibrosis. One may obviously infer the cause if a known disease process is present, such as a large abdominal aortic aneurysm. Multiple, deep biopsies are best for diagnosis.

11. Are percutaneous biopsies adequate?

A specific diagnosis requires multiple biopsies of the mass. Sometimes this can be accomplished with CT-guided needle biopsy; otherwise, open or laparoscopic surgical exploration and biopsy are required.

12. What is the gross appearance of retroperitoneal fibrosis?

Retroperitoneal fibrosis grossly appears as a fibrotic plaque that is grayish-white, like scar tissue. It has a firm, woody consistency. If malignant, it may be almost rock-hard.

13. How about the microscopic appearance?

Early in the disease process, histologic examination of the plaque reveals a cellular immature fibrotic process with many inflammatory cells (primarily lymphocytes and plasma cells) and fibroblasts. Later, as the plaque matures, it becomes relatively acellular and is composed primarily of dense hyalinized collagen. This progresses from the medial aspect of the plaque laterally. Biopsies from the lateral edges may therefore still show a relatively cellular picture late in the disease.

14. How is retroperitoneal fibrosis treated?

Treatment is directed towards the primary process, if one can be identified. Immediate relief of obstruction can be achieved with percutaneous nephrostomy or ureteral stenting. Medications suspected of causation should be stopped, which may result in spontaneous resolution. Malignancies are treated as per their cell type. Idiopathic retroperitoneal fibrosis may respond to corticosteroids and/or additional immunosuppressive medication. However, in advanced disease, a patient may still require surgery to relieve ureteral obstruction and free up other structures blocked by the fibrotic process. This can now be performed with minimally invasive techniques (e.g., laparoscopy) in many instances; but sometimes such is not technically feasible and open surgery is necessary. The ureter(s) is/are freed from the fibrotic process and wrapped in omentum or placed intraperitoneally in an attempt to prevent the fibrosis from recurring. In rare cases, ureteral substitution with segments of intestine (reconnecting one or both kidneys to the bladder) or autotransplantation of one or both kidneys may be required to relieve severe ureteral obstruction.

15. Are steroids alone ever sufficient therapy?

Yes. For a number of years, corticosteroids were thought to be indicated as adjunctive therapy to surgery or used only in patients who were poor surgical risks, but recent reports demonstrate major improvement with steroid therapy alone. This generally requires very high dosing, e.g., methylprednisolone (60 mg daily for 6 weeks) with attendant side effects and risks. During the treatment the patient may require temporary ureteral stenting or percutaneous nephrostomy to relieve ureteral obstruction until the steroids are effective. Definitive surgery may be used when medical treatment fails.

16. What is the prognosis after treatment for retroperitoneal fibrosis?

The prognosis is generally good in cases not involving malignancy. However, patients successfully treated with steroids may relapse, and surgically treated disease may continue to progress as well. Thus, patients require life-long follow-up to be certain that reobstruction does not occur. Obviously, if severe irreversible renal damage (or damage to other organs) has occurred, the patient's prognosis is that of an individual with chronic renal insufficiency.

17. What is the differential diagnosis of retroperitoneal fibrosis?

Other conditions can mimic retroperitoneal fibrosis and can include many of the causes of ureteral obstruction. Bilateral ureteric obstruction in the male may occur with long-standing, severe prostatism, but such does not usually cause medial deviation of the ureters with narrowing of the lumina. A large abdominal or pelvic mass can compress (and may cause medial deviation of) one or both ureters, yet the ureters themselves might not be directly encased or "fibrosed." An acute condition (e.g., trauma) may result in extravasated blood, urine, or some other substance migrating through retroperitoneal tissue planes, causing ureteral compression and deviation, but there would normally be a history of an acute process in such cases. Imaging studies such as CT or MRI can nearly always delineate these and other conditions and enable an accurate diagnosis of retroperitoneal fibrosis.

BIBLIOGRAPHY

1. Amis ES Jr: Retroperitoneal fibrosis: Review article. AJR 157:321–329, 1991.
2. Castilho LN, Iizuka FH, Fugita OE, et al: Laparoscopic treatment of retroperitoneal fibrosis: Report of two cases and review of the literature. Rev Hosp Clin Fac Med Sao Paulo 55:69–76, 2000.
3. Hall MC, von Eschenbach AC, Ames FC: Diseases of the retroperitoneum. In Gillenwater JY, Grayhack JT, Howards SS, Duckett JW (eds): Adult and Pediatric Urology, 3rd ed. St. Louis, Mosby, 1996, pp 1123–1158.
4. Hodge EE: Operations of the ureter. In Novick AC, Streem SB, Pontes JE (eds): Stewart's Operative Urology, 2nd ed. Baltimore, Williams & Wilkins, 1989, pp 369–373.
5. Hughes D, Buckley PJ: Idiopathic retroperitoneal fibrosis is a macrophage-rich process: Implications for its pathogenesis and treatment. Am J Surg Pathol 17:482–490, 1993.
6. Jaffer A, Calabrese L: Severe back and abdominal pain in a 44-year-old woman. Cleveland Clin J Med 65:515–518, 1998.
7. McDougal WS, MacDonell RC Jr: Treatment of idiopathic retroperitoneal fibrosis by immunosuppression. J Urol 145:112–114, 1991.
8. Persky L, Kursh ED, Feldman S, Resnick MI: Diseases of the retroperitoneum: Retroperitoneal fibrosis. In Walsh PC, Retik AB, Stamey TA, Vaughan ED Jr (eds): Campbell's Urology, 6th ed. Philadelphia, W.B. Saunders, 1992, pp 595–613.
9. Resnick MI, Kursh ED: Extrinsic obstruction of the ureter. In Walsh PC, Retik AB, Vaughan ED Jr, Wein AJ (eds): Campbell's Urology, 7th ed. Philadelphia, W.B. Saunders, 1998, pp 387–422.

65. INTERSTITIAL CYSTITIS

Howard B. Goldman, MD

1. What is interstitial cystitis?

Interstitial cystitis (IC) is a complex of voiding symptoms secondary to a functionally diminished bladder capacity. Typically urgency, frequency, nocturia, and suprapubic or bladder pain are noted. In many patients bladder capacity is decreased because of fibrosis. Pain can occur as the bladder fills and stretches. This leads the patient to empty the bladder frequently, which reduces the stretch in the fibrosed bladder and gives pain relief. However, in certain patients the problem is primarily a sensory abnormality and no fibrosis exists. **Interstitial cystitis is a diagnosis of exclusion.** Other known entities can cause a similar symptom complex and it is crucial to rule out all other potential etiologies before labeling a patient as having IC.

2. What is the differential diagnosis for a patient with the above symptom complex?

- **Infectious:** bacterial, viral, fungal, tuberculous, or schistosomal cystitis; urethritis, malacoplakia, active genital herpes, vaginitis
- **Inflammatory:** Cytoxan (cyclophosphamide)- or radiation-induced cystitis; bladder amyloidosis; chemical cystitis, eosinophilic cystitis
- **Neoplastic:** carcinoma in situ; transitional cell carcinoma or squamous cell carcinoma of the bladder; urethral cancer
- **Anatomic:** cystocele; pelvic mass compressing bladder; urethral obstruction

3. How common is interstitial cystitis?

A population-based study conducted in Helsinki, Finland estimated the prevalence of IC to be 18.1 per 100,000 women. With the inclusion of men in this analysis, the prevalence dropped to 10.6 cases per 100,000. Women with IC outnumbered men 10 to 1. An American study reported that in 1987 there were 43,500 diagnosed cases of IC in the United States. However, this may represent a vast underestimate, because many women remain undiagnosed.

4. What diseases are associated with IC?

Multiple allergies, irritable bowel syndrome, and fibromyalgia have all been noted to have an increased prevalence in people with IC.

5. How is IC diagnosed?

As noted earlier, IC is a diagnosis of exclusion. Any patient presenting with the characteristic constellation of symptoms associated with IC must be carefully evaluated to ensure that another process is not the cause of such symptoms.

The characteristic constellation of symptoms includes irritative voiding (urgency, frequency, nocturia) and bladder pain. Usually pain is relieved after voiding. However, many investigators do not consider pain to be a necessary component of the patient's complaints and consider irritative symptoms alone indicative of IC, providing other criteria are met.

A urine culture should be obtained to make sure a bacterial infection is not the cause of these symptoms. Atypical vaginitis (mycoplasma, ureaplasm) should be ruled out as well with specialized cultures and treated if identified. Urine cytology should be obtained to help exclude a malignancy.

A complete examination must be performed to make sure a significant cystocele or pelvic mass is not present. A pelvic ultrasound should be obtained to verify that no other pathology exists that could be causing bladder symptoms.

Urodynamics should be performed to eliminate possible motor detrusor instability. In addition, it will verify that the bladder capacity is diminished and should reproduce an intense urge to void at low bladder volumes (<150 ml).

Cystoscopy is required to rule out potential intravesical or urethral lesions, to identify a Hunner's ulcer, and to perform hydrodistention. If an intravesical or urethral lesion is noted, it should be biopsied. There is some controversy about whether all patients with IC should have bladder biopsies performed. Because there is no pathognomonic pathologic finding for IC, some feel it is unnecessary to biopsy those patients without lesions on cystoscopy.

If all other causes of the patient's symptoms have been ruled out, the characteristic findings of a Hunner's ulcer or glomerulations after hydrodistention are necessary to establish the diagnosis of IC.

6. What is a Hunner's ulcer?

A Hunner's ulcer is a pink ulceration in the bladder mucosa seen in about 10% of people with IC.

7. How is hydrodistention performed?

Hydrodistention is performed with a patient under general or spinal anesthesia, and the bladder is filled to its capacity at a pressure of 80 cm of water. Typically, the fluid bag is hung 80 cm above the level of the patient's pubis and the bladder is filled until leakage occurs around the cystoscope. The bladder is then drained and refilled. The last portion of fluid drained may be blood-tinged. With the bladder refilled, cystoscopic inspection is performed to identify glomerulations.

8. What are glomerulations?

Glomerulations are pinpoint, petechial sites of hemorrhage of the urothelium that are visible after the bladder has been distended, drained, and redistended. Although they are not specific for IC, their diffuse presence in association with appropriate symptoms is required for the diagnosis of IC (except when a Hunner's ulcer is identified, in which case glomerulations are not required to make the diagnosis of IC).

9. What is the National Institute of Arthritis, Diabetes, Digestive and Kidney Diseases (NIADDK) research definition of IC?

The NIADDK established research criteria for the diagnosis of IC in an effort to make sure that patients entered into IC studies at different sites could be compared. Although this was not an effort to actually clinically define the disease, it has been used by many researchers in this way because no other such criteria are available. The criteria are presented below.

Required criteria:
1. Pain associated with the bladder **or** urinary urgency **and**
2. Glomerulations **or** Hunner's ulcer on cystoscopic examination.

Examination of glomerulations should occur after distention of the bladder under anesthesia to a pressure of 80–100 cm H_2O for 1–2 minutes. The bladder may be distended up to two times before evaluation. Glomerulations must be diffuse.

Exclusion criteria:
1. Bladder capacity of greater than 350 ml on awake cystometry
2. Absence of intense urge to void with bladder filled to 100 ml of gas or 150 ml of water during cystometry, using a fill rate of 30–100 ml/min
3. Demonstration of phasic involuntary bladder contractions on cystometry
4. Duration of symptoms <9 months
5. Absence of nocturia
6. Symptoms relieved by antimicrobials, urinary antiseptics, anticholinergics, or antispasmodics
7. Frequency of urination, while awake, of fewer than 8 times/day
8. Diagnosis of bacterial cystitis or prostatitis within a 3-month period
9. Bladder or lower ureteral calculi
10. Active genital herpes
11. Uterine, cervical, vaginal, or urethral cancer

12. Urethral diverticulum
13. Cyclophosphamide or any type of chemical cystitis
14. Tuberculous cystitis
15. Radiation cystitis
16. Benign or malignant bladder tumors
17. Vaginitis
18. Age < 18 years

10. What is the etiology of IC?

Although the definite etiology of IC is unknown, a number of theories may explain the initiation and/or persistence of the disease in certain subpopulations. It is likely that the etiology is multifactorial.

1. A defective glycosaminoglycan (GAG) layer on the urothelium allowing leakage of urine past the luminal surface.

2. An infection that either leads to an autoimmune response or is caused by cryptic organisms that are not appropriately treated.

3. A neurogenic mechanism whereby abnormal sensory impulses lead to an inflammatory response.

4. Reflex sympathetic dystrophy affecting the bladder.

5. Urine that contains substances that the urothelium perceives as toxic, which induces an inflammatory response.

6. Pelvic floor dysfunction

11. How is IC treated?

Hydrodistention may be therapeutic in addition to being diagnostic. Unfortunately, the relief it may provide is usually short-lived. Because up to 50% of patients will experience spontaneous remissions of varying lengths, conservative patient-directed therapy may prove useful. Avoidance of certain foods and beverages, bladder training, and attempts to decrease stress are worth trying. Unfortunately, many patients will require more intensive treatment.

Various oral systemic agents have been used with varying degrees of success. Amitriptyline and other tricyclic antidepressants will provide symptomatic relief, especially of pain, in many patients. They are believed to act through a number of varied mechanisms, including the blocking of histaminergic receptors, anticholinergic actions, and as a sedative. Pentosan polysulfate (Elmiron) has been touted as an effective treatment for IC. It is a semisynthetic polysaccharide that has similar properties to GAG. In addition, it may help stabilize mast cells and prevent histamine release. However, recent studies have demonstrated that although it may provide relief to some patients, the majority do not seem to derive long-term benefit.

Another route of therapy is via intravesical treatments. These may be tried before, after, or concomitantly with systemic treatments. Dimethyl sulfoxide (DMSO) introduced into the bladder via a catheter has been used because of its antiinflammatory, muscle relaxant, and analgesic proprieties. Four to six treatments given at 1 to 2 week intervals are usually required. Intravesical heparin, lidocaine, hydrocortisone, or sodium bicarbonate may augment the effect of the DMSO or may provide symptomatic relief when used without DMSO. Many physicians have their own "cocktail" made up of a combination of the previously listed compounds that they find effective.

12. Is surgical treatment necessary?

Rare patients with a discrete Hunner's ulcer may benefit from transurethral resection, fulguration, or laser coagulation of the lesion. In other patients, all conservative treatment options should be exhausted before surgical therapy is considered. Only a small minority of patients will require surgical treatment. Patients with IC with pain who are unresponsive to other treatments may be considered for a urinary diversion with or without a cystectomy. Either an ileal conduit or a continent diversion may be appropriate, depending on the patient's degree of motivation. Patients who lack pain as a key symptom may do well with an augmentation enterocystoplasty.

13. What new treatments are on the horizon?

Until the exact etiology of IC is elucidated, it may be difficult to find more effective therapies; however, various new systemic and intravesical treatments are currently showing promising results. Systemic cyclosporine or other immunoregulatory substances may provide relief via their immune modulating capabilities. Intravesical bacille Calmette-Guérin (BCG) also is being evaluated and is theorized to provide relief either by increasing nitric oxide production or by stimulating T-helper cells and promoting urothelial repair. Recently, some have attempted to modulate the symptoms of IC via sacral nerve stimulation. Early results in small groups of patients appear promising.

BIBLIOGRAPHY

1. Gillenwater JY, Wein AJ: Summary of the National Institute of Arthritis, Diabetes, Digestive and Kidney Diseases workshop on interstitial cystitis, NIH. J Urol 140:203–206, 1988.
2. Hanno PM: Interstitial cystitis and related diseases. In Walsh PC, Retik AB, Vaughan Jr ED, Wein AJ (eds): Campbell's Urology, 7th ed. Philadelphia, W. B. Saunders, 1998.
3. Held PJ, Hanno PM, Wein AJ, et al: Epidemiology of interstitial cystitis. In Hanno PM, Staskin DR, Krane RJ, Wein AJ (eds): Interstitial Cystitis. London, Springer Verlag, 1990.
4. Jepson JV, Sall M, Rhodes PR, et al: Long-term experience with pentosanpolysulfate in interstitial cystitis. Urology 51:381–387, 1998.
5. Maher CF, Carey MP, Dwyer PL, Schluter PL: Percutaneous sacral nerve root stimulation for intractable interstitial cystitis. J Urol 165: 884–886,2001.
6. Oravisto KJ: Epidemiology of interstitial cystitis. Ann Chir Gynaecol Fenn 64:75–77, 1975.
7. Parsons CL, Hurst RE: Decreased urinary uronic acid levels in individuals with interstitial cystitis. J Urol 143:690–693, 1990.
8. Peters KM, Diokno AC, Steinert BW, Gonzalez JA: The efficacy of intravesical bacillus Calmette-Guérin in the treatment of interstitial cystitis: Long-term follow-up. J Urol 159:1483–1487, 1998.
9. Ueda T, Tamaki M, Ugawa O, et al: Improvement of interstitial cystitis symptoms and problems that developed during treatment with oral IPD-1151-T. J Urol 164:1917–1920,2000.

66. PROSTATITIS

Kurt H. Dinchman, M.D.

1. What is prostatitis?

Prostatitis is a syndrome that presents with symptoms consistent with inflammation and/or infection of the prostate gland, including terminal dysuria, dysfunctional voiding, perineal pain, increased frequency of urination, and pain with ejaculation. Prostatitis is so common that up to 50% of all men may experience symptoms of this syndrome in their lifetime.

2. How is prostatitis classified?

Prostatitis is classified as bacterial or nonbacterial and is characterized as acute or chronic in nature.

3. What is prostadynia?

Patients with prostadynia have symptoms consistent with prostatitis, but cultures of prostatic secretions are negative and white blood cells are absent. The condition is theorized to occur secondary to bladder neck dysfunction (such as high tone or spasms), leading to reflux of urine into the prostatic and ejaculatory ducts.

4. How does acute bacterial prostatitis differ from chronic bacterial prostatitis?

Acute bacterial prostatitis is usually a febrile illness of sudden onset, characterized by severe irritative symptoms, positive urine cultures, and a boggy, enlarged, and tender prostate on physical examination.

Chronic bacterial prostatitis is characterized by persistent bacterial infections with inflammatory cells in prostatic secretions despite multiple regimens of prolonged antibiotic therapy. Patients typically have a long history of irritative symptoms, along with mild obstructive voiding.

5. How is prostatitis diagnosed?

It is difficult to diagnose prostatitis unless it is the acute bacterial variety. It is difficult to differentiate among chronic bacterial prostatitis, nonbacterial prostatitis, and prostadynia, because symptoms and physical findings may be similar.

6. What is the role of examination of prostatic secretions?

Prostatic secretions obtained by prostatic massage may reveal white blood cells from the initially voided specimen; bacterial may be seen in acute prostatitis.

7. What are segmented cultures?

Segmented cultures are quantative cultures aimed at localizing bacteria to a particular segment of the urinary tract. Usually four segments are cultured. The first segment, called VB_1, is the first voided 10 ml of urine. A positive VB_1 culture indicates urethritis and/or prostatitis. A positive VB_2 (midstream urine) culture indicates cystitis. EPS, or expressed positive cultures of VB_3 (first 10 ml of urine voided after prostatic massage), and expressed prostatic secretions (EPS) indicate prostatic infection.

8. What is the most common pathogen in prostatitis?

Escherichia coli by far is the most common. Other agents include *Enterobacter, Proteus, Klebsiella,* and *Pseudomonas* spp.

9. What are the most commonly used antibiotic agents in the treatment of prostatitis? Why?

The most commonly used agent is trimethoprim-sulfamethoxazole, given orally in a dose of 160–180 mg twice a day. In a sulfa-allergic patient, ciprofloxacin (a fluoroquinolone), 500 mg twice a day, is also an excellent choice. Both are superior to other agents because of their 2:1–3:1 concentration in prostatic tissue vs. serum.

10. How do treatment plans differ between acute and chronic prostatitis?

Acute prostatitis often presents with systemic manifestations. The involved pathogen is usually a gram-negative agent and may require parenteral administration of antibiotics, such as an aminoglycoside and ampicillin, followed by a 4-week regimen of oral antibiotics to avert chronic bacterial prostatitis. Chronic bacterial prostatitis may require a prolonged antibiotic schedule. Patients often have prostatic calculi, which may harbor bacteria that present a potential for reinfection; chronic suppression may be required.

11. How is nonbacterial prostatitis treated?

Because no pathogen is isolated, a regimen of a broad-range antibiotic, such as doxycycline, may be tried. Patients with unsatisfactory results may be managed with antiinflammatory agents. Some of these patients may respond to diet modification similar to that recommended for interstitial cystitis patients, i.e., restricting caffeinated, acidic foods with emphasis on hydration.

12. How is prostadynia treated?

Prostadynia is by far the most difficult prostatic syndrome to treat; no infectious or inflammatory process is established. Patients are counseled on the nature of the syndrome, and treatment with an α-adrenergic agent and muscle relaxants, such as diazepam, has proved to be marginally successful. Previously mentioned dietary modification may also benefit these patients as they manage their symptoms.

13. What are the other forms of prostatitis?

Gonococcal prostatitis Mycotic prostatitis
Tuberculous prostatitis Nonspecific granulomatous prostatitis
Parasitic prostatitis

14. What is a prostatic abscess? How is it treated?

A prostatic abscess is a life-threatening infection of the prostate seen in immunocompromised patients, such as those with diabetes and renal failure. Treatment consists of immediate surgical drainage, including transurethral methods and wide-spectrum parenteral antibiotics.

15. What other clinical diagnosis should be considered in patients with a history of acute or chronic prostatitis?

Some patients with a history of prostatitis refractive to conventional therapy should be considered for urodynamic evaluation. Frequently, these patients have bladder dysfunction due to detrusor instability. The possibility of interstitial cystitis also should be considered if the patient does not respond to therapy.

BIBLIOGRAPHY

1. Gillenwater JY, Grayhack JT, Howards SS, Duckett JW (eds): Adult and Pediatric Urology, 3rd ed. St. Louis, Mosby, 1996.
2. Walsh PC, Retik AB, Stamey TA, Vaughan ED Jr, Wein AJ (eds): Campbell's Urology, 8th ed. Philadelphia, W.B. Saunders, 2002.
3. Seidman EJ, Hanno PM (eds): Current Urologic Therapy. Philadelphia, W.B. Saunders, 1994.

67. URINARY TRACT INFECTION IN ADULT FEMALES

Howard B. Goldman, MD

1. What is a urinary tract infection (UTI)?
Urinary tract infection is a broad term used to describe an inflammatory response of urothelium to any infectious agent.

2. What are the common types of UTIs in women?
A UTI can involve either the upper urinary tract (kidneys) or the lower urinary tract (bladder and urethra). **Pyelonephritis** refers to a UTI involving the kidney. Acute pyelonephritis is a syndrome characterized by fever, chills, and flank pain as well as bacteriuria and pyuria. **Cystitis** refers to inflammation of the bladder, usually associated with dysuria (pain during voiding), frequency, urgency, and suprapubic discomfort. In the female, the symptoms of urethritis are very similar to those of cystitis, and it may be difficult to tell the two apart. Primary urethritis is relatively rare in females. The most common UTI in the adult female is acute bacterial cystitis.

3. How are UTIs classified?
UTIs are either uncomplicated or complicated. The clinical distinction is important; complicated UTIs can be much more difficult to treat.

In **uncomplicated** UTIs, patients have no underlying structural or functional abnormalities. These frequently occur in otherwise healthy adult females and usually respond well to treatment with standard, inexpensive antimicrobial therapy. Few complications occur, and the major problem encountered is the morbidity suffered by some women who have recurrent episodes.

In contrast, in **complicated** UTIs, the effectiveness of antimicrobial therapy may be reduced secondary to an underlying structural or functional abnormality. Renal or bladder calculi, urinary obstruction, voiding dysfunction, anatomic abnormalities secondary to previous surgery or of congenital origin, the presence of an indwelling catheter, and other diseases that predispose to infection, such as diabetes mellitus, are but a few abnormalities that can make a UTI "complicated."

In addition, UTIs may be classified as isolated infections, unresolved bacteriuria, bacterial persistence, or reinfection.

Isolated infection is the first UTI a woman has or a UTI isolated from a previous infection by at least 6 months.

Unresolved bacteriuria implies that the urinary tract is not sterilized during therapy, which may be caused by bacteria that are resistant to the antimicrobial therapy selected or secondary to rapid development of resistant bacteria from a previously susceptible population. This also may be secondary to rapid reinfection with another resistant species before the initial species is eradicated.

Bacterial persistence refers to recurrence of infection with the same organism after initial sterilization of the urine. It is caused by a site within the urinary tract that was excluded from the appropriate high level of antimicrobial exposure. Infection stones, urethral diverticula, and enterovesical fistula are but a few of the common sites that are difficult to sterilize with antimicrobial therapy alone.

Reinfections are UTIs in which a new infection occurs with a new organism after a previous infection has been eradicated.

Infections are **recurrent** when more than 2 occur in a 6-month or 3 occur in a 1-year period. The vast majority of recurrent infections are due to reinfection, whereas the minority reflect bacterial persistence.

4. How common are UTIs in adult females?

UTIs occur in approximately 1% of women before the onset of sexual activity. After sexual intercourse has been initiated, the prevalence rises to 3–4%. After the age of 65, 20–30% of women will experience a UTI.

5. How is a UTI diagnosed?

The patient usually will provide a history of signs and symptoms of a UTI (reviewed in question 2). A urinalysis is important: Bacteriuria with pyuria (leukocytes in the urine) should be demonstrated. If pyuria is absent, the diagnosis of a UTI must be questioned. Urine for culture should be carefully collected to reduce possible perineal contamination. In the past it was widely stated that 100,000 colony forming units (CFUs) had to be present to diagnose a UTI. However, the current thinking is that in the symptomatic woman, as few as 100 CFUs/ml represent significant bacteriuria.

6. What are the common organisms that cause UTIs?

The vast majority of UTIs are caused by bacteria, although yeasts and fungi as well as other infectious agents may less frequently cause UTIs.

Escherichia coli (E. coli) accounts for 80–90% of uncomplicated infections. *Staphylococcus saprophyticus* accounts for 10–20%, and other Enterobacteriaceae, such as *Klebsiella, Proteus,* and *Enterobacter,* account for most of the remaining uncomplicated UTIs.

In complicated UTIs, *E. coli* accounts for only about 20% of cases, whereas the other Enterobacteriaceae are much more common. In addition, other gram-negative bacilli, such as *Pseudomonas* and *Acinetobacter*, as well as gram-positive organisms like *Staphylococcus aureus* are more common.

7. What is the pathogenesis of UTIs in women?

Most UTIs in women represent ascending infections. Bacteria from the fecal reservoir may colonize the perineum and after ascending the bladder via the urethra cause a symptomatic UTI. The relatively short length of the female urethra makes the ascent relatively easy.

8. Does sexual intercourse cause UTI?

Sexual intercourse may increase the prevalence of infection in otherwise susceptible women. This is evidenced by the increased prevalence of UTIs after women become sexually active. The theory is that vigorous activity during intercourse "milks" bacteria from the vagina or distal urethra up the length of the urethra and into the bladder. In addition, the activity during intercourse may cause urethral trauma, leaving it more susceptible to infection. Intercourse may play a role in susceptible individuals, but the fact that most sexually active women do not get UTIs argues against its role as a primary mechanism.

9. What makes some otherwise healthy women susceptible to UTIs?

A distinct population of women suffer from recurrent UTIs. Research demonstrates that many of these women have **increased adherence of bacteria to vaginal and urethral surfaces** compared to women without UTIs. In addition, such women are more likely to have a nonsecretor blood group phenotype. Evidently, a protective effect (fewer UTIs) occurs when secretory blood group antigens are present. Thus, genetic differences influence the ability of the genitourinary epithelium to resist bacterial adherence.

10. Are there bacterial characteristics that increase virulence?

Yes. Bacteria have cell surface structures called adhesins that facilitate their binding to epithelial cell-surface receptors. Research demonstrates that certain types of adhesins, in particular certain pili, may contribute to the virulence of an organism. P pili in particular have been shown to be important virulence factors in pyelonephritis.

11. What type of evaluation is necessary for a woman with a UTI?

No additional investigation is required in most women with uncomplicated UTIs. Various studies have examined the yield of cystoscopy, intravenous urography, and cystography in such women and have found it minimal. However, under certain circumstances, these studies are helpful. Indications for urologic evaluation include hematuria, infection with urea-splitting bacteria, or persistent or breakthrough UTIs while on antimicrobial treatment. Any time there is a clinical impression that a complicated UTI is present (e.g., symptoms suggesting a stone, history of previous urologic surgery, diabetes mellitus), a thorough urologic work-up may be called for. The typical evaluation consists of cystoscopy and upper urinary tract imaging with the addition of urodynamics, voiding cystourethrography, retrograde ureteropyelography, and renal scintigraphy when indicated.

12. What is the treatment for an isolated episode of uncomplicated cystitis?

Most such episodes respond very well to a short (3–5 day) course of inexpensive oral antimicrobial therapy. Treatment with trimethoprim-sulfamethoxazole (TMP-sulfa) double-strength twice/day or nitrofurantoin 100 mg 4 times/day usually will provide good coverage and give rapid results. Recent studies though have demonstrated a mild increase in resistance to TMP-sulfa in some geographic areas while the resistance to nitrofurantoin and the quinolones remains low. Thus some now recommend a short course of a quinolone as first-line therapy.

In many of these patients, a pretherapy culture is unnecessary. If symptoms persist, a culture is mandatory and the therapy is adjusted based on susceptibility testing.

13. What is the appropriate therapy for complicated cystitis?

The most important part of successful management of these UTIs is the recognition of complicating factors. Frequently, those factors will be obvious in the history provided by the patient. Occasionally, an atypical presentation or persistence of infection after routine antimicrobial therapy provides clues that a complicated UTI exists.

Correcting any identifiable abnormality is an important step in eradicating these infections. Pretherapy urine culture is also crucial, because many resistant organisms are present in such patients. In addition, because of the different spectra of pathogenic bacteria seen in these patients, more powerful antibiotics (frequently quinolones) given for longer durations (7–14 days) may be necessary.

14. Which patients with pyelonephritis can be treated as outpatients?

Otherwise healthy women with uncomplicated pyelonephritis and only moderate symptoms may be treated with an outpatient oral antimicrobial regimen. However, many women with acute pyelonephritis will require intravenous antimicrobial therapy and hydration and thus require hospitalization. The indications for hospitalization include dehydration, inability to take oral medication, severe pain, hemodynamic instability, and structural or functional complicating factors.

15. How is recurrent uncomplicated cystitis treated?

Three options are available for treating recurrent UTIs. In general, inexpensive oral agents (TMP/TMP-sulfa/nitrofurantoin) may be used.

- **Peri-intercourse prophylaxis:** In patients in whom the UTIs are directly related to sexual intercourse, an oral antimicrobial can be taken just before or after intercourse.
- **Intermittent self-start therapy:** Women with relatively infrequent recurrent UTIs (3–4 per year) may be given a standing prescription for a short course of oral antibiotics that they can start at the first sign of a UTI.
- **Low-dose antimicrobial prophylaxis:** Women with frequent UTIs may benefit from a daily low dose of an oral antimicrobial agent. This will help prevent infection and may lead to the resolution of colonization of the perineum or urethra with uropathic bacterial species. Trimethoprim (TMP) 100 mg, single-strength TMP/sulfa, and nitrofurantoin 100 mg/at bedtime are good choices for prophylactic therapy.

When the above strategies fail to prevent infection, further urologic evaluation may be necessary.

16. Should UTIs be treated during pregnancy?

Yes. Even asymptomatic bacteriuria should be treated: Physiologic and anatomic changes associated with pregnancy increase the risk of pyelonephritis, which may lead to premature delivery and other potential complications.

BIBLIOGRAPHY

1. Fair WR, McClennan BL, Jost RG: Are excretory urograms necessary in evaluating women with urinary tract infection? J Urol 121:313–315, 1979.
2. Kunin CM: Urinary Tract Infections—Detection, Prevention, and Management, 5th ed. Baltimore, Williams & Wilkins, 1997.
3. Gupta K, Scholes D, Stamm WE: Increasing prevalence of antimicrobial resistance among uropathogens causing acute uncomplicated cystitis in women. JAMA 281:736–738, 1999.
4. Nickel JC, Wilson J, Morales A, Heaton J: Value of urologic investigation in a targeted group of women with recurrent urinary tract infections. Can J Surg 34:591–594, 1991.
5. Shaffer AJ, Jones JM, Dunn JK: Association of in-vitro *E. coli* adherence to vaginal and buccal epithelial cells with susceptibility of women to recurrent urinary tract infections. N Engl J Med 304:1062–1066, 1981.
6. Schaeffer AJ: Infection of the urinary tract. In Walsh PC, Retik AB, Vaughan ED Jr, Wein AJ (eds): Campbell's Urology, 7th ed. Philadelphia, W.B. Saunders, 1998.

68. URINARY TRACT INFECTIONS IN CHILDREN

Jeffrey S. Palmer, M.D. and Jack S. Elder, M.D.

1. What is a urinary tract infection?

A urinary tract infection (UTI) is a bacterial infection in the urine. The number of bacteria that must be present to cause a significant urinary infection is 10,000 to 100,000 colony-forming units/ml of voided urine. The infection may involve the kidney (pyelonephritis) or the bladder (cystitis).

2. What is the incidence of bacteriuria in boys and girls?

Childhood UTIs are more common in girls, except during the first few months of life, when they are more common in boys. Between 0.03% and 1.2% of boys develop a UTI during school years; 3–5% of girls develop a UTI during this time.

3. Which sex is more likely to get urinary tract infections?

Boys have a higher incidence of UTI during the first year of life. Girls are more likely to get UTIs after the first year of life.

4. How is UTI diagnosed?

The diagnosis of UTI usually is made from urinalysis and urine culture. In infants and in children who are not toilet trained, a clean bag is placed over the genitalia, which have been washed. This "bag specimen" may be unreliable because of bacterial contamination of the bag itself or contamination from bacteria that have colonized the skin. If the urinalysis from a bag specimen shows significant pyuria, if only one organism is cultured, and if the child is symptomatic, then the bag specimen may be considered to be reliable. However, if any of the three criteria is not met, one may **not** conclude that the child has a UTI. Instead, the infection should be confirmed with either a catheterized urine specimen or a suprapubic tap.

In older patients, diagnosis of a UTI usually is based on a voided specimen, which should grow at least 10,000 and preferably 100,000 colonies of a single organism.

5. At what ages are UTIs most commonly diagnosed?

In boys, UTIs are most common between birth and 6 months, whereas in girls, the peak incidence is at 2–3 years.

6. What are the typical symptoms and signs of UTIs?

Urinary tract infections may be subclassified into cystitis and pyelonephritis. Typically, children with cystitis have dysuria, urgency, frequency, suprapubic pain, and also often have incontinence. An associated symptom is malodorous urine. In some cases, the only manifestation of a UTI may be day and night incontinence or nocturnal enuresis.

Pyelonephritis refers to a renal infection. Typical symptoms include fever and upper abdominal or flank pain localized to the side of the infection; some may experience malaise, nausea and vomiting, and diarrhea.

7. What are typical symptoms of UTIs in infants?

Approximately 66% have fever, 55% have irritability, 40% exhibit poor feeding, 35% have vomiting, and 31% have diarrhea; abdominal distention and jaundice occur in < 10% of patients.

8. How accurate is urinalysis in the diagnosis of a UTI?

Although pyuria, nitrites, and leukocyte esterase are helpful in indicating that a UTI is present, a positive urine culture is necessary to confirm the diagnosis.

9. What is the Griess test?

This test refers to the reagent for the detection of nitrites in solution. Given adequate contact, bacteria convert nitrate normally present in the urine to nitrite. Reagent paper is impregnated with sulfanilic acid and alpha-naphthylamine. In the presence of nitrites, a diazotization reaction occurs, causing the two substances to form a red azo dye. A positive colorimetric reaction implies the presence of bacteria in the urine. Approximately 4 hours is necessary for conversion of nitrate to nitrite. Thus, the first morning urine is the only reliable specimen for this test. The test has a specificity of 92–100% but a sensitivity of 35–85%.

10. What is the leukocyte esterase reaction?

The esterase enzyme, which is released by polymorphonuclear leukocytes, acts on an ester substrate on a test strip to produce the indoxyl compound. Two indoxyl molecules in the presence of oxygen will form indigo, a dark blue shade. The leukocyte esterase activity can thus be substantiated by a positive blue reaction.

11. What is the route of entry for children with cystitis?

The urethra. The bacteria causing cystitis come from stool flora. In uncircumcised males, bacteria that have colonized the glans often are the source of bacteriuria.

12. In children with pyelonephritis, what is the source of bacteria?

Pyelonephritis results from an ascending infection from the bladder, and the bacteria come from the stool flora.

13. What host factors normally resist UTI?

An acidic urine pH, high or low urine osmolality, and high urea and organic acid content resist bacterial growth. Furthermore, the ability of the bladder to empty completely helps resist bacterial colonization of the bladder. Polymorphonuclear leukoyctes, which also resist infection, are present in the bladder mucosal surface.

14. What is bacterial adhesion?

Certain strains of urinary pathogens contain bacterial surface elements called fimbriae (pili), which recognize specific receptors on the epithelial cells. These fimbriae are nonflagellar, proteinaceous appendages that protrude from the bacterial cell surface like tiny hairs. The pili are classified by their ability to agglutinate erythrocytes of different animal species and by sugars that can block this hemagglutination.

Bacterial adhesion may be divided into mannose-sensitive (inhibited by mannose) and mannose-resistant (adhesion not inhibited by mannose). Mannose-sensitive adhesion is mediated by type 1 fimbriae, which agglutinate guinea pig erythrocytes. Type 1 fimbriae are present on most *Escherichia coli* strains, pathogens as well as nonpathogens. Type 2 pili or fimbriae agglutinate human erythrocytes and are mannose-resistant. An example of type 2 pili is P fimbriae, which interacts with a uroepithelial cell receptor that contains a gal-gal disaccharide, which is part of the oligosaccharide chain of the P blood group antigens. *E. coli* with P fimbriae have been identified within 90% of organisms causing pyelonephritis but <20% of *E. coli* causing cystitis.

15. What host factors predispose to the development of UTIs?

Age: During the first few weeks of life, all babies have an increased incidence of UTIs. During this time, the periurethral area of healthy girls and boys is massively colonized with aerobic bacteria, particularly *E. coli,* enterococci, and staphylococci. This colonization decreases during the first year and is unusual in children who do not get recurrent UTIs beyond the age of 5 years.

Voiding dysfunction: Urinary tract infections in girls are particularly common around 2–3 years of age, the peak age of toilet training, presumably because of mild voiding dysfunction that occurs during that time. In children with bladder instability that causes diurnal incontinence beyond the age of 3–4 years, there is a tendency not to empty the bladder completely, leaving residual urine, which also predisposes to UTI.

Vesicoureteral reflux: When urine is transported to the bladder, normally the urine remains in the bladder until it is voided, because a physiologic flap valve prevents it from returning back to the ureter and kidney. Children with reflux have an increased incidence of upper urinary tract infection.

Genitourinary anomalies: Several genitourinary anomalies that cause urinary stasis predispose the child to UTI—ureteropelvic junction obstruction, ureterovesical junction obstruction, retrocaval ureter, ureterocele, and posterior urethral valves.

Sex: Except for the newborn period, girls are more susceptible to UTIs than boys, presumably because the urethra is much shorter in the female.

Fecal colonization: As indicated above, the presence of urinary pathogens in the periurethral area predisposes the child to UTIs.

Chronic constipation: Some children with constipation are predisposed to UTIs because the dilated rectum interferes with voiding and may cause mild retention of urine.

Retention of foreskin: Uncircumcised male infants are much more likely to develop a UTI than boys who are circumcised, because bacteria seem to colonize the glans under the foreskin.

Host receptor activity: Uroepithelial cells from infection-prone girls and women bind *E. coli* more avidly than cells from nonsusceptible girls. Glycolipids characterizing the P blood group system are found in host uroepithelial cells and may serve as bacterial receptors. The P blood group phenotype has been found in 90% of girls with recurrent pyelonephritis.

Immune status: Girls with a normal urinary tract and recurrent UTIs have significantly lower baseline levels of urinary IgA and a blunted response to infection. Lower baseline levels of immunoglobulins in the perineum may diminish the ability to develop a response to infection.

16. At what age are uncircumcised boys most likely to have a urinary tract infection?

They are 10–15 times more likely to have a UTI during the first year of life.

17. What is acute hemorrhagic cystitis?

Hemorrhagic cystitis refers to the passing of blood in the urine during a UTI. In children, this condition may be caused by adenovirus 11. In one series of infants with acute hemorrhagic cystitis, 17% had an adenovirus, 17% had *E. coli,* and the remainder had no infectious agent isolated from their urine.

18. How does pyelonephritis cause renal scarring?

Following intrarenal reflux of infected urine, renal damage may occur by a direct effect of the bacteria, ischemia with reperfusion damage, and/or an inflammatory response. The bacteria may have a direct effect by bacterial adhesion, which brings the bacteria closer to the cell. Bacterial endotoxin is then concentrated adjacent to the cell, which activates the complement system. In addition, ischemic damage may result when the purine pool is consumed during anoxia due to anaerobic metabolism; during reperfusion, the remaining hypoxanthine pool is metabolized to xanthine. In the presence of xanthine oxidase, xanthine is converted to uric acid and superoxide. Superoxide can be converted to peroxide and hydroxyl radicals, both of which are damaging to cells. Within 10 minutes after renal infection occurs, marked granulocyte aggregation may occur, which leads to capillary obstruction. During the inflammatory response, endotoxin causes complement activation, which leads to phagocytosis. This respiratory burst causes the release of superoxide and the formation of peroxide and hydroxyl radicals. All tissues in the body contain superoxide dismutase to degrade rapidly the superoxide. However, urine does not contain superoxide dismutase and thus the hydroxyl radicals act unopposed in the urine.

19. How long should a child with a UTI be treated?

Treatment depends on the age of the child and severity of the illness. In general, in children with a febrile UTI, treatment for 10–14 days is mandatory, whereas for cystitis, treatment for 5–7 days should suffice.

20. How is pyelonephritis diagnosed?

Pyelonephritis may be diagnosed on clinical factors, including fever, malaise, abdominal or flank pain, and irritability. In infants, irritability or poor feeding may be the only sign. The most accurate way of diagnosing true pyelonephritis with renal parenchymal infection is to perform a DMSA renal scan.

21. Which children should undergo radiologic evaluation for a UTI?

AUTI often is the first manifestation of a child's underlying anatomic or functional urinary tract abnormality. Approximately 30% of all children who have bacteriuria, and almost 50% of those under the age of 3 years, have abnormal radiologic studies of the urinary tract. Vesicoureteral reflux is most common. Radiologic investigation is recommended for all children under the age of 5 years with UTI, all boys irrespective of age, all girls with pyelonephritis, and following a second UTI in girls over 5 years old.

22. What does the radiologic evaluation for a UTI consist of?

The initial study is a voiding cystourethrogram to determine whether reflux or a structural abnormality of the lower urinary tract is present. Next, a renal ultrasound should be obtained to determine whether any upper urinary tract abnormalities are present. If both studies are negative, then no further evaluation is necessary. However, if either study shows an abnormality, then further evaluation with an intravenous urogram or renal scan is necessary.

23. Does a voiding cystourethrogram (VCUG) need to be performed after completion of treatment of a UTI to prevent detection of UTI-induced reflux?

UTIs do not cause reflux. Therefore, if the child is on the appropriate antimicrobial based on a urine culture and is responding well to treatment, then the VCUG can be performed during treatment.

24. How does the radiographic work-up of a prepubertal boy with epididymitis and a UTI differ from one without a UTI?

Prepubertal boys with epididymitis are more likely to be related to genitourinary abnormalities. Studies have shown that boys with negative urinary cultures had normal urinary tracts unlike boys with positive cultures. Therefore, prepubertal boys with epididymitis and a UTI should have renal and bladder ultrasound and a VCUG performed. Boys without a UTI do not require any further radiographic testing.

25. How is the child with a UTI managed following antimicrobial therapy, assuming the radiologic evaluation is normal?

The child should have a follow-up urinalysis and/or culture 1–2 weeks following treatment of the infection. In addition, attention to factors predisposing the child to a UTI (e.g., infrequent voiding, hygiene) should be reviewed with the child and family.

26. What is the management for children with recurrent UTI, assuming the radiologic evaluation is normal?

A child who has more than 2 or 3 UTIs in a period of 12 months should be managed with antimicrobial prophylaxis. In general, this consists of either trimethoprim-sulfamethoxazole, trimethoprim alone, or nitrofurantoin. These drugs are chosen because they have little effect on the stool's bacterial flora. In contrast, medications such as amoxicillin and cephalosporins cause alteration of the flora in the stool. The dosage for prophylaxis is ¼ to ⅓ of the normal daily dose used for treatment of a UTI.

27. What is the role of biofeedback in managing children with urinary tract infections?

Discoordination between the bladder detrusor muscle and the external urinary sphincter muscle is a common type of dysfunctional voiding that leads to urinary tract infection in children.

Biofeedback, or pelvic floor retraining, improves detrusor-external sphincter synergy, reducing the incidence of urinary tract infections by more than 90%. In addition, behavior associated with urinary tract infections (e.g., infrequent voiding, large postvoid residuals) is also reduced in more than 90% of children.

28. At what age is a child at greatest risk for renal damage from a UTI?

The child is most likely to develop renal scarring from a UTI during the first year of life. However, renal scarring may occur from pyelonephritis at any age, particularly if the infection is not treated promptly.

29. When should nitrofurantoin and sulfa derivatives be avoided?

These medications should not be administered if the patient is allergic to them. In addition, they should be avoided during the first 2 months of life. Sulfonamides displace protein-bound bilirubin and may interfere with bilirubin excretion, exacerbating neonatal physiologic jaundice. Nitrofurantoin may cause hemolytic anemia because of glutathione instability in the erythrocyte during the first 2 months of life.

30. Which antimicrobials should be used for the treatment of cystitis?

Trimethoprim-sulfamethoxazole, amoxicillin, ampicillin, cephalosporins, and nitrofurantoin often are used. Treatment should be initiated promptly, but the long-term course of therapy should depend on the results of the sensitivity studies.

31. Which antimicrobials should be used in pyelonephritis?

As with cystitis, treatment should be initiated promptly pending sensitivity studies. In neonates or young infants with a complicated UTI (e.g., obstructive hydronephrosis, sepsis, stone disease, abnormal urinary tract, or vomiting), intravenous therapy with an aminoglycoside and cephalosporin or ampicillin is necessary. Otherwise, oral antibiotic therapy with trimethoprim-sulfamethoxazole, amoxicillin, or cephalosporin is satisfactory. Nitrofurantoin should not be given to children with pyelonephritis because tissue levels of the drug in the kidney are low.

32. What is the difference between a relapse and reinfection?

A relapse or persistent UTI refers to a recurrent infection with the same species and strain of organism. Most occur within a week of cessation of therapy. A reinfection refers to recurrent infection with a different organism and is more likely to appear weeks after therapy has ended.

33. What are causes of persistent UTIs?

If the UTI recurs with the same organism following the resolution of bacteriuria and cessation of antibiotics, this suggests that a source of infections may be present within the urinary tract. Causes may include an infected renal calculus, an infected calyceal diverticulum, an infected nonrefluxing ureteral stump following nephrectomy for pyonephrosis, an infected urachal cyst, or an infected necrotic papilla from papillary necrosis. Such conditions are rare.

BIBLIOGRAPHY

1. Benador D, Benador N, Slosman DO, et al: Are younger children at highest risk of renal sequelae after pyelonephritis? Lancet 349:17, 1997.
2. Bourhier D, Abbott GD, Maling TMJ: Radiological abnormalities in infants with urinary tract infections. Arch Dis Child 59: 620, 1984.
3. Burbige KA, Retik AB, Colodny AH, et al: Urinary tract infection in boys. J Urol 132:541, 1984.
4. Coulthard MB, Lambert HJ, Keir MJ: Occurrence of renal scars in children after their first referral for urinary tract infection. BMJ 315:918, 1997.
5. Caldamone AA, Dobkin SF: Prompt treatment, probing follow-up study: Keys to managing pediatric UTI. Contemp Urol December 1989: 49.
6. deMan P, Jodal U, Lincolin K, Svanborg-Eden C: Bacterial attachment and inflammation in the urinary tract. J Infect Dis 158:29, 1988.

7. Ginsburg CM, McCracken GH Jr: Urinary tract infections in young infants. Pediatrics 69:409, 1982.

8. Herndon CDA, DeCambree M, McKenna PH: Interactive computer games for treatment of pelvic floor dysfunction. J Urol 166:1893, 2001.

9. Lee H-J, Pyo J-W, Choi E-H, et al: Isolation of adenovirus type 7 from the urine of children with acute hemorrhagic cystitis. Pediatr Infect Dis J 15:633, 1996.

10. Loening-Baucke V: Urinary incontinence and urinary tract infection and their resolution with treatment of chronic constipation of childhood. Pediatrics 100:228, 1997.

11. Lowe FC, Brendler CB: Evaluation of the urologic patient. In Walsh PC, Retik AB, Stamey TA, Vaughan ED Jr (eds): Campbell's Urology, 6th ed. Philadelphia, W.B. Saunders, 1992, p 307.

12. O'Regan S, Yasbeck S, Schick E: Constipation, bladder instability, urinary tract infection syndrome. Clin Nephrol 23:152, 1985.

13. Roberts JA: Factors predisposing to urinary tract infections in children. Pediatr Nephrol 10:517, 1996.

14. Roberts JA: Vesicoureteral reflux and pyelonephritis in the monkey: A review. J Urol 148:1721, 1992.

15. Rushton HG: The evaluation of acute pyelonephritis and renal scarring with technetium 99m-dimercaptosuccinic acid renal scintigraphy: Evolving concepts and future directions. Pediatr Nephrol 11:108, 1997.

16. Shortliffe LMD: Urinary tract infections in infants and children. In Walsh PC, Retik AB, Vaughan ED Jr, Wein AJ (eds): Campbell's Urology, 7th ed. Philadelphia, W. B. Saunders, 1998, p 1681.

17. Smith EM, Elder JS: Double antimicrobial prophylaxis in girls with breakthrough urinary tract infections. Urology 43:708, 1994.

18. Spencer JR, Shaffer AJ: Pediatric urinary tract infections. Urol Clin North Am 13:661, 1986.

19. Wiswell TE, Roscelli JD: Corroborative evidence for the decreased incidence of urinary tract infections in circumcised male infants. Pediatrics 78:96, 1986.

20. Palmer LS, Franco I, Reda EF, et al: Biofeedback Therapy for Dyssynergistic Voiding: Outcome Analysis by Initial Presentation. Presented at: American Academy of Pediatrics Section on Urology Annual Meeting, San Francisco, October 2001.

69. EPIDIDYMITIS

James C. Ulchaker, M.D.

1. Define acute epididymitis.

Acute epididymitis is inflammation, pain, and swelling of the epididymis of less than 6 weeks' duration. The principal histologic finding is the presence of abundant neutrophils in epididymal tubules, especially those of the tail, sometimes causing abscesses.

2. What is believed to be the most common route of infection in acute epididymitis?

Most cases of epididymitis are believed to occur as a result of ascending infection from the urethra, prostate, or urinary bladder. Infected urine or secretions may enter the ejaculatory ducts and ascend the vas deferens to reach the epididymis.

3. Which microorganisms most commonly cause acute epididymitis?

In men under the age of 35 years, urethritis due to *Chlamydia trachomatis* and *Neisseria gonorrhoeae* is relatively common and accounts for the majority of cases of epididymitis in this age group. In men over the age of 35 years, bacteriuria due to progressive bladder outlet obstruction is more prevalent. In this setting, epididymitis is more often due to coliform bacteria, with *Escherichia coli* being the most common. In immunosuppressed patients, cytomegalovirus (CMV) has been reported to be a causative organism. Granulomatous disease from brucellosis, tuberculosis, and BCG have also been implicated as causes of epididymitis.

4. What are the typical signs and symptoms of acute epididymitis?

Predisposing factors include recent severe physical strain, sexual activity or exposure to sexually transmitted disease, or a history of urethral instrumentation. The most common complaint is rapidly progressive scrotal swelling and pain, which may radiate up the spermatic cord to the lower abdomen. The overlying scrotal skin may be reddened, and the inflammatory process may give rise to a reactive hydrocele. In time, the indurated, enlarged epididymis may be indistinguishable from the testis, forming one large inflammatory mass. Fever is often significant. A urethral discharge or evidence of urinary tract infection may be present. Rectal examination may demonstrate changes consistent with prostatitis. Prostatic massage should not be performed, because it may exacerbate the epididymitis.

5. What laboratory studies may help to identify the causative organism?

If a urethral discharge is present, a Gram stain may reveal the presence of intracellular gram-negative diplococci consistent with *N. gonorrhoeae*. If only white blood cells are seen, the most likely diagnosis is nongonococcal urethritis; the most common organism is *C. trachomatis*. A urinalysis and mid-stream urine culture are routinely performed to identify urinary tract infection as a result of coliform bacteria.

6. What other conditions are included in the differential diagnosis of acute, painful scotal swelling?

The most important condition that must be excluded in diagnosing acute epididymitis is testicular torsion, because delayed diagnosis may result in testicular loss. In adult men, epididymitis is more common than torsion, but the latter must be considered in each instance. With torsion, the testicle is often retracted and may have a firm consistency. The spermatic cord may be thickened and difficult to palpate superior to the testicle. Early in its course, the epididymis may be palpated anterior to the testicle; however, subsequent swelling and inflammation may make this difficult. Doppler ultrasound or radionuclide scanning may provide useful information with regard to testicular bloodflow but should not delay surgical exploration of possible torsion. Other less common conditions in the differential diagnosis include torsion of the testicular or epididymal appendages, testicular tumor, and trauma.

7. What are the potential complications of acute epididymitis?

An epididymal or scrotal abscess may evolve and require operative drainage. Infrequently, an abscess may result in destruction of the testicle. Both the development of chronic scrotal pain and infertility have been associated with epididymitis.

8. What is the treatment of acute epididymitis?

General measures include bed rest, scrotal elevation and support, antinflammatory agents, and initially an ice bag applied to the scrotum to minimize swelling. Patients with acute epididymitis due to sexually transmitted urethritis often may be managed on an outpatient basis. Parenteral ceftriaxone is often administered initially, followed by a 14–21 day course of tetracycline or doxycycline. Sexual partners should be identified and treated. Patients with acute epididymitis secondary to coliform bacteriuria should be promptly treated with broad-spectrum antibiotics. If the infection is severe, hospitalization should be considered and parenteral therapy initiated. In less severe cases, outpatient treatment with trimethoprim-sulfamethoxazole or ciprofloxacin for 28 days is often effective.

9. In which patients with acute epididymitis is subsequent urinary tract evaluation indicated?

Patients with epididymitis due to urethritis infrequently have underlying urologic abnormalities. Men with epididymitis as a result of bacteriuria often have structural abnormalities of the urinary tract and should undergo radiographic and endoscopic evaluation.

10. Are there any special considerations when acute epididymitis occurs in children?

Younger boys usually have epididymitis as a result of bacteriuria, and structural urologic abnormalities are common. One possibility is the presence of an ectopic ureter draining into the epididymis. Conditions causing lower tract obstruction, such as unrecognized posterior urethral valves, also may lead to recurrent infection. Radiographic and endoscopic evaluation is essential.

11. What is chronic epididymitis?

Chronic epididymitis may develop after recurrent episodes of epididymitis; it is characterized by an interstitial lymphocytic infiltrate associated with scarring and induration of the epididymis. Occlusion of epididymal tubules is not uncommon. Some patients may develop recurrent episodes of scrotal discomfort, although this is not always the case. On palpation, the epididymis is thickened, mildly enlarged, and easily distinguished from the testicle. Tenderness may or may not be present during examination. Tuberculous and fungal involvement has been reported.

12. What are the complications of chronic epididymitis?

If clinical epididymitis is bilateral, infertility may result from diffuse scarring and occlusion of the epididymal tubules.

13. How is chronic epididymitis treated?

If clinical findings suggest that an exacerbation of chronic epididymitis is due to an infectious etiology, antibiotic therapy should be initiated. If discomfort or epididymal infection continues to occur in the setting of diffuse epididymal fibrosis, epididymectomy may be indicated; however, epididymectomy does not ensure resolution of scrotal pain.

BIBLIOGRAPHY

1. Berger RE: Sexually transmitted diseases: The classic diseases. In Walsh PC, Reik AB, Vaughn ED Jr, Wein AJ (eds): Campbell's Urology, 7th ed. Philadelphia, W. B. Saunders, 1998, pp 663–684.
2. Berger RE, Alexander ER, Harnish JP, et al: Etiology, manifestations and therapy of acute epididymitis: Prospective study of 50 cases. J Urol 121:750,1979.
3. Meares E: Nonspecific infections of the genitourinary tract. In Tanagho EA, McAninch JW (eds): Smith's General Urology. Norwalk, CT, Appleton & Lange, 1992, pp 228–231.
4. Gord B, Wong TW: Non-neoplastic decrease of the testis and epididymis. In Murphy MM (ed): Urologic Pathology. Philadelphia, W. B. Saunders, 1989, pp 300–301.
5. Kini U, Nirmala V: Post transplantation epididymitis associated with cytomegalovirus. J Pathol Microbiol 39:151, 1996.
6. Padnore DE, Norman RW, Millard OH: Analyses of indications for and outcome of epididymectomy. J Urol 156:95, 1996.
7. Kursh ED, Ulchalcer JC: Office Urology: The Clinician's Guide. Totowa, NJ, Humana Press, 2001.

70. SCROTAL ABSCESS

Donald R. Bodner, M.D.

1. What are the normal contents of the scrotum?

The scrotum is a cutaneous pouch that contains the testis, the epididymis, and the spermatic cord structures. It is divided into two compartments by a septum that is manifest on the scrotal skin as the median raphe.

2. What are the layers of the scrotum and spermatic cord?

The scrotum is a continuation of the abdominal wall. The layers include the scrotal skin; dartos layer, immediately below the skin, which is a continuation of Colles' fasci; external spermatic fascia (continuation of external oblique aponeurosis); cremasteric muscle and fascia (internal oblique muscle); internal spermatic fascia (continuation of transversalis fascia); and tunica vaginalis.

3. How do superficial scrotal abscesses arise?

When superficial scrotal abscesses arise, they generally present as infected hair follicles and infections of scrotal lacerations or minor scrotal surgeries.

4. How do primary intrascrotal abscesses arises?

Intrascrotal abscesses usually arise from bacterial epididymal orchitis. The presumed mechanism includes retrograde passage of bacteria down the vas deferens into the epididymis or via lymphogenous or hematogenous spread to the epididymis. It should be remembered that tuberculous can involve the epididymis and form an abscess. Neurogenic bladder, chronic catheter usage, instrumentation of the lower urinary tract, and neglected epididymitis are risk factors for scrotal abscesses. Abscesses can occasionally occur as a result of extravasation of infected urine from the urethra in patients with stricture and neurogenic bladder using an external collection device.

5. How is scrotal abscess diagnosed?

Scrotal abscess is diagnosed by inspection and palpation of the scrotum. Scrotal ultrasonography is helpful in diagnosing an abscess when an inflammatory mass is present in the scrotum. Ultrasonography also localizes the involvement of the abscess to the scrotal wall, epididymis, and/or testicle. A retrograde urethrogram is indicated if urethral extravasation of urine is suspected as the etiology of the abscess.

6. What is the treatment of a scrotal abscess?

An intrascrotal abscess, regardless of the cause, requires surgical drainage. All abscess cavities must be opened and drained, including the testicle if it is involved. The cavity should be left open and packed. If the contralateral testicle is normal, orchiectomy may be the most expeditious treatment. Epididymal function is often destroyed by the abscess. Broad-spectrum antibiotic coverage also is used, although primary treatment is surgical drainage. If urinary extravastion is the cause of the abscess, placement of a suprapubic cystotomy catheter along with drainage of the scrotum should be considered.

7. What is Fournier's gangrene?

Jean Alfred Fournier, a French venereologist, reported five patients with unexplained gangrene of the penis and scrotum in 1882. Today Fournier's gangrene refers to any gangrenous, infectious process involving the external genitalia and perineum. It is rarely idiopathic and often arises from an infection involving the urinary tract or from direct extension from a perirectal source.

8. How is Fournier's gangrene diagnosed?

Physical examination is diagnostic. Early in the disease, physical findings may be limited to swelling and erythema of the penis and scrotum. As the disease progresses, crepitus may overlie the skin, extending up the abdominal wall along the distribution of Colles' fascia. A foul, feculent odor is often present and indicates an anaerobic infection.

9. What is the treatment of Fournier's gangrene?

Aggressive, broad-spectrum intravenous antibiotics, including coverage of both aerobic and anaerobic organisms, and early, wide surgical débridement are required, because mortality from this infection approaches 50%. Survival can be improved with aggressive surgical and medical management.

BIBLIOGRAPHY

1. Fuchs EF: Scrotal abscess. In Resnick, MI, Kursh ED (eds): Current Therapy in Genitourinary Surgery, 2nd ed. St. Louis, Mosby, 1992, p 392.
2. Kearney GP, Carling PC: Fournier's gangrene: An approach to its management. J Urol 130:695–698, 1983.
3. Papachristodoulou AJ, Zografos GN, Papastratis G, et al: Fournier's gangrene: Still highly lethal. Langenbecks Arch Chir 382:15, 1997.
4. Spirnak JP, Resnick MI, Hampel N, et al: Fournier's gangrene: Report of 20 patients. J Urol 131:289–291, 1984.
5. Yang DM, Yoon MH, Kim HS, et al: Comparison of tuberculous and pyogenic epididymal abscesses: clinical, gray-scale sonographic, and color Doppler sonographic features. AJR 177:1131–1135, 2001.
6. Farriol VG, Comella XP, Agromayor EG, et al: Gray-scale and power Doppler sonographic appearances of acute inflammatory diseases of the scrotum. J Clin Ultrasound 28:67–72, 2000.
7. Corman JM, Moody JA, Aronson WJ: Fournier's gangrene in a modern surgical setting: Improved survival with aggressive management. BJU Int 84:85–88, 1999.

71. GONOCOCCAL AND NONGONOCOCCAL URETHRITIS

Allen D. Seftel, M.D.

1. What is acute urethritis?

Acute inflammation of the urethra.

2. What are its causes?

Ascending infection acquired by inoculation of the external urinary meatus and distal urethra with pathogens during sexual intercourse. Occasionally, acute urethritis results from descending infection from the upper genitourinary tract, bladder, or prostate.

3. Which sexually transmitted diseases are implicated in acute urethritis?

Most commonly, these are divided into two groups: nongonococcal urethritis and gonococcal urethritis.

Gonococcal urethritis is caused by *Neisseria gonorhoeae*. Clinically, there is often a purulent discharge from the urethra. Nonconococcal urethritis can be caused by many different organisms, which are discussed under the section of sexually transmitted diseases (STDs).

4. What diagnostic tests distinguish between nongonococcal and gonococcal urethritis?

The urethral discharge should be examined both stained and unstained. If the unstained wet preparation typically shows 4–5 leukocytes/high-power field, the Gram stain will distinguish between nongonococcal and gonococcal urethritis. If the smear shows polymorphonuclear leukocytes containing gram-negative cocci, then the smear is considered positive and is diagnosed as gonococcal urethritis, with 95% accuracy. A standard urine culture also should be obtained. The smear can also distinguish between trichomoniasis and other types of diseases as well.

5. How is nongonococcal urethritis treated?

Tetracycline or doxycycline may be helpful for all of the organisms except the trichomonads. Ciprofloxacin is also good for chlamydiae. Trichomoniasis is best treated with metronidazole. The sexual partner must be treated as well. Treatment for gonorrhea is with aqueous procaine penicillin or intramuscular ceftriaxone. Another possible treatment for gonorrhea is oral penicillin combined with probenecid, and another alternative is spectinomycin. Recently, HIV has been associated with nongonococcal urethritis. HIV is discussed under the "STD" heading, wherein broader discussion is found of all the STDs.

6. Are there long-term complications of these infections?

These infections could theoretically result in urethral stricture disease or perhaps infertility due to blockage of either the prostate passageway or the urethra. Epididymitis, inflammation of the male epididymis, can occur. Obstruction of the epididymis can result in infertility by blocking egress of sperm from the testis. Other long-term sequelae are unusual and rare.

BIBLIOGRAPHY

1. Ahmed A, Kalayi GD: Urethral stricture at Ahmadu Bello University Teaching Hospital, Zaria. East Afr Med J 75:582–858, 1998.
2. Burstein GR, Zenilman JM: Nongonococcal urethritis—a new paradigm. Clin Infect Dis 28(Suppl): S66–S73, 1999.

3. David N, Wildman G, Rajamanoharan S: Ciprofloxacin 250 mg for treating gonococcal urethritis and cervicitis. Sex Transm Infect 76:495–496, 2000.
4. Sadiq ST, Taylor S, Kaye S, et al: The effects of antiretrovial therapy on HIV-1 RNA loads in seminal plasma in HIV-positive patients with and without urethritis. AIDS 16:219–225, 2002.
5. Massari V, Retel O, Flahault A: A recent increase in the incidence of male urethritis in France. Sex Transm Dis 29:319–323, 2002.

72. SEXUALLY TRANSMITTED DISEASES

Allen D. Seftel, M.D.

MANY DIFFERENT ORGANISMS FALL UNDER THE HEADING OF STD.
ALTHOUGH DISCUSSED PREVIOUSLY GONOCOCCAL
AND NONGONOCOCAL URETHRITIS FALL UNDER THE STD HEADING AS WELL.

BACTERIA

SYPHILIS–(*Treponema pallidum*)

1. What is syphilis?
Primary syphilis is a sexually transmitted genitourinary infection caused by the spirochete *Treponema pallidum*.

2. When does it occur?
It usually occurs 2–4 weeks after sexual exposure.

3. How does it present?
It is usually a painless papule or pustule (chancre) on the glans, corona, foreskin, shaft, or even the pubic area or scrotum. It breaks down to form an indurated, small punched-out ulcer.

4. What are the signs of syphilis?
The patient usually presents because of a painless penile sore. The ulcer is deep, has indurated edges, and a clean base.

5. How is the diagnosis made?
A diagnosis is made by finding the pathogenic spirochetes in the discharge from the ulcer on darkfield examination. Serologic tests for syphilis may remain negative for 1–3 weeks or longer after the appearance of the chancre.

6. What are the complications of syphilis?
Urologic complication of syphilis are rare.

7. How do you treat syphilis?
Penicillin is the first-line therapy. Patients allergic to penicillin should be given tetracycline. Alternatively, erythromycin is a third choice.

8. What is the prognosis?
The prognosis is excellent, if treated. Untreated syphilis may progress to neurosyphilis, tabes dorsalis, Charcot joints, dementia, aortitis, and gummas.

CHANCROID (*Haemophilus ducreyi*)

9. What is chancroid?
A soft chancre. The infecting organism is Haemophilus ducreyi, a short, nonmotile, gram-negative streptobacillus that usually occurs in chains. The incubation period is 1–5 days after sexual contact.

10. How does chancroid present?
Macroscopically, one or several small penile ulcers are present, which are usually painful.

11. What are the clinical findings?

A few days after sexual exposure, one or more painful, dirty-appearing ulcers may be noted, and they gradually enlarge. Often, the inguinal nodes are involved and become large and tender. About 50% of patients usually have a fever, malaise, and headache.

12. What are the laboratory findings?

A smear of Gram's stain may show the *H. ducreyi* organism in 50% of cases. Culture is usually more successful.

13. What are the complications of chancroid?

Genitourinary complications of this organism may include phimosis and paraphimosis or, infrequently, destruction of penile or scrotal tissue. *Haemophilus ducreyi* facilitates the transmission of HIV infection.

14. How is chancroid treated?

Tetracycline, 500 mg every 6 hours for 10 days. Alternatively, erythromycin or trimethoprim-sulfamethoxazole may be used. Penicillin is usually not effective.

LYMPHOGRANULOMA VENEREUM (LGV; *Chlamydia trachomatis*)

15. What organism causes LGV?

Chlamydia trachomatis.

16. How does the disease present?

This disease is characterized by a transient genital lesion, followed by lymphadenitis and, at times, in females or homosexual men, rectal stricture. In men, the lymphatics of the inguinal or subinguinal nodes may become matted or infected.

17. What are the signs and symptoms?

The penile lesion develops 5–21 days after sexual exposure. It heals spontaneously and rapidly and is often not seen. The lesion may be papular or vesicular, although only a superficial erosion may occur. A few days or weeks later, painful enlargement of the inguinal nodes develops because the primary lesion is so often missed. This may be the initial symptom.

18. What are the complications of this disease?

If untreated, multiple sinuses may develop from the involved lymph nodes. Elephantiasis of the genitalia can occur if lymphatic drainage is severely obstructed. Proctitis or rectal stricture may occur occasionally in women and rarely in men.

19. How is it treated?

Tetracycline and erythromycin are usually effective. Sulfonamides can often control a secondary infection.

20. How are the complications treated?

Aspiration of infected or fluctuant lymph nodes is indicated. Draining sinuses may have to be excised. Rectal stenosis may require surgical measures.

21. What is the prognosis?

The prognosis is excellent. Only the late complications present with some difficulties.

22. Are there other sequelae of *Chlamydia* infections?

Chlamydia is found in up to 35–50% of patients, usually young men, with nongonococcal urethritis. The discharge may be purulent, but less purulent than gonococcal urethritis.

23. What are the complications of Chlamydial infections?
Epididymitis and Reiter's syndrome in men; cervicitis and acute salpingitis in women.

GRANULOMA INGUINALE
(*Calymmatobacterium granulomatis*)

24. What is granuloma inguinale?
It is a sexually transmitted chronic infection of the skin and subcutaneous tissues of the genitalia, perineum, or inguinal areas with an incubation period of 2–3 months. The infectious agent is *Calymmatobacterium granulomatis,* a bacterium related to *Klebsiella pneumoniae.*

25. What are the signs of this disease?
The first sign is an elevation of the skin on the genitals, perineum, or groin, which finally breaks down into a superficial painful ulcer that spreads and becomes quite extensive. The base of the ulcer is usually covered by pink granulation tissue that bleeds easily. There is usually a purulent discharge if a secondary infection occurs.

26. Describe the laboratory findings.
Identification of the "Donovan body" in large monocytes on a stained smear makes the diagnosis. Scrapings from the base of the lesion are placed on the slide, fixed in air, and stained. Wright and Giemsa staining techniques are both adequate. In case of doubt, a biopsy may be performed. Complement fixation and skin sensitivity tests are not dependable and are not readily available.

27. What are the complications?
Secondary infection may cause deep ulceration and tissue destruction. Sinuses may result. Marked phimosis may occur, and a rectal stricture may occur as well.

28. How is it treated?
Tetracycline and ampicillin have proved to be effective in a high percentage of cases.

29. What is the treatment of secondary complications?
Secondary infection is effectively combated in most cases by the drugs used to cure the primary disease. Rectal stricture may require surgery.

30. What is the prognosis?
There are a few serious complications, and antibiotics are usually quite effective in treatment. The prognosis is good.

Ureaplasma urealyticum (*Mycoplasma hominis*)

31. How does this present?
Usually as nongonococcal urethritis in men and women.

32. What are the complications?
Prostatitis in men and pelvic inflammatory disease in women.

33. How is this diagnosed?
Routine culture.

34. How is this treated?
Doxycycline or erythromycin.

Mobiluncus species

35. How does this present?
Bacterial vaginosis.

36. What are the complications?
Postpartum endometriosis.

37. How is this diagnosed?
White vaginal discharge, clue cells on microscopic examination, vaginal pH > 4.5, fishy odor after KOH added (Whiff test).

38. What is the treatment?
Metronidazole (oral or gel) or clindamycin cream.

Fungi (*Candida albicans*)

39. What is *Candida albicans*?
A yeast infection.

40. How does it typically present?
Vaginitis—inflammation of the vagina. A white, odorless discharge.

41. How is *Candida* diagnosed?
Fungal elements are identified on KOH preparation.

42. What is the treatment?
The treatment is intravaginal miconazole or clotrimazole.

Viruses (Anogenital Herpes)

43. What is anogenital herpes?
Anogenital herpes is usually due to recurrent herpes virus type 2 and is characterized by grouped vesiculopustular lesions. Secondary adenopathy may be present in the groins. Anogenital herpes can be a painful recurrent condition. It may be associated with cervical carcinoma in women.

44. How is it treated?
Acyclovir ointment (5%) or oral tablets may be helpful for primary attacks or in reduction of severity of recurrences.

45. Does counseling have any role in the treatment plans of STDs?
Patients with sexually transmitted diseases (STDs) need to undergo counseling regarding the use of condoms and the need for continued surveillance. Safe sex is an important component of the treatment plan: Disease recurrence rates rise dramatically if the sexual partners of such patients do not use preventive measures.

Condyloma Acuminata (Human papillomavirus)

46. What is condyloma accuminata?
Genital warts.

47. How does one get this?
Sexual contact with an infected partner.

48. What are the genitourinary manifestations?

These lesions are usually found on the external genitalia and are readily apparent. Occasionally, they are subclinical and are found by staining the penis and scrotum with 3–5% acetic acid with identification of the acetowhite lesions with a hand-held magnifying glass. Less commonly, these lesions can surface in the urethra and produce irritative voiding symptoms or hematuria.

49. How is it treated?

Small external lesions are often treated with topical Aldara (imiquod) cream. Older, less effective remedies include topical podophyllin. Larger external lesions are usually cauterized with a carbon dioxide laser or a hand-held cautery. Urethral lesions are cauterized and occasionally require adjunctive therapy, such as topical 5-fluorouracil.

Long-term issues: In men, left untreated, these lesions can become large and may transform into squamous cell carcinoma (Buschke-Löwenstein tumor). In women, these lesions may be associated with atypia of the cervix, noted on PAP smear, or overt cervical carcinoma.

MOLLUSCUM CONTAGIOSUM (POXVIRUS)

50. What is *Molluscum contagiosum*?

A benign epidermal neoplasm caused by a poxvirus.

51. What is the incubation period?

It can be as long as 6 months.

52. What is the clinical appearance?

A flesh-colored 2–5 mm papule, which may express a "cheese-like material."

53. How is the diagnosis made?

Biopsy or incision of the lesion with expression of the casseous material. Examination of the casseous material should confirm *Molluscum* bodies. Basophilic cytoplasmic inclusions filled with the virion.

54. What is the treatment?

Many lesions resolve on their own. Alternatively, topical podophyllin or cauterization.

HUMAN IMMUNODEFICIENCY VIRUS (HIV—AIDS)

55. What is HIV (human immunodeficiency virus)?

It is a virus that produces a severe immunodeficiency state, manifested by many opportunistic infections.

56. How does one get this?

This virus is usually transmitted by sexual contact. It may also be passed through transmission of infected blood. Maternal-fetal transmission is the third route.

57. What are the genitourinary manifestations?

Nongonococcal urethritis, Kaposi's sarcoma of the external genitalia, nephropathy, testicular abscesses.

58. How is this treated?

Oral therapy with drugs that attack various parts of viral replication is used as a first-line therapy. The oral retrovial drugs indinavir, ritonavir, and saquinavir have been associated with kidney stone formation.

PROTOZOA (*Trichomonas vaginalis*)

59. How does this present?
A profuse yellow-green discharge or pruritus, with a foul odor.

60. How is the diagnosis made?
A wet mount demonstrating trichomonads.

61. What is the treatment?
Metronidazole.

ECTOPARASITES (PEDICULOSIS PUBIS—PUBIC OR CRAB LOUSE— THIS IS CAUSED BY PHTHIRUS PUBIS)

62. What are the symptoms?
Severe itching in the genital area. Nits or eggs are found on the hair shaft. There may be red papules. Occasionally, overt lice can be seen.

SCABIES (SARCOPTES SCABIEI VAR HOMINIS)—SCAB MITE

63. What are the symptoms?
Pruritus, which is worse at night.

64. How is the diagnosis made?
The lesions are pathognomonic—thready, symmetric burrows 1–10 mm long, made by the female mite.

65. What is the treatment?
The treatment for both of these ectoparasites is lindane or permethrin.

BIBLIOGRAPHY

1. Brackbill RM, Sternberg MR, Fishbein M: Where do people go for treatment of sexually transmitted diseases? Fam Plan Perspect 31:10–15, 1999.
2. Steen R, Soliman C, Mujyambwani A, et al: Notes from the field: Practical issues in upgrading STD services based on experience from primary healthcare facilities in two Rwandan towns. Sex Transm Infect 74(Suppl):S159–S165, 1998.
3. van Dam CJ, Becker KM, Ndowa F, Islam MQ: Syndromic approach to STD case management: Where do we go from here? Sex Transm Infect 74(Suppl):S175–S178, 1998.
4. Panel on Clinical Practices for the Treatment of HIV: Guidelines for using antiretroviral agents among HIV-infected adults and adolescents. Recommendations of the Panel on Clinical Practices for Treatment of HIV. MMWR Morb Mortal Wkly Rep 51(RR-7):1–55, 2002.
5. Al-Tawfiq JA, Spinola SM: *Haemophilus ducreyi:* Clinical disease and pathogenesis. Curr Opin Infect Dis 15:43–47, 2002.
6. Roest RW, van der Meijden W: European Branch of the International Union against Sexually Transmitted Infection and the European Office of the World Health Organization. European guideline for the management of tropical genito-ulcerative diseases. Int J STD AIDS 12(Suppl 3):78–83, 2001.
7. Scoular A, Norrie J, Gillespie G, et al: Longitudinal study of genital infection by herpes simplex virus type 1 in western Scotland over 15 years. BMJ 324:1366–1367, 2002.
8. O'Farrel N: Donovanosis: An update. Int J STD AIDS 12:423–427, 2001.

V. Trauma

73. RENAL TRAUMA

J. Patrick Spirnak, M.D.

1. What are the three most common causes of blunt renal trauma?
Motor vehicle accidents, falls, and sports injuries.

2. Blunt trauma causes what percentage of civilian renal injuries?
An estimated 60–90% of all renal injuries occur as a result of blunt trauma.

3. What common clinical findings suggest the presence of a renal injury?
1. Evidence of flank trauma (e.g., rib fracture, flank ecchymosis)
2. Gross hematuria
3. Microscopic hematuria and systolic blood pressure < 90 mm Hg

4. Do all adults with microscopic hematuria and blunt abdominal trauma require a radiographic evaluation of the urinary tract?
No. Adult patients who present with microscopic hematuria, no other associated injuries, and who have stable vital signs do not require urologic evaluation. Patients with microscopic hematuria and shock or other associated injuries requiring hospitalization should undergo radiographic evaluation consisting of either an excretory urogram (IVP) or computed tomography (CT) scan of the abdomen. In many trauma centers, the abdominal CT has replaced the IVP as the initial study of choice, because it is more sensitive in identifying renal injuries and also detects other abdominal injuries.

5. The spiral CT scan has replaced conventional CT scanning in many trauma centers. What precaution should be taken to avoid understaging of renal injuries?
Spiral CT scanning is typically begun 45–60 seconds after contrast administration. The short scan delay time results in improved vascular enhancement and identification of renal parenchymal injuries but often fails to identify injuries to the renal collecting system, which does not have time to opacify. To avoid understaging, a repeat spiral CT performed after completion of the initial scan is recommended.

6. What are the indications for urologic evaluation in the pediatric patient with blunt abdominal trauma?
Hypotension in the pediatric trauma victim with associated microscopic hematuria is an unreliable indicator of major renal injury. Therefore, the indications for evaluation are slightly different than those in the adult trauma victim. Indications include (1) a deceleration–type injury, (2) microscopic hematuria—defined as greater than 50 RBCs per HPF, (3) gross hematuria, (4) rib fracture, and (5) microscopic hematuria associated with multisystem organ injuries.

7. Why are the indications for urologic evaluation different in children?
The pediatric kidneys are at higher risk to sustain renal injury. They are less well protected,

more mobile, and relatively larger than adult kidneys. A congenital anomaly is also more likely in such patients.

8. Does the degree of hematuria correlate with the severity of blunt renal injury?

No. Patients with inconsequential renal contusions may present with gross hematuria, whereas renal pedicle injuries may occur in the absence of hematuria and result in loss of renal function.

9. How should the trauma IVP be performed?

Stable patients are taken to the radiology department, where a high-dose IVP with nephrotomograms will adequately assess the kidneys in up to 90% of patients. Patients who are unable to be transported from the emergency department receive a bolus of intravenous contrast (1 ml/lb body weight up to a maximum of 150 ml), followed by serial abdominal films at 1, 5, and 10 minutes.

10. What is the purpose of the IVP?

The purpose of the trauma IVP is to identify and stage the extent of renal injury (in order to formulate a rational treatment plan) and to document the presence of two functioning kidneys.

11. What is a minor renal injury?

A minor renal injury occurs in up to 90% of all renal trauma patients and includes renal contusion and shallow lacerations limited to the renal cortex.

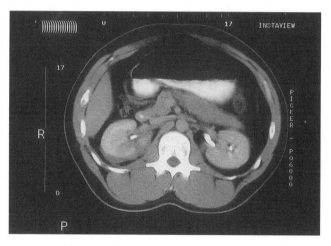

CT scan showing characteristics of a minor right renal injury. Note the shallow posterior laceration and the small subcapsular hematoma.

12. How are minor renal injuries treated?

Patients with minor injuries associated with gross hematuria are hospitalized and placed on bedrest until the urine clears. Patients with microscopic hematuria and a normal IVP require no further evaluation.

13. What is a major renal injury?

Major renal injuries may be classified into pedicle and nonpedicle injuries. Major renal lacerations extend through the corticomedullary junction. If the collecting system is entered, urinary extravasation may be present. Multiple major lacerations will result in a shattered kidney. Pedicle injuries consist of tears or occlusion to segmental or major vascular structures.

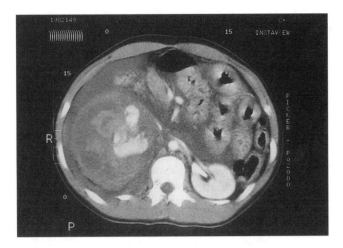

CT scan showing characteristics of a major renal injury. Note the presence of contrast outside the collecting system, the large perinephric hematoma, and the irregular renal outline indicating major lacerations.

14. How are major renal injuries treated?

The treatment of major blunt renal injuries is controversial. Most stable patients with suspected major renal injuries are evaluated with a CT scan to better assess the severity of the injury. Stable patients are hydrated, placed on bedrest until the urine clears, and closely monitored for changes in vital signs that indicate progressive bleeding. Blood transfusions are given as needed, and broad-spectrum antibiotics are administered. Patients with persistent vascular instability despite adequate resuscitative efforts undergo surgical exploration.

15. Does the presence of urinary extravasation require surgical intervention?

The presence of urinary extravasation confirms the diagnosis of major renal injury. Extravasation alone does not require surgical intervention.

These patients are closely observed for signs of sepsis or persistent extravasation that would require surgical exploration and drainage. In addition, it is important to visualize the ureter, because disruption of the ureteropelvic junction can occur and requires immediate exploration and repair.

16. Describe the radiographic findings of renal artery thrombosis.

On IVP, the involved kidney is nonvisualized. The CT scan is characterized by a kidney of normal size and contour, with minimal perirenal hemorrhage and nonenhancement of the renal parenchyma with an absence of excretion of opacified urine.

17. What is the significance of the cortical rim sign?

The cortical rim sign is a CT finding characteristic of renal artery thrombosis. The renal cortex enhances due to persistent perfusion from capsular and collateral vessels.

18. What is the treatment of renal pedicle injuries?

Pedicle lacerations require prompt surgical exploration. Branch vessel occlusion is observed. Bilateral complete renal artery thrombosis requires immediate exploration and revascularization. The treatment of unilateral injuries is controversial. If the contralateral kidney is normal, opinion divides between attempted revascularization or observation. If observation is elected, these patients must be followed closely and their blood pressures monitored. If renal vascular hypertension develops, nephrectomy is performed.

19. What is the treatment of renal gunshot wounds?

All patients with penetrating abdominal gunshot wounds have sustained at least one injury to an abdominal viscus; therefore, surgical exploration is required. If the IVP or CT scan indicates the presence of a renal parenchymal injury, renal exploration, débridement, and reconstruction are performed.

20. Is observation ever indicated in patients with renal gunshot wounds?

If the missile has not penetrated the peritoneal cavity (negative lavage), CT has documented a superficial cortical laceration, and the patient is clinically stable, observation may be appropriate.

21. Must all renal stab wounds be surgically explored?

The management of renal stab wounds depends on the degree of renal parenchymal damage and the presence of other associated intraabdominal injuries. Stab wounds occurring anterior to the mid-axillary line that have penetrated the peritoneal cavity are associated with a significant risk of visceral injury and are explored. At the time of laparotomy, the kidney is explored and repaired. Stab wounds occurring posterior to the mid-axillary line are less likely to be associated with visceral injuries. Observation may be appropriate if the peritoneal lavage is negative, no evidence of severe blood loss is found, and CT findings suggest a superficial laceration.

BIBLIOGRAPHY

1. Bright TC, White K, Peters PC: Significance of hematuria after trauma. J Urol 120:455, 1978.
2. Dixon CM, McAninch JW: Traumatic renal injuries: Part I. Patient assessment and management. AUA Update 10:273, 1991.
3. Smith EM, Elder JS, Spirnak JP: Major blunt renal trauma in the pediatric population: Is a nonoperative approach indicated? J Urol 149:546, 1993.
4. Spirnak JP, Resnick MI: Revascularization of traumatic thrombosis of the renal artery. Surg Gynecol Obstet 164:22, 1987.
5. Spirnak JP: Blunt renal trauma. In Resnick MI, Kursh ED (eds): Current Therapy in Genitourinary Surgery. Toronto, B.C. Decker, 1987, p 355.
6. Spirnak JP: Penetrating renal trauma. In Resnick MI, Kursh ED (eds): Current Therapy in Genitourinary Surgery. Toronto, B.C. Decker, 1992, p 403.
7. Matthews LA, Smith EM, Spirnak JP: Nonoperative treatment of major blunt renal lacerations with urinary extravasation. J Urol 157:2056, 1997.
8. Haas CA, Dinchman KH, Nasrallah PF, Spirnak JP: Traumatic renal artery occlusion: A 15-year review. J Trauma 45:557, 1998.
9. Brown SL, Hoffman DM, Spirnak JP: Limitation of routine spinal computerized tomography in the evaluation of blunt renal trauma. J Urol 160:1979, 1998.
10. Altman AL, Haas C, Dinchman KH, Spirnak JP: Selective nonoperative management of blunt Grade V renal injury. J Urol 164:27, 2000.
11. Brown SI, Spirnak JP, Volsko T, et al: Radiologic evaluation in pediatric blunt renal trauma patients with microscopic hematuria. J Urol 161:14, 1999.

74. URETERAL INJURIES

J. Patrick Spirnak, M.D.

1. What percentage of abdominal gunshot wounds involve the ureter?
About 2.5%.

2. What is the blood supply to the ureter?
The ureter derives its primary blood supply from a branch of the renal artery. In most cases, this artery traverses the entire length of the ureter, running in the outer adventitial sheath. Other sources of ureteral blood supply include branches from the aorta and gonadal, hypogastric, and superior and inferior vesical arteries.

3. Are stab wounds to the ureter more common than gunshot wounds?
No. Gunshot wounds account for greater than 95% of all traumatic ureteral injuries.

4. Is hematuria a reliable finding in patients with suspected ureteral injury?
No. Up to 37% of all traumatic ureteral injuries present with a normal urinalysis.

5. What is the appropriate imaging study to obtain in trauma victims with a suspected ureteral injury?
An intravenous pyelogram (IVP) is obtained in all patients with suspected ureteral injury.

6. What findings on IVP suggest a ureteral injury?
1. Delayed or nonvisualization of the involved renal unit
2. Hydronephrosis
3. Urinary extravasation
4. Incomplete visualization of the entire ureter

7. In the presence of a retroperitoneal hematoma and ureteral contusion, how can one tell if the integrity of the ureter has been compromised?
The intravenous administration of indigo carmine is helpful in identifying urinary extravasation and a devitalized ureter.

8. In the postoperative period, what signs and symptoms are suggestive of a missed ureteral injury?
The findings are nonspecific. The presence of prolonged adynamic ileus, persistent flank or abdominal pain, a palpable abdominal mass, an elevation in blood urea nitrogen, sepsis, and prolonged and persistent drainage from operative drain sites, and/or the development of a spontaneous cutaneous fistula all suggest the diagnosis.

9. What types of iatrogenic ureteral injuries commonly occur?
Ureteral injury can occur as a result of either ligating or crushing the ureter with a clamp or ligature. Surgical transection, avulsion, devascularization, or angulation of the ureter also may occur.

10. What is the incidence of iatrogenic ureteral injury?
Owing to the silent nature of many surgical ureteral injuries, the exact incidence is unknown. However, an incidence ranging from 0.5–30% has been reported following gynecologic surgery.

11. What are the common occasions of iatrogenic ureteral injury associated with gynecologic surgery?

1. During ligation of the infundibulopelvic ligament
2. While clamping or ligating the uterine artery as it crosses the ureter
3. As it lies in the ovarian fossa
4. During extensive pelvic node dissection accompanying radical hysterectomy
5. While attempting to control pelvic hemorrhage

12. When ureteral injury is associated with a vascular reconstructive procedure, is repair indicated?

If the urine is sterile, ureteral repair with the use of indwelling stents, drains, and antibiotics is recommended.

13. What are the goals of ureteral reconstructive surgery?

Restoration of normal anatomy and renal preservation while minimizing patient morbidity.

14. What is the recommended treatment of a ligated ureter?

If noted at the time of injury, simple de-ligation seldom leads to postoperative complications. If the injury is noted and repair undertaken more than 24 hours after injury, de-ligation should be accompanied by stent drainage or resection and primary repair. If the injury is noted more than 72 hours from the time of surgery, resection and primary repair are recommended.

15. How is a proximal or midureteral transection commonly repaired?

Proximal and midureteral injuries are best treated by débridement and ureteroureterostomy. The area is also drained.

16. How should distal ureteral injuries be managed?

Distal injuries are best treated by ureteroneocystostomy.

17. List several relative contraindications to transureteroureterostomy.

- Extensive radiation damage to the ureter
- History of recurrent stone disease
- History of transitional cell carcinoma of the upper urinary tract
- Tuberculosis
- Retroperitoneal fibrosis
- Marked discrepancy in the size of the two ureters
- Anomalies of the recipient ureter

18. If extensive loss of ureteral length has occurred, what adjunctive procedures may be performed to gain length and allow a tension-free repair?

Downward mobilization of the kidney with concomitant nephropexy and/or upward mobilization of the bladder with fixation to the psoas tendon (psoas hitch) performed in conjunction, when necessary, with a Boari bladder flap make it possible to surgically replace nearly the entire ureter.

19. What is an ileal ureter?

An ileal ureter refers to the placement of a damaged ureter with a segment of ileum. It is useful in secondary reconstructive procedures when extensive loss of ureter has occurred.

20. What is the role of cystoscopy with retrograde pyelography and ureteral stent placement in the evaluation and treatment of suspected ureteral injury?

Cystoscopy and retrograde pyelography are indicated when ureteral injury is suspected. They identify the exact point of obstruction and the length of ureter involved. At the same time, an attempt is made to pass a guidewire beyond the point of obstruction over which a double J tent may be therapeutically placed.

21. What is the role of endoscopic repair in the treatment of benign ureteral strictures resulting from unrecognized ureteral trauma?

Endoscopic repair in the form of balloon dilation or endoscopic incision with stenting is a reasonable first-line treatment in patients with strictures < 2 cm in length. If the stricture recurs, open surgical repair is indicated.

BIBLIOGRAPHY

1. Bright TC: Emergency management of the injured ureter. Urol Clin North Am 9:285, 1982.
2. Gurin JI, Garcia RL, Melman A, Leiter E: The pathologic effect of ureteral ligation with clinical implications. J Urol 128:1404, 1982.
3. Hoch WH, Kursh ED, Persky L: Early aggressive management of intraoperative ureteral injuries. J Urol 114:530, 1975.
4. Kerr WS: Effects of complete ureteral obstruction in dogs in kidney function. Am J Physiol 184:521, 1956.
5. Raney AM: Ureteral trauma: Effects of ureteral ligation with and without deligation—experimental studies and case reports. J Urol 119:326, 1978.
6. Spirnak JP, Resnick MI, Persky LP: The management of civilian ureteral gunshot wounds: A review of 8 patients. J Urol 134:733, 1985.
7. Spirnak JP, Hampel N, Resnick MI: Ureteral injuries complicating vascular reconstructive surgery: Is repair indicated? J Urol 141:13, 1989.
8. Selzman AA, Spirnak JP: Iatrogenic ureteral injuries: A 20-year experience in treating 165 injuries. J Urol 155:878, 1996.
9. Armenakas NA: Ureteral trauma. Surgical repair. In Spirnak JP (ed): Atlas of the Urologic Clinics of North America. Urologic Trauma. Philadelphia, W. B. Saunders, 1998, p 71.
10. Kim FJ, Albala DM: Ureteral trauma: Endoscopic repair. In Spirnak JP (ed): Atlas of the Urologic Clinics of North America. Urologic Trauma. Philadelphia, W. B. Saunders, 1998, p 85.

75. BLADDER TRAUMA

J. Patrick Sprinak, M.D.

1. What types of bladder perforation may occur?

Bladder perforation may be intraperitoneal, extraperitoneal, or both.

2. What is the mechanism of intraperitoneal bladder perforation in patients with blunt abdominal trauma?

Intraperitoneal bladder perforation usually occurs during severe, blunt, lower abdominal trauma while the bladder is full or distended with urine. The intravesical pressure becomes acutely elevated, and the bladder perforates at its weakest point, the dome.

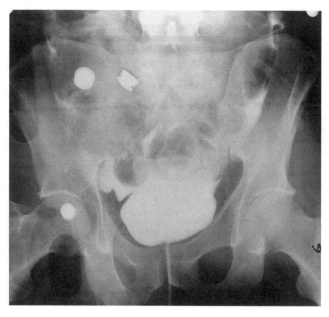

Cystogram showing typical appearance of intraperitoneal bladder rupture. Note the contrast outlining the colon.

3. Explain how extraperitoneal bladder perforation occurs.

Two accepted theories explain how extraperitoneal trauma occurs.

1. When associated with pelvic fracture, extraperitoneal tears are thought to occur as a result of an anterior pubic arch fracture with displacement of bony fragments and bladder perforation near the vesical neck.

2. A second mechanism of injury has been proposed to explain extraperitoneal tears in the absence of pelvic fracture. With the bladder empty, severe lower abdominal trauma may cause a bursting-type injury similar to that which occurs through the dome with the bladder full.

4. What are the indications for bladder evaluation in patients with blunt lower abdominal trauma?

A cystogram is performed in all patients with gross hematuria. If the patient is unable to urinate, has blood at the urethral meatus, or has perineal ecchymosis with swelling or a nonpalpable prostate, a urethrogram must be performed prior to performing a cystogram.

5. How often does bladder rupture occur in patients with pelvic fracture?

Bladder rupture occurs in approximately 5–10% of patients with pelvic fracture. The perforation can be extraperitoneal (50–85%), intraperitoneal (15–45%), or rarely both (0–12%).

6. Do patients with pelvic fracture and microscopic hematuria require bladder evaluation?

Studies have shown a low incidence of bladder injury in the absence of gross hematuria, and thus urologic evaluation is not performed in the absence of other signs suggestive of a urologic injury.

7. How is a cystogram performed?

An 18F Foley catheter is placed into the bladder, and contrast material is administered under gravity to fill the bladder (300–500 ml). After the inflow of contrast material has stopped, an additional 10–15 ml of contrast is injected under slight pressure to ensure complete bladder filling and to avoid a false-negative study. With the catheter clamped, an abdominal radiograph is obtained. A complete bladder study requires oblique and drainage films.

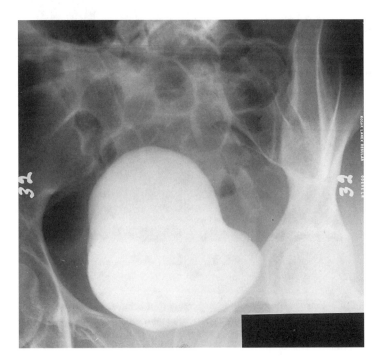

Normal cystogram.

8. What are the cystographic findings suggestive of an extraperitoneal bladder perforation?

Radiographic findings include a teardrop-shaped bladder secondary to compression by a pelvic hematoma associated with extravasation confined to the pelvis. The pattern of extravasation may range from flame-like wisps or linear streaks to a large stellate or sunburst pattern that may be more obvious on drainage film.

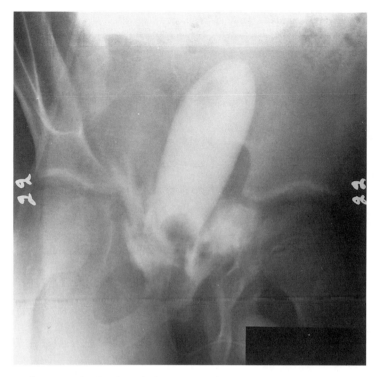

Cystogram showing the typical appearance of extraperitoneal bladder rupture.

9. What cystographic findings suggest intraperitoneal bladder perforation?

Intraperitoneal perforation may produce diffuse extravasation of contrast material through the peritoneal cavity with no filling of the bladder. Contrast material may accumulate in the dependent portion of the pelvis, obscuring the superior aspect of the bladder and resulting in an hourglass configuration. Contrast material also may extend into the paracolic gutters to the diaphragm.

10. What is CT cystography and how is it performed?

A CT cystogram is an alternative to traditional retrograde cystography. Before performing a pelvic CT scan, 350 ml of contrast is injected into the bladder and the catheter is clamped. The pelvic CT scan is performed with the bladder full. There is no need for a drainage study.

11. What is the appropriate treatment of an intraperitoneal bladder rupture?

All patients with intraperitoneal bladder perforation undergo surgical exploration and watertight bladder closure.

12. How are extraperitoneal bladder perforations treated?

The treatment of extraperitoneal bladder perforation is controversial. If surgical exploration is performed for other associated injuries, the bladder is explored and repaired. If the patient has an isolated extraperitoneal bladder injury, a nonoperative approach consisting of catheter drainage and broad-spectrum antibiotics is recommended. A cystogram is performed prior to catheter removal, usually after 7–14 days. Severe bleeding with clots, sepsis, and persistent urinary extravasation is an indication for exploration.

13. How are gunshot wounds to the bladder treated?

Penetrating wounds to the abdomen and bladder are surgically explored. The bladder is repaired and the area drained.

BIBLIOGRAPHY

1. Bodner DR, Selzman AA, Spirnak JP: Evaluation and treatment of bladder rupture. Semin Urol 13:62, 1995.
2. Brosman SA, Fay R: Diagnosis and management of bladder trauma. J Trauma 13:929, 1973.
3. Carroll PR, McAninch JW: Major bladder trauma: Mechanism of injury and a unified method of diagnosis and repair. J Urol 132:254, 1984.
4. Spirnak JP: Lower urinary tract trauma. In Resnick MI, Kursh ED (eds): Urology Problems in Primary Care. Oradell, NJ, Medical Economics, 1987, pp 303–306.
5. Spirnak JP: Pelvic fracture and injury to the lower urinary tract. Surg Clin North Am 68:1057, 1988.
6. Spirnak JP, Resnick MI: Intraoperative consultation for the bladder. Urol Clin North Am 12:439, 1985.
7. Walsh PC, Retik AB, Vaughan ED Jr, Wein AJ (eds): Campbell's Urology, 7th ed. Philadelphia, W. B. Saunders, 1998.
8. Lis LE, Cohen AJ: CT cystography in the evaluation of bladder trauma. J Comput Assist Tomogr 14:386, 1990.

76. URETHRAL INJURY

Kenneth W. Angermeier, M.D.

1. Define the components of the anterior and posterior urethra in the male.

The anterior urethra consists of the glanular, pendulous (penile), and bulbous portions of the urethra. It extends from the urethral meatus to the perineal membrane and is surrounded by the corpus spongiosum throughout its course. The posterior urethra consists of the membranous and prostatic portions of the urethra and extends from the perineal membrane to the bladder neck. The membranous urethra is encompassed by the striated urethral sphincter and the prostatic urethra by the prostate gland.

2. What is the most common cause of traumatic injury to the anterior urethra?

Blunt perineal trauma, usually in the form of a straddle injury, is the most common cause of disruptive anterior urethral injuries. Other causes include penetrating injury as a result of gunshot or stab wound, urethral instrumentation such as catheterization or endoscopy, disruption in association with a penile fracture, and iatrogenic injury during penile surgery.

3. In what setting are injuries to the posterior urethra most commonly encountered?

Virtually all posterior urethral injuries occur in association with traumatic pelvic fracture, as in a motor vehicle accident. Penetrating trauma to the posterior urethra is seen infrequently.

4. When should one suspect a urethral injury?

Patients with a history of perineal or pelvic trauma, particularly in the presence of a pelvic fracture, should be suspected of having a urethral injury. Blood at the urethral meatus is a common finding, and the patient may be unable to void. These signs are not always present, however, and a high level of suspicion is necessary. Severe urethral injuries may be associated with swelling and ecchymosis of the penis and/or perineum.

5. Describe the fascial layers and attachments that may contain extravasated urine or blood from a urethral injury.

The deep penile fascia (Buck's fascia) is the layer immediately surrounding the corpora cavernosa and corpus spongiosum. It is attached distally to the undersurface of the glans penis at the corona. Proximally, Buck's fascia encloses each crus of the corpora cavernosa and the bulb of the corpus spongiosum. Injuries to the anterior urethra with extravasation confined to Buck's fascia may result in swelling and ecchymosis of the penis alone. The superficial fascia of the perineum (Colles' fascia) curves around the superficial transverse perinei muscles and attaches laterally to the ischia and inferior rami of the pubis as well as the fascia lata of the thigh. Anteriorly, Colles' fascia is continuous with the dartos layer of the scrotum and Scarpa's fascia of the abdominal wall until its superior attachment to the coracoclavicular fascia. Extravasation penetrating through Buck's fascia and confined by Colles' fascia may result in a "butterfly" perineal and scrotal hematoma and potentially may extend along the anterior abdominal wall to the level of the clavicles.

6. What finding on rectal examination is associated with pelvic fracture and a posterior urethral distraction injury?

A superiorly displaced, "high-riding" prostate on rectal examination is helpful in the diagnosis of a posterior urethral distraction injury. Distraction and separation of the membranous urethra in association with pelvic fracture allow the prostate to be displaced superiorly by the pelvic hematoma that fills the surrounding area.

7. How often does a pelvic fracture result in urethral injury?

Approximately 10% of pelvic fractures are associated with injuries to the lower urinary tract. Urethral injuries are present in approximately 3.5–5.0% of cases.

8. What is the evaluation of the patient with possible urethral injury?

Retrograde urethrography is the first step in the diagnosis of urethral injury. It is important to use contrast suitable for intravenous administration, because extravasation into the corpus spongiosum and surrounding tissues may occur. A Foley catheter should not be passed until a retrograde urethrogram has confirmed that the urethra is normal; the catheter may disrupt or worsen an incomplete urethral injury if present.

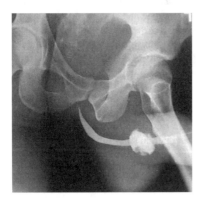
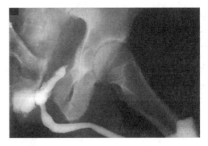

Retrograde urethrogram demonstrating extravasation resulting from penile fracture with partial urethral disruption.

Extravasation from membranous urethra following motor vehicle accident with pelvic fracture.

9. Describe the different types of posterior urethral injury.

The vast majority of posterior urethral injuries occur within the membranous urethra. The developed prostate gland tends to protect the prostatic urethra, and distraction injuries are primarily located distal to the prostatic apex. Injury may involve the proximal, mid, or distal membranous urethra. In the mildest case, the membranous urethra is stretched by surrounding hematoma without disruption, as radiography demonstrates. Partial disruptions of the membranous urethra demonstrate varying degrees of contrast extravasation with visualization of the more proximal prostatic urethra. Complete posterior urethral distraction injuries are the most severe and demonstrate complete extravasation of contrast into the pelvis and/or perineum.

10. How is an injury to the anterior urethra managed?

Blunt injury to the anterior urethra that results either in partial disruption with significant extravasation of contrast or in complete disruption should be managed with placement of a suprapubic catheter to divert the urine. After several weeks, the patient is evaluated with urethrography and endoscopy. If a significant urethral stricture has developed, the area is allowed to completely heal over several months, and urethral reconstruction is undertaken as described in chapter 45. Penetrating injury to the anterior urethra should be explored, and associated injuries should be repaired. If tissue loss is minimal, primary urethral repair may be accomplished. The urethra is stented, and a suprapubic catheter is placed for urinary diversion. If tissue loss is extensive, a suprapubic catheter is placed, and the injury is débrided, with care to preserve as much viable tissue as possible. Urethral reconstruction is accomplished at a later date.

11. What are the initial steps in the management of the patient with a posterior urethral distraction injury?

At the time of the acute injury, suprapubic cystotomy is performed. The bladder is inspected for evidence of injury, and repair is undertaken if necessary. If the patient is stable, an attempt to place an aligning urethral catheter is reasonable. This procedure is often accomplished with a combination of retrograde and antegrade passage of catheters, with or without endoscopy. If the procedure is successful, the urethral catheter is capped, and a suprapubic catheter is secured into position. If the patient is unstable, a suprapubic catheter alone is placed in the most expeditious manner possible. In general, placement of an aligning urethral catheter does not prevent formation of a urethral stricture but may help to align the prostatic apex with the distal urethra and may facilitate subsequent posterior urethral reconstruction.

12. What is the timing of posterior urethral reconstruction after a posterior urethral distraction injury?

In general, posterior urethral reconstruction is delayed for approximately 4–6 months to allow complete healing of the perineum and resolution of the pelvic hematoma. In most instances, resolution of the hematoma allows the prostate to return near its original location, with a resulting scar defect of approximately 1.5–2 cm between the ends of the urethra.

13. What operative approach is used for posterior urethral reconstruction?

Posterior urethral reconstruction almost always can be performed through a perineal incision with the patient in the exaggerated lithotomy position. Excision of the scar with a primary urethral anastomosis affords the best chance for success and is technically feasible in most cases.

14. Describe several techniques that may be used to gain length on the anterior urethra to allow a tension-free primary urethral anastomosis.

After excising the scar and preparing the proximal urethral opening, the anterior urethra is mobilized away from the corpora cavernosa to the level of the suspensory ligaments of the penis. Buck's fascia is completely dissected from the corpus spongiosum to allow maximal extension of the urethra. Subsequently, the corporal bodies may be divided proximally in the midline to shorten the distance to the proximal urethral opening. This distance may be further shortened by performing an inferior pubectomy, with or without supracrural rerouting of the urethra. Using such maneuvers in a progressive fashion allows a tension-free primary urethral anastomosis in the majority of cases.

15. Are there any concerns about subsequent transurethral resection of the prostate (TURP) after posterior urethral reconstruction?

Yes. By their nature, posterior urethral distraction injuries often result in damage to the striated urethral sphincter mechanism. After posterior urethral reconstruction, urinary continence is maintained primarily by the smooth muscle at the level of the bladder neck. TURP results in resection and obliteration of this continence mechanism. Patients undergoing this procedure after posterior urethral reconstruction are at high risk for significant urinary incontinence. Therefore, symptomatic benign prostatic hyperplasia in such patients is best managed with medical therapy or, if necessary, by intermittent self-catheterization.

BIBLIOGRAPHY

1. Angermeier KW, Devine CJ Jr: Anatomy of the penis and male perineum. Part 2. American Urological Association Update Series. Vol. 13, Lesson 3, 1994.
2. Corriere JN Jr: Trauma to the lower urinary tract. In Gillenwater JY, Grayhack JT, Howards SS, Duckett JW (eds): Adult and Pediatric Urology, 3rd ed. St. Louis, Mosby, 1996, pp 563–585.
3. Devine CJ Jr, Angermeier KW: Anatomy of the penis and male perineum. Part 1 American Urological Association Update Series. Vol. 13, Lesson 2, 1994.

4. Jordan GH: Treatment of urethral stricture disease. In Stein BS (ed): Practice of Urology. New York, Norton, 1993, pp 1–38.
5. Lowe MA, Mason JT, Luna GK, et al: Risk factors for urethral injuries in men with traumatic pelvic fractures. J Urol 140:506, 1988.
6. Morey AF, Hernandez J, McAninch JW: Reconstructive surgery for trauma of the lower urinary tract. Urol Clin North Am 26:49, 1999.
7. Pierce JM Jr: Disruptions of the anterior urethra. Urol Clin North Am 16:329, 1989.
8. Sagalowsky AI, Peters PC: Genitourinary trauma. In Walsh PC, Retik AB, Vaughan ED Jr, Wein AJ (eds): Campbell's Urology, 7th ed. Philadelphia, W. B. Saunders, 1998, pp 3108–3114.

77. TESTICULAR TRAUMA

James A. Daitch, M.D., and Anthony J. Thomas, Jr., M.D.

1. What types of injury befall the testicles?

Probably every man over the age of 18 years has experienced some form of testicular trauma. Although most instances are not severe enough to require medical attention, at the time of even relatively minor injury, many a strong man has been brought to his knees. Blunt trauma is by far the most common cause of testicular injury, followed by penetrating, self-inflicted, and, finally, dislocation injuries. Testicular trauma has been reported to occur during breech delivery, but most instances occur in the adolescent and young adult , ≤40 years of age. Most are solitary testicular injuries, although some, particularly those caused by a penetrating object, may involve the contralateral testis or penis and urethra.

2. What is the goal of treatment for a serious testicular injury?

With any testicular injury, the primary objective is to preserve as much functional tissue as possible. The spermatogenic portion is the most sensitive to insult compared with the more resilient Leydig cells, fibrous tissue, and blood vessels. Numerous studies indicate that early surgical exploration and repair of a significant testicular rupture lead to a higher salvage rate and lower morbidity than a more conservative watchful-waiting approach.

3. Can testicular torsion or tumors occur as a result of trauma?

Direct trauma causes neither torsion nor tumor. Torsion may be associated with strenuous physical activity, including contact sports (e.g., football, rugby, martial arts), and the physician must differentiate by taking a careful history to determine whether there was a direct hit to the scrotum. Swelling due to traumatic hematocele is generally greater than that found with torsion. Minor trauma may bring a patient with a testicular neoplasm to the attention of a physician. If the degree of swelling is out of proportion to the type of injury reported, the presence of a testicular neoplasm should be considered, and appropriate evaluation and treatment should be carried out.

4. What action should be taken when a patient has sustained blunt testicular trauma?

If possible, an accurate history should be obtained to determine the cause of the injury and thus to allow a fuller appreciation of the severity of the incident. Blunt trauma causes testicular rupture when a significantly strong blow forces the testis abruptly against the pubic bone. If the testis is still palpable and the swelling is not excessive, gentle examination of the testis, epididymis, and, finally, the cord structures should be undertaken. Any defect that can be palpated in the tunica albuginea is large enough to require surgical repair. Often a thorough examination of the scrotum and its contents is difficult, because the area may be quite swollen and exquisitely sensitive. If scrotal swelling is marked and the testis is not palpable, and if the patient's condition is otherwise stable, an ultrasound examination is helpful in determining the extent of the injury. With a high degree of suspicion that the tunica been ruptured with or without ultrasound confirmation, surgical intervention should be considered. In the operating room, the testis is examined. If a tunica tear is found, the loosely extruded tubules may be cut sharply from the healthy tissue, which is gently pushed back into the confines of the tunica albuginea, and the albuginea is closed with absorbable sutures. The tunica vaginalis should be closed over the testis, if possible, leaving within the tunica vaginalis a small (¼-inch diameter) Penrose drain that exits through the inferior portion of the scrotum.

5. How does the evaluation of the testis after penetrating injury differ from evaluation after blunt trauma?

Penetrating injuries within an urban setting are caused most commonly by knives or bullets.

Falls onto sharp objects also may damage the testis, but they are a more rare occurrence. Little diagnostic skill is needed to identify the type and severity of the injury caused by a sharp object or projectile. Most, if not all, injuries need to be explored carefully. Large hematomas should be evacuated, the testis débrided, and viable tissues saved, and the tunic closed with absorbable sutures. With injuries from a bullet, cloth fragments from the victim's clothes often are brought into the wound and imbedded in the tissue. Such fragments should be removed, the wounds cleansed thoroughly, and the scrotal contents drained, as with blunt injuries. High-velocity projectiles may cause particularly severe injuries that are not initially appreciated. Delayed tissue necrosis may occur at the area of injury. In most instances, if a high-velocity bullet strikes the testis, little is left to be repaired. The cord structures may need to be débrided, the open vessels secured, and the wound adequately drained and closed.

6. Are antibiotics needed for the treatment of blunt or penetrating testicular injury?

Penetrating injuries require broad-spectrum antibiotic coverage. Blunt injuries, particularly those that cause only a contusion and do not require surgery, generally do not require antibiotics unless significant hematocele is associated with the injury. In some reports, subsequent infection has been associated with hematocele. If operative intervention is performed for a blunt injury, of course, it may be prudent to administer antibiotics before and after the procedure.

7. What is a dislocation injury? How serious is it?

Blunt trauma does not always result in contusion or rupture. Sudden force may push the testicle upward toward or through the inguinal canal. It may then be held in position at the external ring, within the inguinal canal or even in the abdomen. This dislocation injury can be extremely painful. At times, the testis may twist on its cord, compromising circulatory integrity, or the tunica albuginea may rupture. Such injuries appear to be more frequent during motorcycle accidents, perhaps as a result of a sudden impact against the wide gas tank, which the driver straddles. Most serious motorcycle accidents result in multiple organ injury, and the "missing testis" may not be noticed. If the patient is conscious, he may complain of severe inguinal pain. Examination reveals the empty hemiscotum, and often the testis can be palpated in the groin area. If no more serious injuries are present and if the testis is palpably normal, the patient is given intravenous analgesia for sedation and pain relief. With gentle massage, an attempt is made to push the testis back into the scrotum. If this approach fails or if the structural integrity of the testis is in question, the patient is taken to the operating room for a formal exploration; the testis is repaired and replaced in the scrotum.

8. If the cord structures are damaged, should an attempt be made to revascularize the testis?

Blunt injury to the cord structures is relatively uncommon. The cord is fairly well protected, and generally the injuries are limited to contusions that do not require surgery unless a large hematoma is present. Gunshot wounds of the cord usually destroy the vasculature and require orchiectomy and ligation of the vessels. Injuries that may require microsurgical expertise either result from accidental avulsion of the scrotum and testes or are self-inflicted by mentally disturbed men. The patient with accidental avulsion usually reports working with a large piece of machinery when his pants get trapped in the gears or teeth and drag parts of him into the machinery before it can be shut down. Certain types of farm equipment are notorious for such mutilating injuries. In most instances, the testis is damaged beyond repair. Self-inflicted injuries are often cleaner, and if the testis is brought in with or by the patient, an attempt at reimplantation may be considered, depending on the condition of the patient, the time lapse between injury and presentation, and, of course, the condition of the testis(es).

9. Can testicular trauma adversely affect fertility?

Immediately following any significant traumatic event, sperm production may be altered adversely, at times to an azoospermic state. Most patients resume active spermatogenesis in time, but recovery may take 3–9 months after injury. Data from laboratory experiments suggest that unilateral testicular injury may cause permanent changes in both the ipsilateral and contralateral testes. Indeed, preliminary evidence indicates that men who sustain significant testicular trauma do have impaired semen analyses even upon long-term follow-up. Whether all patients who have sustained significant trauma to a testis should be followed with subsequent semen analysis remains to be seen. Men presenting with infertility problems, however, should be questioned about a past history of testicular trauma.

10. What are the basic principles for treatment of a traumatic testicular injury?
1. Identify the cause of the injury, if possible.

2. Use ultrasound, if available, to look at the testis and help to determine if the tunica albuginea is ruptured.

3. Do not depend totally on ultrasound to give the right answer every time. Use clinical judgment.

4. Surgery may result in less morbidity than watchful waiting if there is any doubt that more than a simple contusion is present.

5. Universal precautions should be followed in all patients; among patients who sustain penetrating scrotal trauma, such precautions should be re-emphasized, because the prevalence of hepatitis B and C is high (approximately 38%) in this population.

BIBLIOGRAPHY

 1. Altarac S: A case of testicular replanatation. J Urol 150(5 pt 1):1507–1508, 1993.
 2. Bhandary P, Abbitt PL, Watson L: Ultrasound diagnosis of testicular rupture. J Clin Ultrasound 20:436–438, 1992.
 3. Cass AS, Luxenberg M: Testicular injuries. Urology 37:528–530, 1991.
 4. Cline KJ, Mata JA, Venable DD, et al: Penetrating trauma to the male external genitalia. J Trauma 44:492–494, 1998.
 5. Corrales JG, Corbel L, Cipolla B, et al: Accuracy of ultrasound diagnosis after blunt testicular trauma. J Urol 150:1834–1836, 1993.
 6. Gomez RG, Castanheira AC, McAninch JW: Gun shot wounds of the male external genitalia. J Urol 150:1147–1149, 1993.
 7. Kukadia AN, Ercole CJ, Gleich P, et al: Testicular trauma: Potential impact on reproductive function. J Urol 156:1643–1646, 1996.
 8. Learch TJ, Hansch LP, Ralls PW: Sonography in patients with gunshot wounds to the scrotum: Imaging findings and their value. Am J Roentgenol 165:879–883, 1995.
 9. Masui Y, Ueda K, Ootaguro K: Traumatic dislocation of the testis: A case report. Hinyokika Kiyo 35: 1417–1420, 1989.
10. Sauvage P, Geiss S, Leculee R, Hideux S: Injuries of the testis in children. Chirurgie Pediatrique 29:136–141, 1988.
11. Singer AJ, Das S, Gavrell GJ: Traumatic dislocation of the testes. Urology 35:310–312, 1990.
12. Tiwary CM: Testicular injury in breech delivery: Possible implications. Urology 34:210–212, 1989.

78. PRIAPISM

Drogo K. Montague, M.D., and Milton M. Lakin, M.D.

1. What is priapism?

Priapism is a prolonged, usually painful erection not associated with sexual desire.

2. Describe the types of priapism.

- Low-flow (ischemic) priapism
- High-flow (nonischemic) priapism

3. What are the causes of priapism?

1. **High-flow priapism** is secondary to penile or perineal trauma and results when injury creates an arterial-sinusoidal shunt within the corpus cavernosum.

2. **Low-flow priapism** may result from sickle cell disease, leukemia, anticoagulants, spinal cord lesions, fat emboli, malignant penile inflammation, autonomic neuropathy, penile injection therapy for erectile dysfunction, and drugs. Many cases have unknown etiologies. Low-flow priapism, which is painful, is much more common than nonpainful high-flow priapism.

4. How do drugs cause priapism?

- **Psychotropic agents** may have peripheral α-blocking activity and/or central serotonin-like activity. A commonly used antidepressant associated with priapism is trazodone (Desyrel).
- **Intracavernous pharmacotherapy** is a technique used to treat erectile dysfunction (impotence). Drugs commonly injected into the corpora cavernosa for this purpose include papaverine, phentolamine, and prostaglandin E_1. Although this technique is very effective in the treatment of erectile dysfunction, it is associated with low-flow priapism in a small percentage of cases.

5. Does priapism have any distinctive features on physical examination?

Yes. A normal erection involves both corpora cavernosa, the corpus spongiosum, and the glans penis. With priapism, only the corpora cavernosa are erect. The glans penis is small and flaccid and the ventral surface of the erect penis is flat, since the bulge of erect corpus spongiosum that surrounds the urethra in normal erection is absent. With ischemic priapism, the erection is abnormally rigid and cannot be bent. With arterial priapism, the erection is almost full and can be bent.

6. Is priapism an emergency?

Yes. Most cases of priapism are of the low-flow, ischemic variety. When oxygen levels in the blood trapped within the corpora drop, pain occurs and time-dependent damage to cavernosal smooth muscle ensues. Treatment of the less common form of priapism, arterial priapism, is not an emergency.

7. What are the consequences of delayed or nontreatment of ischemic priapism?

Cavernosal fibrosis results, and subsequent ability to obtain normal erections is lost.

8. How soon should priapism be treated?

Ideally, any painful, fully rigid erection lasting 4 hours should cause a man to seek prompt urologic attention. In reality, most patients present with an erection of at least 24 hours' duration. Successful reversal of the priapism at this point may still preserve subsequent erectile function, but with increasing duration of priapism, the incidence of erectile dysfunction rises sharply.

9. Describe the initial encounter with the patient who has low-flow ischemic priapism.

The history should document the duration of the priapism and elicit factors that may be responsible. Physical examination confirms the presence of priapism by its characteristic findings. The patient, and whenever possible the partner or family, are then counseled regarding the possibility of permanent erectile dysfunction (impotence) regardless of success in the treatment of the priapism.

10. What is the first step in the treatment of low-flow, ischemic priapism?

Nonoperative treatment should always be tried first. A 19-gauge butterfly needle is inserted into one corpus cavernosum. (The septum between the corpora is incomplete and entry into one side provides access to both corporeal bodies.) Blood is aspirated and sent for blood gas determination to document the degree of ischemia. Blood is then aspirated from the corpora (10–15 ml), discarded, and then replaced with an equal amount of normal saline. This process is repeated until the aspirate is bright red. A solution of phenylephrine is prepared by taking 1 ml containing 10 mg and diluting it to 100 ml with normal saline. Three to 5 ml of this dilute solution are then injected into the corpora, and this process is repeated at 10-minute intervals until the erection subsides. The patient's pulse and blood pressure should be monitored during this procedure.

11. Why is phenylephrine used to reverse priapism?

Any sympathomimetic amine can be used to reverse priapism. However, when the priapism subsides, the sympathomimetic drug that was injected into the corpora is released into the systemic circulation. If epinephrine is used, tachycardia and arrhythmia often result. If metaraminol is used, severe hypertension often results. Phenylephrine has minimal systemic side effects.

12. How does operative treatment play a role in the treatment of low-flow, ischemic priapism?

If nonoperative treatment of priapism fails, prompt operative intervention is indicated. Surgical treatment of priapism involves establishing a shunt between the erect corpora cavernosa and the glans penis, or corpus spongiosum, or saphenous vein system.

13. How is the presence of high-flow, nonischemic priapism established?

A history of penile or perineal trauma is invariably present. Color duplex ultrasonography is useful in revealing the presence of an arterial-sinusoidal shunt.

14. Describe the treatment of high-flow, nonischemic priapism.

Selective internal pudendal arteriography confirms the presence of the arterial-sinusoidal shunt, and then selective embolization of the artery feeding the shunt is performed. Alternatively, the artery feeding the shunt may be surgically ligated.

15. What is stuttering priapism?

Stuttering priapism consists of recurrent episodes of ischemic priapism, which either subside spontaneously after several hours or are successfully reversed by corporeal aspiration and phenylephrine injection. These episodes occur frequently, often daily.

16. Describe the treatment of stuttering priapism.

Stuttering priapism has been treated by all of the following methods:

- Systemic sympathomimetic amines (phenylpropanolamine, pseudoephedrine, or terbutaline)
- Monthly injections of a luteinizing hormone-releasing hormone agonist, leuprolide acetate (Lupron)
- Self-administered intracorporeal injections of a sympathomimetic amine
- Oral administration of digoxin

BIBLIOGRAPHY

1. Brock G, Breza J, Lue TF, Tanagho EA: High flow priapism: A spectrum of disease. J Urol 150:968–971, 1993.
2. Carson CC, Mino RD: Priapism associated with trazodone therapy. J Urol 139:369–370, 1988.
3. Dittrich A, Albrecht K, Bar-Moshe O, Vandendris M: Treatment of pharmacological priapism with phenylephrine. J Urol 146:323–324, 1991.
4. Fouda A, Hassouna M, Beddoe E, et al: Priapism: An avoidable complication of pharmacologically induced erection. J Urol 142:995–997, 1989.
5. Fowler JE, Koshy M, Strub M, Chinn SK: Priapism associated with the sickle cell hemoglobinopathies: Prevalence, natural history and sequelae. J Urol 145:65–68, 1991.
6. Gupta S, Salimpour P, Saenz de Tejada I, et al: A possible mechanism for alteration of human erectile function by digoxin: Inhibition of corpus cavernosum sodium/potassium adenosine triphosphatase activity. J Urol 159:1529–1536, 1998.
7. Klein EA, Montague DK, Steiger E: Priapism associated with the use of intravenous fat emulsion: Case reports and postulated pathogenesis. J Urol 133:857–859, 1985.
8. Levine LA, Guss SP: Gondadotropin-releasing hormone analogues in the treatment of sickle cell anemia-associated priapism. J Urol 150:475–477, 1993.
9. Lue TF, Hellstrom WJG, McAninch JW, Tanagho EA: Priapism: A refined approach to diagnosis and treatment. J Urol 136:104–108, 1986.
10. Molina L, Bejany D, Lynne CM, Politano VA: Diluted epinephrine solution for the treatment of priapism. J Urol 141:1127–1128, 1989.
11. Shantha TR, Finnerty DP, Rodriquez AP: Treatment of persistent penile erection and priapism using terbutaline. J Urol 141:1427–1429, 1989.
12. Shapiro RH, Berger RE: Post-traumatic priapism treated with selective cavernosal artery ligation. Urology 49:638–643, 1997.
13. Winter CC, McDowell G: Experience with 105 patients with priapism: Update and review of all aspects. J Urol 140:980–983, 1988.

VI. Calculus Disease

79. RENAL CALCULI

J. Patrick Spirnak, M.D.

1. What causes renal calculi to form?

Many theories have been proposed to explain the cause of renal stone formation. Unfortunately, no one mechanism fully explains the cause in all stone formers.

In one commonly accepted model of stone formation, a period of abnormal crystalluria is required. For crystals to form and grow, the urine must be supersaturated with the salt of the stone-forming crystal. Urinary substances that act as inhibitors to crystal formation must be reduced or absent from the urine, and certain proteins that act as the framework for crystal depositions must be present in the urine.

2. What risk factors enhance stone formation?
1. Metabolic state (influenced by patient's genetic background)
2. Hormonal imbalances
3. Environmental factors
4. Dietary excesses
5. Anatomic abnormalities leading to chronic infection or stasis

3. Where do renal stones form?

Stones form in the collecting tubules and pass into the calyces, renal pelvis, and ureter.

4. List the four most common types of stones found in North America.
1. Calcium-containing stones (calcium oxalate, calcium phosphate, mixed), 70%
2. Infection stones (struvite, magnesium ammonium phosphate), 15–20%
3. Uric acid stones, 5–10%
4. Cystine stones, 1–5%

5. What is the composition of the most common stone found in American men?

Calcium stones occurring in combination with either oxalate or phosphate.

6. Name the most common stone found in American women. Why?

Infection stones. Women are more prone to urinary tract infections than men.

7. What stone is inherited as an autosomal-recessive trait?

Cystine.

8. How does the typical patient present with a nonobstructing caliceal stone?

Nonobstructing caliceal stones are usually discovered as incidental findings on radiographs obtained for the evaluation of other organ systems or during the evaluation of hematuria.

9. Describe the typical presentation of a patient with an obstructing renal pelvic stone.

Obstruction occurring at the level of the ureteropelvic junction causes sharp, intermittent colicky pain localized to the flank or costovertebral angle. The pain is not related to activity and may be accompanied by nausea and vomiting.

10. What are the expected urinalysis findings in patients with renal colic?

Microscopic or gross hematuria is common. However, the absence does not exclude renal stone disease. Pyuria may be present without infection. Crystals may be seen.

11. Is urine pH important in determining the type of stone present?

Yes. An acid urine (pH <5.5) is suggestive of a uric acid stone, whereas a pH of 8 suggests an infectious stone.

12. Is a KUB film sufficient to diagnose a renal stone?

No. Only 90% of stones are radiopaque. Pure uric acid stones are usually radiolucent and do not appear on a plain film of the abdomen.

13. What x-ray study should be performed?

An excretory urogram (IVP) is obtained in all patients suspected of having a renal stone, unless they are allergic to the contrast.

14. List the indications for surgical stone removal.
- Persistent pain
- Recurrent, gross hematuria
- Obstruction with progressive renal damage
- Recurrent urinary tract infection

15. What type of stone can be consistently dissolved by taking oral medication?

Pure (100%) uric acid stones can almost always be dissolved by oral alkalinization therapy. Potassium citrate and sodium bicarbonate are two oral agents that may be used to alkalinize the urine to a pH range of 6.5–7.

16. What treatment options currently exist to treat renal calculi and what are the indications for each?

(1) Extracorporeal shock-wave lithotripsy (ESWL) is indicated to treat the majority of renal calculi less than or equal to 2.5 cm. in largest diameter; (2) percutaneous nephrostolithotomy is recommended as the treatment of choice in the majority of stones greater than or equal to 2.5 cm in diameter or to treat stones refractory to ESWL therapy; and (3) open stone removal is reserved for patients who fail less invasive forms of therapy or those with anatomic abnormalites requiring reconstruction at the time of stone removal.

17. Is pyelolithotomy the treatment of choice in managing a 1-cm obstructing calcium pelvic stone?

No. ESWL is the treatment of choice and is successful in >90% of cases.

18. Can all renal stones be treated by ESWL?

Cystine stones are usually refractory to ESWL therapy. In addition, stones of other composition >2.5 cm in diameter are frequently associated with obstruction following ESWL treatment. Such patients may be best managed by either percutaneous or open surgical stone removal.

BIBLIOGRAPHY

1. Niall O, Russell J, MacGregor R, et al: A comparison of noncontrast computerized tomography with excretory urography in the assessment of acute flank pain. J Urol 161:534, 1999.
2. Pak CYC: Medical management of nephrolithiasis. J Urol 128:1157, 1982.
3. Resnick MI, Spirnak JP: Calculus disease: General considerations. In Pollack HM (ed): Clinical Urography. Philadelphia, W. B. Saunders, 1990, p 1752.
4. Sarmina I, Spirnak JP, Resnick MI: Urinary lithiasis in the black population: An epidemiologic study and review of the literature. J Urol 138:14, 1987.
5. Spirnak JP, Resnick MI: ESWL. In Pak C, Resnick MI (eds): Urolithiasis. Philadelphia, W. B. Saunders, 1990, pp 321–362.
6. Spirnak JP, Resnick MI: Urinary stones. In Tanagho EA, McAninch JW (eds): Smith's General Urology. Norwalk, CT, Appleton & Lange, 1992, p 271, 298.
7. Vieneg J, Ten C, Freed K, et al: Unenhanced helical computerized tomography for the evaluation of patients with acute flank pain. J Urol 160:679, 1998.
8. Paik ML, Wainstein MA, Spirnak JP, et al: Current indications for open stone surgery in the treatment of renal and ureteral calculi. J. Urol 159:374, 1998.

80. STAGHORN CALCULI

Stevan B. Streem, M.D.

1. How did staghorn calculi get their name?
Here is a plain abdominal x-ray in a patient with bilateral staghorn calculi. Now you know.

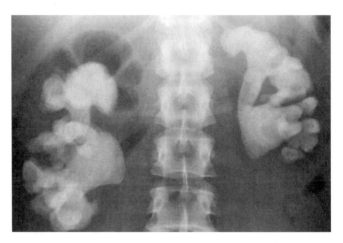

Plain abdominal radiograph in a woman with documented recurrent *Proteus* urinary tract infections reveals bilateral staghorn calculi.

2. What causes them?
Most stones of "staghorn" size and shape are infection-related and composed of magnesium-ammonium phosphate (struvite) along with calcium phosphate. These minerals precipitate on a matrix "cast" of the pyelocalyceal system in a branched staghorn configuration. The basic abnormality in these patients is a chronically alkaline urine that results from infection with urease-producing urinary pathogens.

3. Are all staghorn stones related to infection?
Most stones of staghorn size and shape are infection-related. However, uric acid stones and cystine stones also may develop in a staghorn configuration. Calcium oxalate and calcium phosphate stones, the most common stones, only rarely grow in a staghorn shape or to such a large size.

4. Do staghorn stones need to be removed even if they are not causing symptoms?
Many studies have shown that the natural history of these stones is progressive obstruction, infection, and loss of kidney function. Therefore, the presence of this type of stone is itself an indication for intervention, even in the absence of symptoms.

5. How are they removed?
In the past, a "kidney-splitting" operation called anatrophic nephrolithotomy was often performed. Currently, various combinations of percutaneous stone removal and extracorporeal shock-wave lithotripsy (SWL) may be used as an alternative to such surgery.

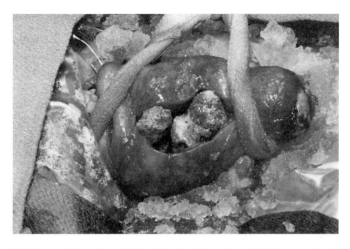

Anatrophic nephrolithotomy is performed by incising the kidney in a relatively avascular plane. The renal artery is clamped during this time to allow the surgery to be performed in a bloodless field. Renal ischemia is prevented by introperative cooling of the kidney while the artery is clamped. (From Novick AC, Streem SB: Surgery of the kidney. In Walsh PC, et al (eds). Campbell's Urology, 6th ed. Philadelphia, W.B. Saunders, 1992, p 2461; with permission).

BIBLIOGRAPHY

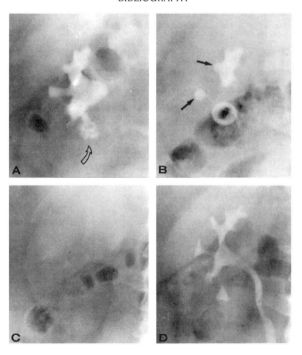

A. Plain abdominal radiograph reveals a staghorn calculus. **B.** Most of the stone has been removed by percutaneous ultrasonic nephrostolithotomy. Residual fragments inaccessible to the percutaneous tract (*arrows*) are treated with extracorporeal shock-wave lithotripsy (ESWL). **C.** Follow-up plain x-ray shows no residual stones. **D.** Follow-up pyelogram reveals an excellent functional and anatomic result.

BIBLIOGRAPHY

1. Blandy JP, Singh M: The case for a more aggressive approach to staghorn stones. J Urol 115:505, 1976.
2. Boyce WH, Elkins IB: Reconstructive renal surgery following anatrophic nephrolithotomy: Followup of 100 consecutive cases. J Urol 111:307, 1974.
3. Gil-Vernet J: New surgical concepts in removing renal calculi. Urol Int 20:255, 1965.
4. Nickel JC, Emtage J, Costerton JW: Ultrastructural microbial etiology of infection induced urinary stones. J Urol 133:622, 1985.
5. Novick AC, Streem SB: Surgery of the kidney. In Walsh PC, Retik AB, Vaughan ED Jr, Wein AJ (eds): Campbell's Urology, 7th edition. Philadelphia, W. B. Saunders, 1998, pp 2973–3061.
6. Kahnoski RJ, Lingeman JE, Coury TA, et al: Combined percutaneous and extracorporeal shock wave lithotripsy for staghorn calculi: An alternative to anatrophic nephrolithotomy. J Urol 135:679, 1986.
7. Segura JW, Preminger GM, Assimos DG, et al: Nephrolithiasis clinical guidelines panel summary report on the management of staghorn calculi. J Urol 151:1648, 1994.
8. Smith MJ, Boyce WH: Anatrophic nephrotomy and plastic calyrhaphy. J Urol 99:521, 1968.
9. Streem SB, Yost A, Dolmatch B: Combination "sandwich" therapy for extensive renal calculi in 100 consecutive patients: Immediate, long term, and stratified results from a ten year experience. J Urol 158:342, 1997.
10. Vargas AB, Bragin SR, Mendez R: Staghorn calculus: Its clinical presentation, complications and management. J Urol 127:860, 1982.

81. URETERAL CALCULI

Martin I. Resnick, M.D.

1. Where in the collecting system do ureteral calculi become impacted?
Uroliths create symptoms when they become trapped in a segment of the upper urinary tract. To become impacted, a calculus must have a diameter greater than 2 mm. Areas where a calculus may become impacted include:

    1. **Ureteropelvic junction.** Here, the large diameter of the renal pelvis decreases to that of the ureter (2–3 mm). Beyond the ureteropelvic junction, the ureter develops a diameter of 10 mm (30F), and small calculi can pass distally to the iliac vessels.

    2. **Ureters cross the pelvic brim.** As the ureters arch over the iliac vessels, they narrow to approximately 4 mm (12F).

    3. **Ureterovesical junction.** The ureter narrows at this point to a diameter of 1–5 mm and it is here where most ureteral stones lodge. In women, another area is in the posterior pelvis, where the ureter is crossed anteriorly by the pelvic blood vessels and the broad ligament.

2. What variables affect spontaneous passage of ureteral calculi?
The size and location of the calculus are the two most important variables in planning therapy. Ninety percent of stones in the distal ureter measuring 4 mm in diameter will pass spontaneously, compared to only 50% of stones 4–5.9 mm in diameter. Only 20% of stones 6 mm will pass without surgical intervention. Proximal ureteral stones are less likely to pass than distal ureteral stones.

3. What is Steinstrasse?
Steinstrasse is a term meaning "stone street"; it describes the fragments of a urinary calculus created after extracorporeal shock-wave lithotripsy (ESWL), which stack up and may obstruct the ureter. Some pass spontaneously whereas others require intervention to effect removal.

4. How do calculi create symptoms?
Ureteral calculi create symptoms when they become trapped and obstruct the flow of urine from the upper collecting system. Ureteral pain (or colic) is characterized as an extremely intense pain, sudden in onset and stabbing in nature. The pain and associated symptoms often are related to the location of the calculus within the ureter.

5. Describe the symptoms stones produce according to their location.
Caliceal calculi. Small nonobstructing caliceal calculi are usually asymptomatic but are detected when a patient develops gross hematuria or incidentally on a radiograph. These calculi can result in urinary tract infections, persistent hematuria, or flank pain if they become large enough to obstruct an infundibulum.

Renal pelvic stones. Small renal pelvic calculi are usually asymptomatic. If they become impacted at the ureteropelvic junction or pass into the proximal ureter, the resultant obstruction of urine may cause symptoms of localized flank or costovertebral angle tenderness. If urinary infection is associated, the patient may develop pyelonephritis or even florid sepsis.

Proximal ureteral calculi. Patients experience sharp intermittent flank pain of acute onset associated with either gross or microscopic hematuria. As the stone passes distally to the pelvic brim, pain may radiate to the lateral flank of the abdominal region.

Distal ureter. As the stone enters the distal ureter, pain frequently radiates along the inguinal canal into the corresponding groin and genitals. Calculi lodged at the ureterovesical junction create symptoms of vesical irritability, including urinary urgency, frequency, and dysuria.

6. What are the indications for hospitalizing a patient with a ureteral calculus?
1. A stone in a solitary kidney
2. Fever, leukocytosis, or bacteriuria
3. Azotemia
4. Colic and associated nausea and vomiting too severe to be managed on an outpatient basis
5. Uncontrollable pain requiring parenteral analgesics
6. Complete obstruction of the kidney

7. Where do ureteral calculi form?
Ureteral stones originate in the collecting ducts of the kidney and likely grow in the renal pelvis and pass into the ureter, where they frequently become lodged. Calculi that primarily develop in the ureter are rare. Instances in which they may develop in the ureter have been seen in association with ureteroceles, neoplasms, ectopic ureters, ureteral strictures, and foreign bodies such as a stent or suture in the ureter. Right and left ureteral calculi occur with equal frequency.

8. How are stones diagnosed?
Typically stones are diagnosed either with x-ray (KUB, IVP), ultrasound, or CT scanning. Patients often present with acute pain and are initially seen in an emergency room. Commonly, spiral CT scans are obtained without the administration of intravenous contrast agents.

9. What is the composition of ureteral calculi?
Because most ureteral calculi originate in the kidney, they possess the same composition as renal calculi. Calcium oxalate stones are the most frequent.

10. How quickly do ureteral calculi need to be treated?
If infection exists behind an obstructed ureter, the obstruction must be relieved as soon as possible. If no infection is present but the patient is experiencing minimal discomfort, clinical judgment should be used. With complete obstruction (in dog studies), renal deterioration begins within 18–24 hours. Within 5 days to 2 weeks, some irreversible changes in function have occurred. After 16 weeks of obstruction, only partial return of function is expected. Partial obstruction, of course, modifies these values. Studies have indicated that chronic partial obstruction results in significant renal damage, and therefore early intervention is recommended.

11. What are phleboliths? How are they different from ureteral calculi?
Phleboliths are calcifications within pelvic veins. They differ from ureteral calculi in that they are rounder, cast shadows lateral to the course of the ureter, and have radiolucent centers. At times, they can be difficult to distinguish from distal ureteral stones when viewed with x-ray (KUB) or CT imaging.

12. Describe the expectant strategy for ureteral calculi.
Most calculi ≤ 5 mm in diameter will pass spontaneously. Expectant management consists of hydration, analgesia, and serial abdominal x-rays obtained at 1–2 week intervals to assess stone passage. Patients should be instructed to strain all their urine and save the stone for analysis. The patient should be instructed to watch for signs of fever, urinary tract infection, increasing pain unresponsive to oral medications, or severe nausea or vomiting.

13. What are the indications for surgical intervention?
- Infection unresponsive to antibiotics
- Severe colic unresponsive to oral medications
- Complete urinary obstruction of a solitary kidney
- Impaction
- Hydronephrosis that fails to imrpove with observation

14. Describe the invasive treatment options for ureteral calculi.

Treatment options for ureteral calculi include extracorporeal shock-wave lithotripsy, endourologic stone extraction, and rarely open surgery. No single modality is superior for treating all ureteral calculi. The choice of treatment needs to be individualized to the patient as well as the experience of the surgeon.

Extracorporeal shock-wave lithotripsy (ESWL). Since its introduction in 1980, ESWL has become the noninvasive treatment of choice for upper ureteral and most renal calculi. Response rates are much higher for upper ureteral (98%) compared to iliac (70%) and distal ureteral (85%) calculi. Calculi in the lower ureter are more difficult to localize and are thus treated with ESWL. Other factors influencing the success of ESWL include stone composition, size, and degree of impaction.

Ureteroscopy. Although ESWL is effective in managing most urinary calculi, a significant proportion of patients do not respond to this therapy alone. With the advent of ureteroscopes with significantly reduced diameters (5–11F), endourologic intervention has become an increasingly safe and effective means of therapy for ureteral calculi. Success rates of 97% have been reported with ureteroscopic techniques. Calculi ≥ 6 mm require fragmentation before extraction, usually by ultrasound, electrohydraulic, laser, or impact lithotripsy.

Ureterolithotomy. Ureterolithotomy is now used in 2% of patients, when ESWL or endourologic intervention has failed. Indications for ureterolithotomy include conditions requiring concomitant surgical correction of an anatomic abnormality, such as ureteral stricture, ureterovesical obstruction, and vesicoureteral reflux.

15. When is chemolysis used?

In chemolysis, urinary calculi are dissolved by alterations in the urinary environment. This process can be accomplished systemically by oral or parenteral therapy (systemic chemolysis) or by direct irrigation of the renal pelvis (direct contact chemolysis). Cystine, struvite, and uric acid calculi are all amenable to this therapy. The success of ESWL and endourologic intervention has limited the role of this therapy. Currently, percutaneous chemolysis is used as adjunctive therapy for residual stones after ESWL, open stone surgery, and endourologic procedures.

BIBLIOGRAPHY

1. Frauscher F, Klauser A, Halpern EJ: Recurrent renal stone disease. Lancet 359:79–80, 2002.
2. Coll DM, Varanelli MJ, Smith RC: Relationship of spontaneous passage of ureteral calculi to stone size and location as revealed by unenhanced helical CT. AJR 178:101–103, 2002.
3. Tiselius HG, Ackermann D, Alken P, et al: Guidelines on urolithiasis. Eur Urol 40:362–371, 2001.
4. Reilly AJ, Addison J: Evaluation of a nonenhanced helical CT protocol for detecting ureteric stones. Radiology 221:558–559, discussion 559–61, 2001.
5. Chang CP, Huang SH, Tai HL, et al: Optimal treatment for distal ureteral calculi: Extracorporeal shock-wave lithotripsy versus ureteroscopy. J Endourol 15:563–566, 2001.
6. Hollenbeck BK, Schuster TG, Faerber GJ, Wolf JS Jr: Comparison of outcomes of ureteroscopy for ureteral calculi located above and below the pelvic brim. Urology 58:351–356, 2001.
7. Painter DJ, Keeley FX Jr: New concepts in the treatment of ureteral calculi. Curr Opin Urol 11:373–378, 2001.

82. BLADDER CALCULI

Nehemia Hampel, M.D.

1. Who is most affected with bladder calculi?
Bladder calculi are most commonly found in adult males with bladder outlet obstruction and in male children who live in underdeveloped countries.

2. What are primary and secondary bladder calculi?
Primary bladder calculi are endemic and involve only children. Secondary bladder calculi occur primarily in adults and are secondary to urinary stasis with or without associated infection or foreign bodies. Whenever foreign bodies are present, such as chronic indwelling catheters, bladder calculi should be suspected.

3. Has the incidence of bladder calculi in children changed?
In the past, bladder calculi in children were more common than in adults. With industrialization, increase in the average income, and dietary and nutritional progress, bladder calculi are disappearing from previously afflicted areas. They continue to occur in some underdeveloped countries.

4. What is the composition of pediatric bladder calculi?
In endemic areas, most calculi are composed of ammonium acid urate, calcium oxalate, or mixtures of both.

5. What is the chemical composition of bladder calculi in adults?
The chemical composition of bladder calculi is similar to the spectrum seen in the upper tract calculi. Calcium oxalate is the most common constituent of calculi in the United States. In Europe, uric acid and urate stones are more prevalent.

6. What is the sex distribution of bladder calculi?
They are predominantly a disease of males of all ages and all nationalities. The most important factor for male preponderance is associated with urine stasis due to obstruction.

7. What are the symptoms of bladder calculi?
Patients with bladder calculi may be free from any specific symptoms, particularly in the pediatric age group. However, patient history may provide a clue to diagnosis. The symptoms in most cases are bladder outlet obstruction and urinary infection. Typical symptoms of bladder calculi are intermittent voiding with sudden painful interruptions. They may be associated with terminal hematuria. The pain may be in the lower abdomen and referred to the tip of the penis, along the course of the second to the fourth sacral nerves. Irritating voiding symptoms of frequency, urgency, and dysuria are usually present.

8. Are there specific laboratory findings?
No specific laboratory tests can identify bladder calculi. Proteins, erythrocytes, and leukocytes are usually found in the urine, and urine cultures may be positive in the presence of infection. None of these findings are specific to bladder calculi.

9. How do you establish the diagnosis of bladder calculi?
The absence of shadow on the plain roentgenogram does not exclude bladder calculus. About 50% of calculi are missed on plain x-rays. Cystogram may detect those radiolucent calculi. The

best and surest method for detecting bladder calculi is cystoscopy. No stones should be missed on direct inspection of the bladder.

10. How do treatment plans for primary and secondary bladder calculi differ?

Primary and secondary bladder calculi present different problems and require individual approaches. In primary (endemic) calculi, the stones have to be removed, and the patient should be followed with proper dietary correction. In secondary calculi, eradication of the calculi does not prevent recurrences. The underlying obstructive lesion and infection should be corrected. Foreign bodies should be removed whenever possible.

11. Describe the treatment options to eliminate bladder calculi.

Standard treatment options include chemodissolution, transurethral extraction, fragmentation with mechanical electrohydraulic or ultrasonic instruments, and evacuation or surgical removal (open or percutaneous surgery). Chemodissolution, although an attractive option, requires long periods of time, and therefore is impractical compared with other options. Most calculi can be removed transurethrally and open surgery is seldom required. Because of the relatively large stones at presentation and a narrow urethra, stones in boys are usually surgically removed.

12. What is the prognosis for patients with bladder calculi?

Primary bladder calculi are gradually being eliminated in developed countries. They are more of a socioeconomic problem than medical. Recurrence of secondary bladder calculi is mostly related to the correction of the underlying obstruction and infection and the elimination of catheters. With proper care and regular urologic follow-up, there should be few recurrences.

BIBLIOGRAPHY

1. Dalton DC, Hughes J, Glenn JF: Foreign bodies and urinary stones. Urology 6:1, 1975.
2. Gillenwater JY, Grayhack JT, Howards SS, Duckett JW (eds): Adult and Pediatric Urology, 3rd ed. St. Louis, Mosby, 1996.
3. Menon M, Parulkar BG, Drach GW: Urinary lithiasis: Etiology, diagnosis and medical management. In Walsh PC, Retik AB, Vaughan ED Jr, Wein AJ (eds): Campbell's Urology, 7th ed. Philadelphia, W. B. Saunders, 1998 pp 2661–2733.
4. Rous SN: Stone disease, diagnosis and management. Orlando, Grune and Stratton, 1987.
5. Salah MA, Holman E, Toth C: Percutaneous suprapubic cystolithotripsy for pediatric bladder stones in a developing country. Eur Urol 39:466–470, 2001
6. Schwartz BF, Stoller ML: The vesical calculus. Urol Clin North Am 27:333–346, 2000.

83. CALCIUM OXALATE STONES

Stevan B. Streem, M.D.

1. How common are calcium oxalate stones?

In the United States, the incidence of urinary stone disease has been estimated to be 0.1 to 0.3 percent. Therefore, 240,000–720,000 Americans suffer a kidney stone event each year, with men more frequently affected than women. The prevalence of stone disease has been estimated to be 5–10%. In other words, in the United States alone, 12–24 million people will develop a stone at some time during their lives.

Calcium oxalate stones, with or without a calcium phosphate component, account for approximately 75% of all urinary calculi. Obviously then, calcium oxalate stones pose a significant health care problem in the United States.

2. What are the usual presenting symptoms and signs of calcium oxalate stones?

Calcium oxalate calculi may first come to medical attention when they cause pain or hematuria. The symptoms usually result from acute obstruction, such as when a stone moves to the ureter. Occasionally, otherwise asymptomatic patients with calcium stones may be found serendipitously at the time of radiographic evaluation for unrelated abdominal or musculoskeletal disorders. Radiographic evaluation of asymptomatic stones also may be prompted by microhematuria or pyuria found at the time of a routine urinalysis.

3. What do calcium oxalate stones look like radiographically?

On a plain x-ray, calcium oxalate stones are opaque with a radiodensity similar to that of bone or iodinated contrast. Therefore, after contrast is administered for an intravenous urogram or during a retrograde study, the stone may be obscured. Ultrasound and CT scan also can identify stones, although in vivo, calcium oxalate calculi cannot be reliably distinguished from stones of other chemical composition with those studies.

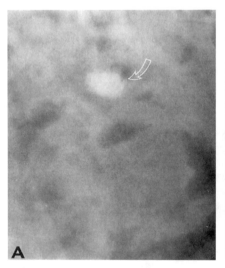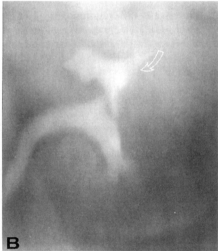

A. A plain x-ray reveals opacity overlying the renal shadow, consistent with a calcium stone. **B.** During intravenous urography, the stone itself is obscured by radiographic contrast media, which has the same radiodensity.

4. What causes calcium oxalate stones?

In simplest terms, calcium oxalate stones form when the urine is supersaturated with calcium oxalate—i.e., when the concentration of calcium oxalate in the urine exceeds its solubility.

5. What specific risk factors predispose people to calcium oxalate stone formation?

Hereditary, environmental, and metabolic risk factors have all been identified.

6. What are some of the important environmental factors?

A low urine volume is clearly associated with an increased risk of stones. Although not well documented, patients in hotter climates or hot working conditions appear to be at increased risk, at least during an initial acclimatization period.

7. It has been said that people with calcium oxalate stones should avoid dairy products. Is this true?

Probably not. Although it may seem reasonable that the relatively high calcium content of dairy products may predispose to calcium oxalate stones, little scientific evidence supports this theory. In fact, in otherwise healthy people as well as in stone formers, a diet high in calcium may provide protection from such stones. One possible explanation is that the dietary calcium is needed to bind oxalate in the intestinal tract, which then prevents intestinal absorption of the oxalate. The risk for calcium oxalate stone formation is thus reduced.

8. What kind of dietary advice should be given to prevent calcium oxalate stones?

High fluid intake is most important, because it increases urinary volume and decreases the concentration of calcium oxalate. A diet low in oxalates is more reasonable than a calcium-restricted diet and may be beneficial in some affected patients. Studies also have shown a benefit in restriction of salt and fat intake as well as increased dietary fiber. An overall healthy, balanced diet may help to prevent stone formation.

9. When should a patient be evaluated for metabolic risk factors?

Opinion varies, but certainly any patient with recurrent calcium stones should be offered a metabolic evaluation. A single kidney stone event in a pediatric patient should prompt metabolic evaluation.

10. What should the evaluation include?

Serum studies should be obtained for calcium, phosphate, uric acid, electrolytes, and creatinine. These results are generally combined with a 24-hour urine study to determine volume, calcium, oxalate, uric acid, citrate, sodium, and, to ensure an adequate collection, creatinine. During the course of the evaluation, a fasting urine pH should be obtained.

11. What can the laboratory evaluation reveal?

The most frequent cause of recurrent calcium oxalate stones is **"idiopathic" hypercalciuria.** A reasonable definition for this is a 24-hour urinary calcium excretion exceeding 300 mg/day in men or 250 mg/day in women. Others define hypercalciuria as 24-hour urinary excretion in excess of 4 mg/kg/day. The uric acid level is important even for calcium stones; hyperuricosuria is clearly associated with an increased risk of calcium oxalate stones. The citrate levels are important, because hypocitraturia is a well known risk factor for recurrent calcium stones and also may be associated with renal tubular acidosis. Sodium excretion is an important marker of sodium intake, and elevated salt intake is associated with increased calcium excretion.

12. What type of treatment is used to prevent stones?

Treatment depends on the result of the metabolic evaluation. Hypercalciuria is usually treated with diuretics that decrease urinary calcium excretion. The most frequently used and perhaps best studied diuretics for this purpose are the **thiazides,** which are very effective in these cases. Patients with hyperuricosuria may benefit to some degree from a purine-restricted diet, although dietary restriction alone may not be adequate. In such cases, **allopurinol** is used to decrease urinary uric acid excretion and has proven effective in reducing the recurrence rate of calcium oxalate stones. Patients with hypocitraturia can be treated with **citrate supplements.** Patients with renal tubular acidosis require large doses of **alkalinizing agents.**

13. Some stones can be dissolved. Is this true for calcium stones?
No.

14. When is intervention indicated for calcium stones?

Indications for Intervention for Calcium Oxalate Calculi

Progressive obstruction
Intractable pain
Associated infection
Significant hematuria
Stone growth
Socioeconomic concerns
Stone too large to pass

Basically, stones require intervention whenever they cause progressive obstruction or intractable pain. When stones are associated with infection or significant hematuria, they also require intervention, although calcium oxalate stones are only rarely infection-related. Stones that increase in size despite appropriate medical management also require intervention. Some patients have stones that may pass spontaneously; however, they may opt for early intervention to allow them to return to work. Finally, any calcium stone in the ureter judged too large to pass on its own requires intervention. Stones smaller than 4 mm generally will pass spontaneously, whereas those between 4 and 7 mm have a 50% chance of passing. Stones in the ureter larger than 7 mm are unlikely to pass spontaneously.

15. What forms of treatment are available for such intervention?
Currently, most stones in the kidney and upper ureter are treated with extracorporeal shock-wave lithotripsy (SWL), an effective, safe treatment that generally can be done on an outpatient basis. Occasionally though, stones in the kidney are best treated percutaneously. This approach is generally reserved for patients in whom SWL fails or is contraindicated, or in whom the stone is larger than 2 cm in size. Stones in the lower ureter may be managed with SWL or with ureteroscopy, at which time they can be either removed intact or fragmented using laser, electrohydraulic, or electromechanical lithotripsy. **Open surgical intervention** is only rarely indicated for management of calcium stones. Specific indications for open operative intervention include the failure of or contraindication to less invasive forms of management, or an associated anatomic abnormality requiring open operative reconstruction.

BIBLIOGRAPHY

1. Barcelo P, Wuhl O, Servitge E, et al: Randomized double-blind study of potassium citrate in idiopathic hypocitraturic calcium nephrolithiasis. J Urol 150:1761, 1993.
2. Borghi L, Meschi T, Amato F, et al: Hot occupation and nephrolithiasis. J Urol 150:1757, 1993.
3. Curhan GC, Willett WC, Rimm EB, Stampfer MJ: A prospective study of dietary calcium and other nutrients and the risk of symptomatic kidney stones. N Engl J Med 328:833, 1993.
4. Laminski NA, Meyers AM, Kruger M, et al: Hyperoxaluria in patients with recurrent calcium oxalate calculi: Dietary and other risk factors. Br J Urol 68:454, 1991.

5. National Institutes of Health Consensus Development Conference on Prevention and Treatment of Kidney Stones. J Urol 141:705–808, 1989.
6. Pak CYC, Resnick MI: Urolithiasis: A Medical and Surgical Reference. Philadelphia, W. B. Saunders, 1990.
7. Sakhaee K, Harvey JA, Padalino PK, et al: The potential role of salt abuse on the risk for kidney stone formation. J Urol 150:310, 1993.
8. Segura JW, Preminger GM, Assimos DG, et al: Nephrolithiasis clinical guidelines panel summary report on the management of ureteral calculi. J Urol 158:1915, 1997.

84. URIC ACID CALCULI

Martin I. Resnick, M.D.

1. What percentage of urinary calculi are uric acid stones?

Uric acid stones account for 5–10% of all urinary calculi in the United States. The incidence varies among other countries, with the Middle Eastern countries, such as Israel, having an incidence as high as 25%. Very likely, both genetic and environmental factors influence these differences.

2. In what other mammal do uric acid calculi form?

Dalmatian coach dog is the only mammal, other than humans, that is at risk for formation of uric acid urinary lithiasis. Its risk is roughly equal to that of humans and relates to metabolic pathways unique to the species. (See question 3.)

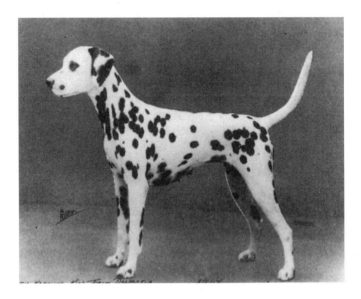

3. Why are humans affected but not other mammals?

Humans do not possess the hepatic enzyme **uricase** found in other mammals, which transforms the water-insoluble uric acid into allantoin, which is freely soluble and excreted by the kidney. The consequence of this enzymatic defect is that humans (and Dalmatian dogs) have urinary uric acid levels that are 10 times greater than those of other mammals.

4. What are the four categories of uric acid nephrolithiasis?

1. **Idiopathic uric acid lithiasis.** Patients have normal serum and urinary levels of uric acid, but a chronically low urinary pH. Patients with a gouty diathesis, chronic diarrhea, ileostomies, and on medications that acidify their urine are included in this category.

2. **Hyperuricemia associated with uric acid calculi.** Approximately 25% of patients with uric acid calculi are hyperuricemic, including those with gout, myeloproliferative disorders, and Lesch-Nyhan syndrome. Approximately 25% of patients with symptomatic gout form uric acid calculi, and 25% of patients who form uric acid calculi will prove to have gout. Patients with myeloproliferative disease, including lymphoma, develop elevated serum levels of uric acid, presumably from increased cell turnover. In addition, patients receiving chemotherapy for neoplastic disease

may develop increased serum and urinary levels of uric acid. Lesch-Nyhan syndrome, an X-linked genetic deficiency of the enzyme hypoxanthine-guanine-phosphoribosyl transferase (HGPRT), is characterized by choreoathetosis, striking growth, mental retardation, spasticity, and compulsion for self-mutilation. Patients with this syndrome develop both uric acid calculi and gouty arthritis.

3. **Uric acid calculi associated with chronic dehydration.** Patients have concentrated and acidic urine as a result of chronic diarrhea, ileostomies, inflammatory bowel disease, or excessive perspiration.

4. **Uric acid calculi-associated hyperuricosuria without hyperuricosemia.** Patients in this group include those who ingest uricosuric medications (salicylates, thiazides, sulfinpyrazone, probenecid) have a dietary excess of purine-rich foods (organ meats and sardines), or excrete excessive uric acid secondary to specific metabolic pathways.

5. Describe the etiology of uric acid calculi formation.

Uric acid is the end product of purine metabolism, and the supersaturation of urine with the undissociated uric acid is needed for the development of uric acid crystals. Normal 24-hour urinary excretion of uric acid is 800 mg in males and 750 mg in women.

Uric acid exists in the urine in two forms: uric acid and urate salt. The salt form complexes with sodium and is 20 times more soluble than free uric acid. Uric acid is a weak acid with a pKa of 5.75. At this pH, half of the molecules exist in the insoluble acid form, and the other half in the soluble salt form. As the urine becomes more acidic, more ions dissociate into the insoluble form. Many patients with uric acid calculi have persistently acidic urine with urine pH <6 and often at 5.0. The mechanism for this disturbance is a deficiency in renal production of ammonium, which is available for urinary buffering.

6. What factors are responsible for the formation of uric acid calculi?

1. Urinary pH
2. Low urine volume
3. Uric acid concentration

Probably the most important factor, and the most commonly encountered problem related to uric acid formation, is a persistently acid urine in the presence of normal urinary uric acid. The interaction of all three of these variables, however, influences uric acid crystallization and subsequent stone formation.

7. What is the differential diagnosis of a stone or obstruction seen on intravenous urography?

Filling Defect of the Renal Pelvis	Radiolucent Stone
Urothelial tumor	Uric acid calculi
Blood clot	Sodium urate stones
Sloughed renal papilla	Ammonium urate stones
Fungal ball	Xanthine stones
	2,8-Dihydroxyadenine stones (rare)
	Indinevar stones

8. What diagnostic tests are typically used for evaluating possible uric acid calculi?

Urinalysis will typically show a urine pH of <5.5 and uric acid crystals that appear as needles under ordinary light microscopy. Under polarized light, these crystals appear as strongly negatively birefringent.

Intravenous urogram demonstrates a radiolucent filling defect.

Ultrasound is a noninvasive study that can detect calculi as small as 0.5–1.0 cm. With this technique, the uric calculus produces a negative shadow that is not seen with blood clots or tumor but is seen with stones of other chemical composition.

Computed tomography, done without intravenous contrast, is simple and can detect calculi as small as 0.5 cm. It can clearly differentiate uric acid calculi from nonopaque masses (the density of a uric acid calculus is 350–400 Hounsfield units on a ±1000 scale). It also provides greater density discrimination than conventional radiography as well as a means to follow stone dissolution therapy.

Other more **invasive measures** include retrograde pyelography and retrograde brushing in association with urinary cytology. Ureteroscopy may be required to visualize a defect and to obtain a biopsy.

Biochemical values measured include serum levels of uric acid and a 24-hour uric acid. The upper limit of normal for serum uric acid is 7 mg/dl in male and 5.5 mg/dl in females. Most patients with uric calculi have normal levels of uric acid excretion and normal serum levels. Patients with evidence of hyperuricemia should undergo a brief evaluation to rule out the possibility of myeloproliferative or neoplastic disease.

9. How are patients with uric acid calculi managed?

Uric acid calculi are unique in that of all calculi of the urinary tract, they are the most easily dissolved with appropriate diet and pharmacologic therapy. Goals of management include raising urinary pH and lowering the urinary uric acid concentration by decreasing excretion and increasing urinary volume.

Hydration. Patients must increase their oral fluid intake to ensure their urine output is >1500–2000 ml/day. Higher urinary output also results in some increase in urinary pH secondary to the diuretic effects of the water.

Alkalinization. Uric acid stone formers typically have low urinary pH of 5.0–5.5. Various agents may be used to alkalinize the urine, and the choice depends on the clinical situation. Nitrazine paper may be used to monitor and maintain urinary pH between 6.5 and 7.0. Excessive alkalinization can be detrimental, because patients may begin to form stones that precipitate in an alkaline solution, especially calcium oxalate.

10. What agents are used to achieve urinary alkalinization?

1. **Oral agents.** Sodium bicarbonate (650 mg or more every 6–8 hours) or potassium citrate (15 mEq 3–4 times/day). In patients with malabsorption problems or chronic diarrhea, a liquid preparation of potassium citrate or sodium-potassium citrate is of particular value. The liquid preparation allows for better absorption in patients with rapid intestinal transit time.

2. **Intravenous agents.** If the patient requires hospitalization because of nausea, vomiting, and pain, intravenous infusion of 1/6 molar lactate provides rapid alkalinization. A disadvantage of this treatment is that because of the increased sodium load, patients must be monitored for signs of congestive heart failure.

11. Is invasive therapy ever warranted?

Chemolysis of uric acid stones can be accomplished with direct irrigation of the renal pelvis with sodium bicarbonate solution via a transureteral or percutaneous catheter. Although of limited use it has application in debilitated patients who are poor candidates for operative procedures. ESWL and percutaneous procedures also may be used to render these patients stone-free.

12. What is the role of allopurinol?

If the patient is hyperuricosuric, efforts should be made to reduce uric acid excretion. Aside from dietary measures already described, medications such as allopurinol (100–300 mg/day) may be given. Allopurinol decreases uric acid synthesis by inhibiting the enzyme xanthine oxidase, which catalyzes the conversion of hypoxanthine to uric acid.

BIBLIOGRAPHY

1. Coe FJ, Favus MJ, Pak CYC, et al (eds): Kidney Stones, Medical and Surgical Management. Philadelphia, Lippincott-Raven, 1996.
2. Gillenwater JY, Grayhack WT, Howard SS, Mitchell ME (eds): Adult and Pediatric Urology, 4th ed., Philadelphia, Lippincott William & Wilkins, 2002.

3. Pak CYC, Resnick MI, Preminger GM (eds): Urolithiasis 1996 Symposium of 8th International Symposium on Urolithiasis. Dallas, TX, Millett, September 29–October 2, 1996.

4. Walsh PC, Retik AB, Vaughan ED Jr, Wein AJ (eds): Campbell's Urology, 7th ed. Philadelphia, W. B. Saunders, 1998.

5. Pak CY, Sakhaee K, Peterson RD, et al: Biochemical profile of idiopathic uric acide nephrolithiasis. Kidney Int 60:757–761, 2001.

6. Moran ME, Abrahams HM, Burday DE, Greene TD: Utility of oral dissolution therapy in the management of referred patients with secondarily treated uric acid stones. Urology 59:206–210, 2002.

85. STRUVITE STONES

J. Patrick Spirnak, M.D.

1. What is a struvite stone?
A struvite stone is an infectious stone.

2. What does a struvite stone consist of?
A mixture of magnesium ammonium phosphate and carbonate apatite.

3. What percentage of all stones are struvite?
Approximately 15–20%.

4. Are struvite stones more common in men or women?
Women, by an approximate ratio of 2:1. Women have a higher incidence of urinary tract infections, which predispose them to stone formation.

5. How does infection cause struvite stone formation?
The association between struvite stone formation and urinary tract infection has long been recognized, but it is still unclear whether the stone or the infection is the initiating factor.

The presence of a struvite stone is evidence for either a past or current infection with urea-splitting bacteria. The enzymatic breakdown of urea by urease increases the bicarbonate and ammonia concentrations with a resultant increase in urinary pH above 7.0. When alkaline, the urine becomes supersaturated with magnesium, ammonium, phosphate, and carbonate apatite, leading to stone formation.

6. Can struvite stones form in the absence of an alkaline urine?
No. A pH >7.0 is necessary for stone formation to occur.

7. Name three common bacteria that are known to produce urease.
Proteus, Pseudomonas, and *Klebsiella.*

8. List three conditions predisposing to struvite stone formation.
1. Congenital anomalies such as ureteropelvic junction obstruction, duplication anomalies, or vesicoureteral reflux are associated with a higher incidence of urinary tract infection and struvite stone formation.
2. Neurogenic bladder or an enlarged prostate may prevent patients from emptying the bladder completely, making them prone to infection and struvite stone formation.
3. Urinary diversion or chronic catheter drainage also make patients prone to struvite stone formation.

9. What is a staghorn stone?
It is a large branched stone that may grow to fill the entire renal collecting system. About 60–90% of staghorn stones are struvite. (See also chapter 78.)

10. Do asymptomatic struvite stones in a healthy individual require treatment?
Large struvite stones should be surgically removed in order to avoid the potential infectious complication of perinephric abscess and sepsis. Loss of renal function and patient mortality are also increased if the stone is not removed.

11. What role do antibiotics play in the treatment of struvite stones?

Antibiotics are important in controlling the acute infection. They also are used to sterilize the urine in the perioperative period. Antibiotics may be used prophylactically once the stone has been removed if an anatomic abnormality is present that may predispose to future infection and stone formation.

12. Why are patients with struvite stones susceptible to recurrent infections?

Bacteria exist in the stone itself and persist even after the patient completes a course of culture-specific antibiotics. It is possible to sterilize the urine temporarily, but once the antibiotic is stopped, the bacteria re-emerge from the stone to reinfect the urine.

13. What surgical interventions are used to treat struvite stones?

Open surgical procedures, such as **anatrophic nephrolithotomy,** have long been the primary means to eradicate struvite stones. More recently, a combined approach using percutaneous lithotripsy and **extracorporeal shock-wave lithotripsy** (ESWL) has proven successful in eradicating struvite stones.

14. Are fragments left after treatment significant?

If a large (>1 cm) struvite stone fragment is left after treatment, the most likely outcome will be recurrent urinary tract infection and stone formation.

15. Is it possible to dissolve struvite calculi?

Yes. The use of 10% hemiacidrin irrigation has been used to dissolve struvite calculi. When combined with percutaneous and ESWL techniques, hemiacidrin use may enhance stone-free rates.

16. Does hemiacidrin use have any contraindications?

The presence of an uncontrolled urinary tract infection is an absolute contraindication. In the presence of an infection, sepsis may occur.

17. What are urease inhibitors?

Urease inhibitors (acetohydroxamic acid) inhibit the bacterial enzyme urease, thereby reducing the alkalinity of the urine and the subsequent precipitation of struvite.

18. When is the use of urease inhibitors indicated?

The primary indications are patients who have residual stone fragments after incomplete surgical removal and patients with intractable urinary tract infections that cannot be eradicated (e.g., cutaneous urinary diversion).

BIBLIOGRAPHY

1. Blandy JP, Singh M: The case for a more aggressive approach to staghorn stones. J Urol 115:505, 1976.
2. Griffith DP: Struvite stones. Kidney Int 13:372, 1978.
3. Menon M, Parulklar BG, Drach GW: Urinary lithiasis: Etiology, diagnosis, and medical management. In Walsh PC, Retik AB, Vaughan ED Jr, Wein AJ (eds): Campbell's Urology, 7th ed. Philadelphia, W. B. Saunders, 1998, pp 2661–2733.
4. Resnick MI: Evaluation and management of infection stones. Urol Clin North Am 8:265, 1981.
5. Spirnak JP, Resnick MI: Urinary stones. Prim Care 12:735–104, 1985.
6. Spirnak JP, DeBaz BP, Green HY, Resnick MI: Complex struvite calculi treated by primary extracorporeal shock wave lithotripsy and chemolysis with hemiacidrin irrigation. J Urol 140:1356, 1988.
7. Wang LP, Wong HY, Griffin DP: Treatment options in struvite stones. Urol Clin North Am 24:149, 1997.
8. Saltzman B, Vaughan ED: Staghorn calculi: Is intervention always indicated? 1987.
9. Lingeman JE: Staghorn Stones: The Continued Challenge. 1993.
10. American Urological Association: The Management of Staghorn Kidney Stones: A Patient's Guide. Clinical Practice Guidelines. ?yr.

86. CYSTINE STONES

Stevan B. Streem, M.D.

1. About how many patients with cystine stones is a busy family practitioner likely to see each year?
None.

2. How common are cystine stones?
Cystine stones are rare. Only 1–2% of all stone patients have cystine stones.

3. What causes them?
Cystine stones result from an inherited defect of renal tubular reabsorption of cystine. Actually, the tubular defect affects the reabsorption of the four dibasic amino acids.

4. How can I remember which four?
With the mnemonic **COLA:**
Cystine
Ornithine
Lysine
Arginine

5. Why aren't there ornithine, lysine, or arginine stones?
Those three amino acids are very soluble over the normal range of urinary pH. Only cystine is relatively insoluble and will precipitate in urine to form stones.

6. How is the propensity to form cystine stones inherited?
Cystine stones are inherited in a complex autosomal recessive fashion. If both parents are carriers or if one sibling has cystine stones, a person has a 25% chance of being affected.

7. Is there a specific radiographic appearance that is suggestive of cystine stones?
Cystine stones are opaque, although not as opaque as most calcium stones. They may have a homogenous, "ground glass" appearance. Because they are less opaque than radi-

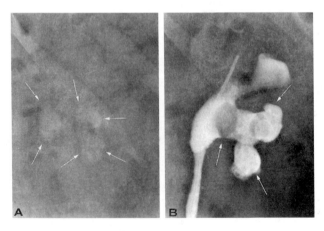

A. A plain abdominal radiograph reveals multiple, lightly opaque, homogeneous calculi (*arrows*) suggestive of cystine stones. **B.** After retrograde injection of contrast, the stones are visualized as filling defects. Although cystine stones are opaque, they are relatively lucent compared to contrast material.

ographic contrast, they may appear to be relatively lucent during intravenous or retrograde pyelography.

8. How does urinalysis specify the presence of cystine stones in a patient with stones?

Often, the urinanalysis will reveal classic hexagonal crystals—this finding alone is diagnostic of cystinuria. A 24-hour urine study for cystine excretion should always be done in these patients. Normal individuals excrete less than 100 mg cystine/day. Heterozygotes excrete 150–300 mg cystine/day, but generally do not get cystine stones. Homozygous cystinurics excrete more than 400 mg cystine/day.

9. Although cystine stones are a genetic problem, can they be prevented?

For many affected patients, cystine stones can be prevented or even dissolved with medical management.

10. What is the best treatment?

Three to 4 quarts of oral fluids/day should be ingested to decrease the urinary concentration of cystine. Also, the urine should be alkalinized because cystine is more soluble in an alkaline urine. When cystine stones form or increase in size with fluid and alkalinization therapy, drugs that bind with cystine to form the more-soluble cysteine should be prescribed. These drugs include d-penicillamine and alpha-mercaptopropionylglycine (MPG).

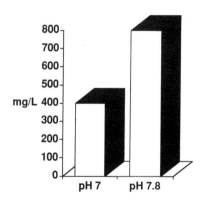

11. Why aren't cystine-binding drugs used as preventive therapy in all patients?

Unfortunately, they are associated with a 30–50% incidence of significant side effects, necessitating discontinuation of the drug.

12. What is the best way to remove cystine stones?

Of all stone types, cystine stones are the least amenable to extracorporeal shock-wave lithotripsy (SWL). However, they do fragment well with ultrasonic lithotripsy or holmium lasers. Therefore, patients with cystine stones are now treated preferentially with percutaneous or ureteroscopic procedures combined with one of these forms of intracorporeal lithotripsy. "Open" surgery should be avoided whenever possible because of the high rates of recurrence that necessitate repeated intervention.

BIBLIOGRAPHY

1. Chow GK, Streem SB: Medical management of cystinuria: Results of contemporary clinical practice. J Urol 156:1572, 1996.

2. Chow GK, Streem SB: Contemporary urologic intervention for cystinuric patients: Immediate and long-term impact and implications. J Urol 160:341, 1998.
3. Crawhall JC, Scowen EF, Watts RWE: Effect of penicillamine on cystinuria. BMJ 1:585, 1963.
4. Crawhall JC, Watts RWE: Cystinuria. Am J Med 45:736, 1968.
5. Dent CE, Rose GA: Amino acid metabolism in cystinuria. QJM 20:205, 1951.
6. Dent CE, Senior B: Studies on the treatment of cystinuria. Br J Urol 27:317, 1955.
7. Evans WP, Resnick MI, Boyce WH: Homozygous cystinuria—evaluation of 35 patients. J Urol 127:707, 1982.
8. Giugliani R, Ferrari I, Greene LJ: Heterozygous cystinuria and urinary lithiasis. Am J Med Genet 22:703, 1985.
9. Harris H, Mittwoch U, Robson EB, et al: Phenotypes and genotypes in cystinuria. Ann Hum Genet 20:57–91, 1955.
10. Kachel TA, Vijan SR, Dretler SP: Endourological experience with cystine calculi and a treatment algorithm. J Urol 145:25, 1991.
11. Knoll LD, Segura JW, Patterson DE, et al: Long-term followup in patients with cystine urinary calculi treated with percutaneous ultrasonic lithotripsy. J Urol 140:246, 1988.
12. Pak CYC, Fuller C, Sakhaee K, et al: Management of cystine nephrolithiasis with alpha-mercaptopropionylglycine. J Urol 136:1003, 1986.
13. Sakhaee K, Poindexter JR, Pak CYC: The spectrum of metabolic abnormalities in patients with cystine nephrolithiasis. J Urol 141:819, 1989.

INDEX

Page numbers in **boldface type** indicate complete chapters.